A
W
L
S

ADVANCED
WILDERNESS
LIFE
SUPPORT®

SENIOR EDITORS
DAVID DELLA-GIUSTINA, MD, FAWM
RICHARD INGEBRETSEN, MD, PhD

WITH INTRODUCTION BY
RICHARD INGEBRETSEN, MD, PhD

Licensed from the University of Utah

Accreditation through Wilderness Medical Society

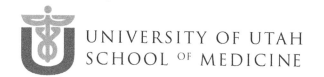

UNIVERSITY OF UTAH
SCHOOL OF MEDICINE

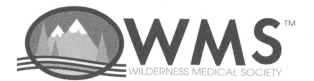

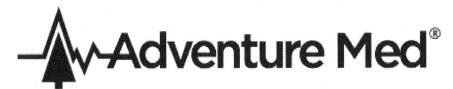

Wilderness Medicine Education

ISBN: 0615496083
ISBN 13: 9780615496085

CONTRIBUTORS

Jerome Bidinger, JD, PhD
Faculty, Advanced Wilderness Life Support
Wilderness Medicine Attorney
Castle Valley, Utah

Jane Bowman, MD, FAWM
University of Utah School of Medicine
Western Gynecological Clinic
Salt Lake City, Utah

Lauke Bisschops, MD
Emergency Physician
Resident Elderly Care Medicine
Founder: *Outdoor Medicine*
The Netherlands

Anne Brants, MD, FAWM, DIMM
Emergency Physician
Founder: *Outdoor Medicine*
The Netherlands

Jon Christensen, PA-C, FAWM
Department of Emergency Medicine
Madigan Army Medical Center
Tacoma, Washington

David Della-Giustina, MD, FAWM
EM Residency Program Director
Chief of Education Section
Department of Emergency Medicine
Yale School of Medicine
New Haven, Connecticut

Karen Della-Giustina, MD
Department of Emergency Medicine
Bridgeport Hospital
Bridgeport, Connecticut

Jillian Franklin, MD
Department of Emergency Medicine
Madigan Army Medical Center
Tacoma, Washington

Katja Goldflam, MD
EM Residency Associate Program Director
Department of Emergency Medicine
Yale School of Medicine
New Haven, Connecticut

Jennifer Harris, MS, RDN
Department of Nutrition and Integrative Physiology, University of Utah
Cottonwood Medical Clinic
Salt Lake City, Utah

David Hile, MD, FAWM
Department of Emergency Medicine
Yale School of Medicine
New Haven, CT

Lisa Hile, MD, FAWM
Department of Emergency Medicine
Yale School of Medicine
New Haven, CT

Richard J. Ingebretsen, MD, PhD
Adjunct Instructor, Department of Medicine
Associate Dean, College of Science
University of Utah School of Medicine
Salt Lake City, Utah
Clinical Assistant Professor
Department of Emergency Medicine
Ohio State University **College of Medicine**
Columbus, Ohio

Christopher Kang, MD, FAWM
Department of Emergency Medicine
Madigan Army Medical Center
University of Washington
Tacoma, Washington

Tristan Knutson, MD
Department of Emergency Medicine
Madigan Army Medical Center
Tacoma, Washington

Maybritt I. Kuypers, MD, FAWM
Emergency Physician
Founder: *Outdoor Medicine*
The Netherlands

Owen McGrane, MD
Department of Emergency Medicine
Madigan Army Medical Center
Tacoma, Washington

Robert Quinn MD, FAWM
Professor and Department Chairman
Residency Program Director
Department of Orthopedic Surgery
UT Health Science Center San Antonio
San Antonio, Texas

Paul Schmutz, DDS

Faculty, Advanced Wilderness Life Support
Wilderness Dentistry
Bountiful, Utah

Julian Speight, MBBS, BSc, FRCS(Ed), FRACS
Consultant General Surgeon
Southland Hospital
Invercargill, New Zealand

Gerald W. Surrett MD, FAWM
Flight Surgeon/Dive Medical Officer
Department of Emergency Medicine
Madigan Army Medical Center

Anthony Tomassoni, MD
Department of Emergency Medicine
Yale School of Medicine
New Haven, Connecticut

Martin Watts, MB, ChB, FACEM
Emergency Medicine Specialist
Southland Hospital
Invercargill, New Zealand

Ian Wedmore, MD, FAWM
Director of Austere and Wilderness Medicine
Fellowship
Department of Emergency Medicine,
Madigan Army Medical Center
Tacoma, Washington

PREVIOUS CONTRIBUTORS

We would like to acknowledge the following contributors to previous editions of this textbook and course:

Paul S. Auerbach, MD, MS, FAWM

Michael Adams, MD

E. Wayne Askew, Ph.D.

Vince Ball, MD

Justin Coles, DO

Andrew Crockett, MD

Sarah Crockett MD

Paul Frandsen, MD

Joey Fyans, MD

Andrew J. Gregory, MD

Colin Grissom, MD, FAWM

DeVon Hale, MD

Harland Hayes, MD

David Hughes, MD

Stein H. Ingebretsen MD

Adam Johnson, MD

Nate Kofford, MD

Jackson Lever, MD

Emily Luerssen, MD

William Mackie, MD

Andre Pennardt, MD, FAWM

Beth Phillips, MD

William A Shakespeare, MD

Christian Smith, MD

Gregory Stiller, MD, FAWM

Scott Young, DO

TABLE OF CONTENTS

Section 4: Bites, Stings, and Infections

Section 5: Tools and Techniques

Section 6: Appendix – Additional Educational Material

Section 7: Index

INTRODUCTION

The History of Advanced Wilderness Life Support

As more people venture into the backcountry, injuries are increasing. There has been no branch of medicine devoted to teaching medical professionals how to treat or prevent such injuries. Wilderness medicine encompasses the prevention, diagnosis, and treatment of injuries and medical conditions that may occur during activities in remote territories away from cities, ambulances and hospitals. It covers how to practice medicine where there is no medical support and where a person might have to improvise care.

In 1993 while biking in the mountains near Salt Lake City, Utah, USA, I witnessed a serious mountain bicycle accident. The unhelmeted young rider hit his head on the ground and was knocked unconscious. Then, a week later, while rafting with Boy Scouts on the Colorado River, in the Western United States, one of the participants lacerated his leg. I realized that both times I felt unsure of how I could help someone injured in the backcountry, away from modern medical equipment. I knew that wilderness medicine instruction was not offered at any medical school and the majority of physicians did not receive this type of training. As a doctor, and an active hiker, biker, and river

1

runner, I knew that people would turn to me for guidance if they were injured in a remote area and I felt that doctors needed to be prepared.

I contacted the Wilderness Medical Society (WMS) to see what I would need to do to be trained in wilderness medical care. This society was formed in 1983 to institute sound principles of medical practice in wilderness settings. Through association with the WMS I began to study wilderness medicine while in residency, and in 1998 as a faculty member of the University of Utah's medical school, I approached the curriculum committee about teaching a course to the medical students. They approved the course. While this was great news, I realized that this had not been done before, so now, I had to decide what was going to be taught. I approached a number of doctors and sources to get their ideas. After all, there are literally dozens of topics that might be incorporated. Which of these would be the most important or even essential to include? The University of Utah already had several exceptional physicians on its faculty who had done work in wilderness medicine areas such as high altitude medicine. Their ideas formed the basis of this first medical school wilderness medicine course. It was taught in the spring of 1998. The course was an instant success and the students loved it, primarily because so many of the principles that we taught were so very practical and useful.

But the course still lacked structure and a formal teaching and testing process and furthermore, I felt that we had not really developed protocols for treating people in the backcountry. At this point, a number of wilderness medicine experts from across the country and military joined the program. We worked on setting up a testing process where students could learn standards and protocols. A committee was formed and we established the Advanced Wilderness Life Support (AWLS) certification.

The first step was to list all of the possible subjects that a wilderness medicine certification process could teach. Then we ranked these subjects, listing at the top the most important subjects and at the bottom, the least important. For example, how important is it to teach about spelunking versus water treatment. Is it absolutely necessary to teach high altitude disease? What about children in the wilderness? It was clear to our committee at the outset which of the subjects was the most important and the core curriculum was established.

Now we turned our attention to treatment protocols. On the surface, this seemed like a simple task as so many of protocols have been established for hospital medicine. But we quickly realized that the situation was so different in the backcountry that it would be a much larger task. For example, how are burns treated when you are days away from help? Should you close a wound using sutures or just keep it covered? Should you evacuate all patients with abdominal pain or let some remain in the backcountry? These questions and protocols are very important and took a significant amount of time and research to develop. Working as a team with medical students and rescue personal with broad knowledge treating people away from a hospital setting, we formulated backcountry medical treatment protocols.

But it did not end there. One of the earliest discoveries was that there were many misconceptions among the general public and medical professionals as to how back country injuries should be treated. We needed to dispel these erroneous notions. For example, many people thought that making an incision in a snakebite with a knife and trying to extract the venom from the wound was standard protocol. Actually, there are no effective methods for treating snakebites in the wilderness and it is crucial to evacuate the patient to a hospital as soon a possible. Incredibly, we found that everyone had a different method for removing a tick – almost all of which are ineffective. The most effective method was to simply pull the tick straight off from the victim.

Appropriate evacuation was another issue that we needed to work on. Evacuation is often dangerous, costly and difficult, and if someone does not need to be taken for definitive care, then it should not be risked. However, there were no guidelines to follow. So in 2001 several enterprising medical students began a literature search, spoke with numerous specialists and developed the first guidelines to help backcountry medical providers decide if a patient needed to be evacuated.

Another early concern was what to include in a first aid kit. We developed an algorithm to help people determine what first aid kits would be best depending upon the number of people, the length of the trip, as well as the location of the adventure. It is now the industry standard.

With all of this done it became necessary to formalize all of this in a textbook format. This was no easy task. Dozens of experts from multiple fields and expertise were employed to write, edit and review chapters in this new text. Then these needed to be reviewed again for consistency and accuracy. Illustrations needed to be created. After many months of lengthy work, the AWLS textbook was created and published. Today AWLS has achieved international certification status for medical professionals studying wilderness medicine. The protocols and guidelines that have been developed are considered the standard of care in backcountry medicine. Since its inception, thousands of medical professionals in all parts of the world have certified with the AWLS program.

Richard Ingebretsen, MD, PhD
Advanced Wilderness Life Support

CHAPTER 1

Patient Assessment

In this chapter you will learn to safely and effectively approach and assess patients in wilderness settings by meeting these objectives:

- Recognize possible threats to the rescuer(s) and patient(s) and identify resources through adequately surveying the scene.
- Rapidly determine the presence of any immediately life-threatening conditions while making appropriate interventions during the primary survey.
- Obtain a thorough history and perform an appropriate physical exam as part of the secondary survey.
- Understand the importance of the following acronyms in evaluating and treating patients in the wilderness: MARCH, CARTS, AVPU, SAMPLE, COLD-ERR, and AEIOU-TIPS.

SCENE SURVEY

The scene survey consists of several components with the most important being an evaluation of the scene for safety of the rescuer and victims. Placing a rescuer at undue risk can exponentially complicate the situation, if not create additional patients. Surveying the scene also requires the rescuer to identify the number of patients with a quick estimate of each patient's condition, and note the presence of bystanders, equipment, and other clues that may be useful in determining the mechanism of injury (MOI) and/or the nature of illness (NOI). This phase of the patient assessment may also require triage of several patients to effectively utilize limited resources.

Scene Safety

Is the scene safe for me and my assistants to enter? Consider external hazards such as:
- ☐ Physical dangers (rocks, snow/ice, water, trees, fires, wildlife, etc.)
- ☐ Weather/environment (hot/cold temperatures, lightning, altitude, etc.)
- ☐ Other people (bikers on single track, climbers above you, hunters, etc.)

Will the scene remain safe? If not, what is my plan?
- ☐ Safe zones
- ☐ Moving patients (drags, carries, and litters)

Is it safe for me to physically care for the patient(s)? Body substance isolation (BSI) should be considered in every victim to help prevent disease transmission.

How many patients are there? Which one(s) need help first? (See Triage section below.)
- ☐ The victim's equipment may provide information about medical conditions or the MOI/NOI.
- ☐ Bystanders may have witnessed the victim's demise or may be able to assist with patient care.

Are there resources near the scene that may be useful in treating or evacuating the patient?

Approaching, Identifying, and Getting Permission to Treat the Victim(s)

When approaching the victim, use caution so that you do not expose them to additional hazards such as rock or icefall. Consider marking the route to the scene if additional rescuers are to follow.

Attempt to approach the patient from the side and in a direction so that they can see you approaching. That will make it less frightening for the victim and they may not have to turn their head and neck to see you are and what you are doing.

Immediately identify yourself as a medical professional and request the victim's permission to treat. If the victim is unconscious or has an altered level of responsiveness, their consent to treatment is implied. Otherwise, the victim has the right to decline treatment.

Ask the victim's name and say, "Can you tell me what happened?" In addition to defining the MOI/NOI, this will almost always elicit the chief complaint. If the patient cannot answer these questions, they are either unconscious or have an altered level of responsiveness; commence with the primary survey.

Triage

- When multiple victims are present, it may be necessary to determine the severity of each patient in order to effectively utilize resources.
- Initially, this is done as part of the scene survey by quickly looking over the patients and determining which "look" the worst.
- There are several methods of triaging patients. A common method is to triage them into different color categories based on the victims' severity of illness or injury.
    - ☐ BLACK: Dead on arrival. Patient lacking ABCs despite opening airway.
    - ☐ RED: Critical, immediately life-threatening injury, notable finding during Primary Survey.
    - ☐ YELLOW: Severe injury(s) that is not immediately life threatening.
    - ☐ GREEN: Minor injuries, non-emergent, "walking wounded."
- The color assigned to each patient determines the priority (in order): RED-YELLOW-GREEN-BLACK.
- One key exception is for lightning victims; the BLACK coded patients should be cared for first (see lightning chapter).

INITIAL ASSESSMENT

Assessing Responsiveness

The initial assessment focuses on determining the responsiveness of the victims using **AVPU** (Alert, Verbal Painful, Unresponsive). Is the patient alert and oriented, responsive only to verbal stimulation, responsive only to painful stimulation or unresponsive? If the victim shows any signs of life such as movement, moaning, or talking, then you move on to the primary survey (below). For those victims who are unresponsive, the rescuer must quickly move forward with cardiopulmonary resuscitation (CPR) and Basic Life Support (BLS). This is especially important if the situation involves a lightning strike, drowning or avalanche event with snow burial because these are situations where immediate CPR may save a victim's life. See the box below for more information on the use of CPR and wilderness considerations.

PRIMARY SURVEY

Primary Survey: MARCH

The objective of the primary survey is to identify and treat conditions that pose an immediate threat to life. Approaching the victim using the acronym **M A R C H** allows the rescuer to address the life-threatening issues in order of importance. Why **M A R C H** instead of the more common ABCDE? We teach **M A R C H** as the initial approach because the management of victims in the wilderness is different than the hospital setting. In the wilderness, a victim may have to exert themselves in their rescue, which could include walking out on their own. The fact that they may lose a significant amount of blood in a matter of minutes could be detrimental towards them being able to assist in their rescue. There is no way to replace the blood lost in the wilderness. Because this portion of the assessment is searching for critical conditions, it is most applicable to patients who have an altered level of consciousness or have a significant injury. However, this survey should be utilized in *every* victim for whom one cares for in the wilderness. In those victims who are alert and appear well, this assessment may be brief.

Primary Survey

M – Massive hemorrhage management
A – Airway with cervical spine stabilization
R – Respiration
C – Circulation
H – Hypothermia / Hyperthermia and
   Hike vs. Helicopter

M – Massive hemorrhage management
- The first objective is to stop massive hemorrhage rapidly because a victim can lose most of their blood volume in a matter of minutes with major arterial or venous bleeding.
- In the wilderness, you cannot replace this blood, and the victim may be required to be much more active than the typical hospitalized patient.
- This step is applicable only for major bleeding and does not include injuries with only minor oozing that will be addressed later in the secondary survey. Generally, these types of injuries are rare in the wilderness but can have fatal consequences if not treated rapidly.
- Treatment usually consists of the placement of a tourniquet if it is an extremity injury. If one does not have a tourniquet or if the injury is not amenable to the use of a tourniquet (e.g. facial or torso wound), then a pressure dressing directly on the area of bleeding is the best option.
- The placement of the tourniquet does not mandate that the tourniquet stay in place until the patient reaches definitive medical care. The expectation is that that the rescuer will reassess the wound and the bleeding after the patient has been stabilized in the secondary survey and ongoing assessment stage. The use of tourniquets and their management is covered in depth in the wound management chapter.

A – Airway with cervical spine stabilization
- There are two issues in the assessment of the victim's airway:

- ☐ Is the airway currently open?
- ☐ Is the victim able to maintain their airway?

■ First, is the airway open and is the patient able to move air in and out of their airway with minimal obstruction?

- ☐ If the awake victim is moving air but has sonorous or noisy breathing, then they will generally place themselves in the best position that allows them to keep their airway open. Do not force them into a position that they do not want to go to. In medicine, we prefer to place patients on their back, but you should not force a victim to this position if they cannot tolerate it.
- ☐ If the victim has a decreased level of consciousness, roll them onto their back as a single unit, being careful not to twist or jerk the spine or neck. Once the victim is on their back, attempt to open the airway using the **head tilt-chin lift** maneuver unless trauma is the MOI.
- ☐ If you suspect that the victim has head or spinal injuries, use the **jaw-thrust** technique to minimize neck movement by placing one hand on each side of the victim's head and grasping the angles of the victim's lower jaw and lifting up and forward with both hands.
- ☐ If the victim with a decreased level of consciousness is not moving air well with initial positioning, then inspect for and remove any foreign objects from their mouth. In victims of avalanches or major trauma, it is not unusual to see snow, teeth, dirt and/or leaves in their mouths.

■ The second issue is whether the patient is going to maintain their airway throughout the rescue.

- ☐ There are potential airway issues, especially trauma and allergic reactions, where the patient will have a worsening obstruction to their airway.
- ☐ This is a major consideration when you evaluate evacuation options and the urgency of evacuation.

■ The evaluation and clearing of the cervical spine is fully covered later in this course. However, the rescuer must have a great deal of caution for potential spinal injuries when they first approach and care for a wilderness victim, especially if that victim is unconscious or has an altered level of consciousness. If there is any concern of a spinal injury, then treat that victim as if they have a spinal injury until you have evaluated the patient more thoroughly in the secondary survey.

R – Respiration

■ Respiration involves the evaluation of how well the patient is breathing and whether there is any potential for respiratory compromise in the future.

■ If the victim does not start breathing after the airway has been opened, begin rescue breathing as described for basic CPR using current guidelines.

- ☐ Each breath should be delivered over one second with enough air to see the chest rise.
- ☐ If the breath does not go in, reposition the airway and try again.

■ If the victim is breathing, briefly assess the quality of the respirations. Does the patient appear to be working hard to breathe, are they breathing rapidly/slowly, is their breathing appropriate, etc.?

C – Circulation

Any patient who is awake or showing any sign of life will have a heartbeat. This step is to assess the victim's cardiovascular status with a focus on the heart rate, pulse strength and to treat non-massive hemorrhage.

You can assess the pulse at the pedal/tibial, radial, brachial, femoral or carotid arteries.

☐ Assess the quality of the pulse. Is it weak/thready, bounding, rapid, or irregular?

☐ Check for bleeding by performing a blood sweep. This is a rapid (5 - 10 seconds) full, head-to-toe check for blood, wet clothing, swelling or other signs of significant bleeding.

☐ A blood sweep also affords the rescuer the opportunity to simultaneously note major deformities.

H – Hypothermia / Hyperthermia and Hike vs. Helicopter

At this point in the primary survey, the rescuer has treated any immediate threats to the patient's life and has taken steps to mitigate those threats. Wilderness medicine presents an additional issue that one must consider: the environment and its potential to worsen the victim's medical course.

Recognize that whatever the environment, the victim has likely been exposed to it for a longer period and has not been compensating as well as the rescuers.

A victim in a cold/hot environment will likely be colder/hotter than the rescuer.

Steps should be taken to limit the victim's exposure to the environment.

Hypothermia in trauma can lead to the cascade of acidosis and coagulopathy with increased mortality.

Think about the evacuation plan (hike vs. helicopter).

☐ The life-threatening injuries have been identified at this point.

☐ What types of resources will you need and how can you get them to you to help your victims?

☐ This is also a point to consider sending someone to go get help depending on the situation. This can be helpful because that individual can relay more valuable information beyond the initial "someone's unconscious."

☐ If you are going to send somebody ahead to get help, you should send two people to help ensure that help is reached and that something does not occur to that single person sent out.

As a general rule, especially when dealing with possible injuries to the spinal column, perform first aid on the victim where he or she lies. However, there are special circumstances under which there is potential for more severe injury or death if the victim is not moved.

Primary Survey in Conscious Patients

When the patient is conscious, the rescuer may be able to substitute portions of the complete primary survey with questions. For example:

☐ A talking patient has, for the time being, intact airway, breathing and circulation. The rescuer should still assess the quality of the breathing and pulse.

☐ Asking a patient about what happened and if they are bleeding may eliminate the need for a blood sweep and spinal immobilization.

CPR – Cardiopulmonary Resuscitation

CPR Guideline Update

The American Heart Association guidelines emphasize chest compressions during CPR by re-ordering the initial A-B-C to C-A-B and stating compressions should begin within the first 10 seconds of patient contact.

The professional rescuer is still instructed to check for a pulse prior to beginning compressions, while the lay rescuer is advised to only briefly (5-10 seconds) check for signs of movement or breathing.

The compression rate remains 100 per minute with a 30:2 compression-to-breath ratio for adult one- and two-rescuer as well as child/infant single-rescuer.

Two-rescuer CPR for children/infants should be done at a 15:2 compression-to-breath ratio.

The lay rescuer may also elect to employ "hands-only CPR," wherein no rescue breaths are delivered. Note that this should only be done for witnessed adult arrests in urban locations.

Hand positioning remains in the center of the patient's sternum, with a greater emphasis on ensuring adequate compression depth of at least 2 inches in adult patients and at least 1/3 of the depth of the patient's chest in children/infants.

The professional rescuer should use judgment for those cases when airway and breathing should precede compressions: drowning, lightning strike, and avalanche burial.

Wilderness CPR Considerations

Even in urban settings, CPR with delayed use of an automated external defibrillator (AED) or delayed access to advanced medical care has success rates that are only 1-6%.

CPR should not be initiated in patients who have obvious signs of death such as lividity, rigor mortis, or decapitation.

Consider that CPR is exhausting to a rescuer, particularly in extreme conditions where energy may be required for self-evacuation. Safety of the rescuers must be considered in decisions regarding initiation and duration of CPR attempts.

Current AHA guidelines advise discontinuing CPR in patients who have sustained non-traumatic or blunt traumatic cardiac arrest with the exception of special situations such as lightning or hypothermia after a trial of advanced cardiac life support (ACLS) has been given.

Since ACLS is generally unavailable in the wilderness, if a patient has been pulseless for longer than 15 minutes, with or without CPR, further attempts at resuscitation should not be made (exceptions are lightning and hypothermia victims).

A hypothermic patient is "not dead until warm and dead" and requires longer time for determining the absence of a pulse (30-60 seconds).

These considerations should not prevent initiating CPR in situations where a helicopter or ACLS is accessible within 15-30 minutes, even if a prolonged evacuation may follow resuscitation.

- Rescue breathing is vital and necessary in patients with lightning strike, drowning and avalanche with snow burial.
- The European Rescue Council recommends giving 5 breaths at the beginning of CPR for a drowning victim instead of the 2 breaths recommended by the AHA.

SECONDARY SURVEY

- The goal of the secondary survey is to identify and treat any remaining less-critical injuries and illnesses.
- These conditions may become problems if left unnoticed or require advanced medical attention. This portion of the patient assessment is comprised of two key elements:
  - ☐ An abbreviated medical history
  - ☐ A physical exam
- The individual scenario should dictate the order in which these components are performed. For example, a fallen rock climber should typically have the physical exam portion of the secondary survey performed first to identify any other traumatic injuries, whereas an abbreviated history from a camper who has developed abdominal pain may be more useful. To reinforce the flexibility of the order, we will discuss the physical exam first.

Physical Exam

- The physical exam during the secondary survey is a more detailed **head-to-toe** examination where the rescuer should visibly inspect and palpate the victim from the head to toe, including the back.
- Use the mnemonic **CARTS** (see below) to assist in evaluating for potential sources of bleeding that are both internal and external.
- A general guide for areas to inspect include the following:
  - ☐ Pupils should be equal, round, and reactive to light (PERRL).
  - ☐ Blood or fluid draining from the ears or nose could suggest a head injury.
  - ☐ Look inside the mouth for loose teeth or other debris that may compromise the airway.
  - ☐ Palpate the cervical spine for tenderness and deformities.
  - ☐ Palpate the chest examining for tenderness, crepitance, and subcutaneous air.
  - ☐ Palpate all four quadrants of the abdomen.
  - ☐ Apply pressure to the pelvis in anterior-posterior and lateral-medial directions.
  - ☐ Examine all four extremities for deformities, tenderness, pulses, and, if the patient is conscious, strength and sensation.
- When an abnormality is found, ask the patient if this is an old or new problem.
- Use caution when assessing an area that is suspected to have an injury. Causing pain may impede your ability to obtain an accurate remainder of the exam. You should examine obvious areas of injury last in order to better facilitate your full evaluation of the patient.
- When examining an area the patient identifies as painful, begin by assessing above and below the injury, thereby determining the extent of the injury prior to touching the focus of the pain.
- Be aware of "distracting injuries" that cause so much pain that the patient does not notice that they have additional injuries. Determining a detailed MOI can help you anticipate other injuries.
- Examine the back of the patient at opportune times (e.g., when log-rolling the patient) to minimize movement.

Remember that with an alert and oriented patient, portions of the exam may be substituted for a reliable recollection of the MOI, such as, "I rolled my ankle, didn't fall, and just sat down here on this rock." Such a patient may only require a focused exam instead of a complete head-to-toe exam.

Abbreviated History

Most of the patient's history is obtained immediately by asking, "What happened?" But a few other key questions must be answered to ensure proper care is delivered.

The acronym **SAMPLE** will help you to remember the essential points of a patient's history.

For critical patients, you may be the only person who gets to talk to the patient while they are conscious. Therefore, if an initially unconscious patient regains consciousness, immediately obtain a history.

In patients with an altered level of responsiveness, other clues may be needed to obtain the history. A few examples of clues:

- ☐ Medical alert tags can be found in the form of necklaces, bracelets, anklets, tattoos, etc.
- ☐ List of medications or medical problems may be found in a wallet.
- ☐ Medications or devices such as a glucometer (blood sugar meter) or epinephrine auto-injector may be found in a victim's bag/tent/pocket/etc.
- ☐ Bystanders or family members may be familiar with a victim's past or present medical history.

To assist you in characterizing a victim's pain, employ the acronym **COLDERR**. Notice that this is most helpful in patients with pain from medical problems rather than traumatic injuries.

ONGOING SURVEY

Monitoring and Vitals

A unique aspect of wilderness medicine is that the rescuer may continue to care for a victim for several hours to days. This wide range of time requires adaptation of the usual patient assessment to include ongoing care. The ongoing survey is heavily dictated by patient's condition, and as such, is quite dynamic.

The initial set of vitals should generally be obtained during the secondary survey.

Vital signs may include:

- ☐ Pulse
- ☐ Respirations
- ☐ Level of Responsiveness (AVPU)
- ☐ Blood Pressure
- ☐ Skin Color, Temperature, Moisture

- ☐ Temperature
- ☐ Circulation, Sensation, Motor (CSM)
- ☐ Pain Level
- ☐ Blood Sugar

■ Reevaluate the vital signs depending on patient severity and if there is any change in their status.

■ As changes occur, for example, patient condition, level of responsiveness, or environment, go back to the beginning of the patient assessment.

■ If the rescuer has the time and appropriate materials, he or she should try to document the pertinent portions of the evaluation so that this can be handed off to the next level of care so that they have a better understanding of the victim's history.

■ To help in formulating your assessment of patients with an altered level of responsiveness, consider the acronym **AEIOU-TIPS**.

Primary Survey
Level of Responsiveness

A   Alert and Oriented x 1, 2, 3, 4 out of 4
       Person (self), Place, Time, Event
V   Verbal – Awakens briefly, withdraws, or moans when spoken to (A+O x 0/4)
P   Pain – Awakens briefly, withdraws, or moans in response to painful stimuli
U   Unresponsive – No response to any stimuli

Secondary Survey:
A Brief History

S   Signs and Symptoms (chief complaint)
A   Allergies - to anything
M   Medications / Medical alert tags
P   Past medical / surgical history (illness and injuries)
L   Last meal
E   Events leading up to and causing the accident / injury (what happened?)

Secondary Survey:
Characterizing the Pain

C   Character: What does the pain feel like?
O   Onset: When did the pain start?
L   Location: Where is the pain located? Have the victim point with one finger.
D   Duration: How long does the pain last?
E   Exacerbation: What makes the pain worse?
R   Relief: What makes the pain better?
R   Radiation: Does the pain move anywhere?

Secondary Survey: CARTS
Potential Areas of Major Bleeding

CHEST	The chest is a common source of bleeding, particularly in high-energy trauma. Look for shortness of breath, pain with breathing and coughing up blood. Examine for chest tenderness, crepitance over the ribs and sternum, flail chest, and crackling noises over the chest consistent with subcutaneous air.
ABDOMEN / PELVIS	Assume abdominal and/or pelvis bleeding in every trauma victim until proven otherwise. Look for bruising over the abdomen and pelvis. Palpate for abdominal and pelvic tenderness on compression.
RENAL / RETROPERITONEAL	Usually the bleeding is from the kidneys. Look for blood in the urine if you have a prolonged time with the victim. Examine for tenderness of the spine and chest at the level of the lowest ribs.
THIGH	This may occur if there is femur fracture. Look for deformity, swelling and bruising of the thigh. Palpate for tenderness and crepitance of the thigh.
SKIN / STREET	This is the most obvious place for a rescuer to detect blood. A common error in the wilderness setting is the failure to remove clothing or to roll the patient to look for bleeding. Also, ensure that you survey the area immediately surrounding the victim for a large amount of blood on the ground that may have come from the victim. Specifically, an arterial injury that bleeds significantly may be in spasm at the time you are evaluating the victim and not be an obvious source of bleeding.

GLASGOW COMA SCALE

Adults	#	Infants/Children
EYE OPENING		
spontaneous	4	spontaneous
to voice	3	to voice
to pain	2	to pain
none	1	none
VERBAL RESPONSE		
oriented	5	alert
confused	4	cries
inappropriate words	3	irritable
incomprehensible words	2	restless, moaning
none	1	none
MOTOR RESPONSE		
obeys commands	6	spontaneous
localizes pain	5	localizes pain
withdraws	4	withdraws
abnormal flexion	3	abnormal flexion
abnormal extension	2	abnormal extension
none	1	none

Formulating the Assessment:
Altered Mental Status Patients

A   Allergies (anaphylaxis) / Altitude
E   Environment (hyper or hypothermia) / Epilepsy (seizure) – active or postictal
I   Infection (sepsis, meningitis)
O   Overdose (alcohol, medicine)
U   Underdose (medicines)
T   Trauma / Toxins
I   Insulin (diabetes)
P   Psychological disorder
S   Stroke

QUESTIONS

1. **What is the purpose of the blood sweep during the primary survey?**
   a. To clear the scene of blood by sweeping it away
   b. To identify sites of major bleeding
   c. To stop bleeding from most wounds
   d. All of the above

2. **You are rock climbing with several of your friends when there is a rock slide and 3 of your friends fall 10 to 20 feet to the bottom of the cliff. There are also 2 other people who were injured by falling debris soon afterwards while standing at the bottom of the cliff and looking up. Which one of the following is correct in terms of managing this situation?**
   a. You should move all of the injured people away from the base of the cliff
   b. You should not move anybody as there is a risk of spinal injury by moving them
   c. You should put an overhead shade over those at the base of the cliff but not move them
   d. You should leave all patients where they are lying and leave immediately to get help

3. **A hiker falls down a steep embankment 100 feet and lands at the bottom. She is pale but awake. She has a thready carotid pulse of 130 beats / minute and complains of feeling very thirsty. Which one of the following best explains her increased heart rate, paleness and thready pulse?**
   a. Abrasions on her lower legs and hands that are dirty but have no active bleeding
   b. Deformity of her left wrist without any significant swelling.
   c. Deformity, pain and swelling in her right ankle
   d. Severe tenderness on palpation of her abdomen

4. **Which one of the following is NOT correct in regards to obtaining a history from a patient in the secondary survey?**
   a. S = Signs and Symptoms
   b. A = Allergies
   c. M = Medications
   d. P = Past medical history
   e. L = Last meal
   f. E = Exposure to elements

5. **You are three days into a weeklong backpacking trip when someone in your group develops worsening abdominal pain. After performing a thorough assessment, you suspect constipation to be the cause and elect to watch the patient overnight. How frequently should you re-assess the victim?**
   a. Every 15 minutes
   b. Just reassess in the morning
   c. Never, you already made your assessment
   d. Whenever a change in patient condition or environment occurs

6. **Which one of the following is NOT an area that is concerning for occult blood loss in the trauma victim?**
   a. Abdomen
   b. Buttocks
   c. Chest
   d. Pelvis

7. **You are snowshoeing in the mountains during winter. It has been in the mid 20's most of the day when you come upon a 35 year-old man off to the side of the trail. He is breathing and has a strong regular pulse but is very confused and slow to respond to you. He does not complain of anything. Which one of the following is a potential etiology for his altered mental status?**
   a. Hypoglycemia due to too much insulin
   b. Seizure with a post-seizure confusion
   c. Intoxication with alcohol
   d. All of the above should be considered

8. **You arrive at the scene of a drowning event. The victim has been pulled from the water and is lying on his back. On your initial assessment the victim is completely unresponsive without any sign of life. Which one of the following is the most appropriate next step in the management of the victim?**
   a. Initiate CPR with chest compressions only
   b. Initiate CPR starting with 2-rescue breaths
   c. Perform a blood sweep
   d. Start rewarming the patient using blankets and body heat

9. **Which one of the following is not correct for the Primary Assessment?**

    a. M – Massive hemorrhage management
    b. A – Airway with cervical spine stabilization
    c. R – Respiration
    d. C – Circulation
    e. H – Hemorrhage assessment

Answers:

1. b
2. a
3. d
4. f
5. d
6. b
7. d
8. b
9. e

CHAPTER 2

Wound Management

This chapter describes the assessment and treatment of injuries to the skin that occur in the wilderness.

Objectives:

- Recognize the importance of identification and thorough examination of wounds in the wilderness
- Classify the different types of wounds and burns
- Describe the actions necessary for hemostasis
- Discuss methods to prevent infection
- Understand closure options for wounds in the wilderness
- Differentiate wounds that may require evacuation from the backcountry

CASE 1

You are the medical expert in a group on a multi-day trek. You come across an individual who has a blood-soaked shirt wrapped around his forearm. He states that he fell six hours ago while free climbing. You examine his forearm and note some continued bleeding from a four-centimeter laceration includes exposed and injured muscle.

1. What are the examination principles for this wound?
2. What steps should you take to attempt to achieve hemostasis?
3. What is the most important step to prevent infection?
4. If you have the appropriate supplies, should you close the wound?
5. Does the patient require evacuation?
6. What factors determine the need to evacuate wounded patients from the backcountry?

CASE 2

You are the medical expert on a mountaineering expedition when one of the individuals suffers a splash burn from the oil in a kerosene lamp. You assess the patient, beginning with a primary survey. You note no airway compromise or respiratory distress. The rest of the examination is normal, except for a full circumference burn of the left forearm, totaling about 5% total body surface area (TBSA). Most of the burn is erythematous with blisters, but about 2% TBSA is off-white and insensate.

1. What is the proper initial treatment for this burn?
2. Should you initiate evacuation procedures for this individual?
3. Which burns require evacuation?
4. When is an escharotomy necessary?

BACKGROUND

- Injuries to the skin are among the most common problems encountered in the wilderness.
- In the wilderness, where it may be difficult to keep an injury clean or properly covered, even a simple abrasion can become a serious problem.
- When evaluating any wound, it is important to thoroughly examine the wound. Areas of consideration include the following:

- [ ] Type of wound (abrasion, laceration, etc.)
- [ ] Location
- [ ] Dimensions (width, length, and depth)
- [ ] Severity of contamination
- [ ] Presence or absence of foreign body
- [ ] Bone, tendon, joint, muscle and nerve involvement

■ If the wound is overlying or adjacent to a joint, it must be examined through a full range of motion of the joint to look for evidence of disruption of the joint capsule. Other principles to consider:
  - [ ] Full exposure of affected area
  - [ ] Hemostasis
  - [ ] Examination of distal neurovascular and musculoskeletal function
  - [ ] Cleaning and control of infection
  - [ ] Definitive wound care to preserve function of the injured part

■ Examination in the wilderness can be challenging; lighting may not be adequate. A headlamp is an excellent hands-free tool to improve visualization in the wilderness.

PATHOPHYSIOLOGY

General

■ An understanding of the processes involved in wound formation and repair is essential to properly direct treatment and to determine the need for evacuation.

■ When skin is disrupted, the wound becomes invaded with potentially infectious bacteria. Contaminants may include skin flora (especially concerning if the patient is colonized with methicillin-resistant *S. aureus* (MRSA)), or bacteria that reside on the surface of the penetrating object. Other virulent organisms include *Clostridium* species from soil, *Pseudomonas* residing in footwear or water sources, and oral flora from various bites, including *Pasteurella*, *Eikenella*, and *Streptococcus*.

■ Early thorough irrigation and protection from the environment are essential to wound management. This may be difficult in the wilderness. As time elapses without intervention for the wound, bacteria growth quickly increases to a point where primary closure may no longer be a reasonable approach. This is a common dilemma in the wilderness, as an injured individual may not have access to immediate and adequate treatment. There is no single time limit that best determines whether a wound may be closed primarily or by delayed primary closure or should be left open to heal by secondary intention. Instead, familiarity with the multiple factors associated with wound infections and scarring should be considered when evaluating and treating a wound.

■ Factors to consider when treating a wound:

- ☐ Time elapsed since injury
- ☐ Location of injury
- ☐ Degree of contamination
- ☐ Severity of injury and involvement of underlying tissue
- ☐ Type of forces applied
- ☐ Immunocompetency of the patient

Head and facial wounds heal especially well, even with closure up to 100 hours from the initial time of injury.

Abrasions

Abrasions are superficial injuries to the skin typically caused by friction against a hard or rough surface resulting in injury to or loss of the upper layers of the skin.

A well-known example of an abrasion is "road rash."

Blisters

Blisters are intradermal pockets of fluid that result from frictional forces exerted on the skin surface.

If friction continues without intervention, the blisters enlarge and rupture, leading to painfully exposed sensitive lower dermal layers.

Lacerations

Lacerations are caused by multiple different types of forces.

Wounds created by shear forces are most common; a sharp object cuts through the skin. Shear force injuries also have the best healing properties, as underlying tissue is minimally disrupted.

A puncture wound is a focal, potentially deep injury from a penetrating object where the depth is greater than the length of the wound. Because of the concentrated force and potential depth involved, puncture wounds are associated with a higher rate of infection.

A crush injury occurs when one strikes a blunt object, as in the forehead striking the ground. This leads to tissue devitalization and increased risk for infection.

Burns

Burns lead to local necrosis and release of inflammatory mediators. When more than 15–20% of the total body surface area is involved, the effects become systemic.

Wilderness causes of burns with varying degrees of severity include the following:

- ☐ Scald burns due to splashes or immersion in hot liquid

- ☐ Flame burns
- ☐ Flash burns due to explosions
- ☐ Thermal burns from contact with hot materials

CLINICAL PRESENTATION

Abrasions

These "road rash" injuries can range from minor scrapes that involve the epidermis only and require minimal attention to injuries that cause major skin disruption, as seen in high-speed crashes.

More serious injuries may involve muscle tissue and be serious enough to require skin grafting.

Most abrasions result in minimal blood loss but can be very painful due to the exposure of many nerve endings.

Blisters

Blisters that develop in the backcountry most commonly form due to repetitive frictional forces.

Hiking in improperly broken-in or poorly fitting shoes is a common etiology.

A blister is typically preceded by a "hot spot," which is a tender, erythematous area formed from frictional forces.

Presentation may range from minor and even painless fluid collections to debilitating injuries that may require evacuation.

Complications include cellulitis and osteomyelitis; occasionally resulting in systemic infections.

Lacerations

Cuts of the skin have multiple presentations:

- ☐ Linear or abnormal lacerations due to shear, blunt, or stretching forces
- ☐ Puncture wounds are lacerations with depth greater than length. These have a higher risk of infection and retained foreign bodies. Due to the depth and unknown pathway, adequate examination is difficult.
- ☐ Avulsion and amputation are lacerations in which tissue is excised. Some tissue avulsions may be minor or involve the very distal extremities. In such minor cases, re-implantation is neither possible nor necessary.
- ☐ Animal bites may cause puncture wounds and lacerations. Due to the oral flora of the animal and the tissue damage from the teeth, these are at high risk for infection.

Burns

■ Burns are categorized by size, quantified as the percentage of body surface area involved, depth, and location.

Burn Size

The "Rule of Nines" can be used to estimate the percentage of the total body surface area (TBSA) that has been burned.

- ☐ Each arm: 9% of TBSA
- ☐ Each leg: 18% of TBSA
- ☐ Front of trunk: 18% of TBSA
- ☐ Back of trunk: 18% of TBSA
- ☐ Head and neck: 9% of TBSA
- ☐ Groin: 1% of TBSA

Another, sometimes easier to use, estimation guide is the patient's palm, which represents approximately 1% TBSA.

Burn Depth

Burns have classically been described in terms of degrees (1st, 2nd, 3rd, 4th). However, the currently accepted classification is based according to need for surgical intervention: superficial, superficial partial-thickness, deep partial-thickness, and full-thickness burns.

Superficial Burns

The epidermis is reddened and mildly tender. A common example is sunburn.
■ Although painful, this is the easiest type of burn to treat, and evacuation is generally unnecessary.

Partial Thickness Burns

Superficial partial-thickness

The epidermis and superficial dermis are injured.
The skin is blistered and the exposed dermis is red.

Deep partial-thickness

■ Extends into deeper layers of the dermis, damaging hair follicles and sweat glands.
The skin is blistered and the exposed dermis is pale white to yellow.
Similar to full-thickness burns, the center of the burn may be insensate.

Full Thickness Burns

- All layers of the skin have been burned including blood vessels and nerves.
- The flesh may be charred, but the victim feels little or no pain because the nerve endings have been destroyed.
- Painful partial thickness burns may surround the full-thickness burn.
- Full-thickness burns require skin grafting.
- These injuries may extend through the skin to the subcutaneous fat, muscle, or bone.

WOUND TREATMENT

General Considerations

Exposure

- Adequate exposure and visualization of the entire wound.
- Areas immediately adjacent to the injury should also be exposed, including associated joints.

Hemostasis

First line of action: Direct pressure
- ☐ Application of direct pressure controls bleeding from most wounds.
- ☐ Using the cleanest material available, control the bleeding by applying direct pressure to the source of bleeding.
- ☐ Larger wounds may require direct pressure for several minutes.
- ☐ Scalp wounds may require continuous direct pressure for 30 to 60 minutes in order to achieve hemostasis.

Second line of action: Pressure dressing +/- a hemostatic bandage
- ☐ If after 10 minutes the wound is continuing to bleed, then you must move on to more significant measures.
- ☐ You should apply a pressure dressing and a hemostatic bandage if you have one available.
- ☐ The key is to add additional pressure and dressings over the initial dressing, rather than removing it, otherwise removal will likely worsen the bleeding. The one time where one should remove the initial dressing is if it is not a hemostatic bandage and you have a hemostatic bandage available to put directly on the wound.
- ☐ How to apply a pressure dressing:
  - Place the dressing over the wound or the initial dressing.

- Wrap and hold that dressing in place with an elastic bandage (Ace® wrap) or tape that is wrapped circumferentially around the extremity.
- If you have a special "hemostatic" dressing which is specifically designed to stop bleeding then you should apply this directly to the wound and then wrap it with a pressure dressing.
- If the patient continues to bleed through the pressure dressing, then you should remove the elastic bandage and place additional dressing on top of the dressing that is already on the wound.
    - Do not remove that initial dressing
    - Wrap this additional dressing with elastic bandage
    - Apply direct pressure with your hand on top of this pressure dressing. This step is often skipped as the provider feels that the pressure dressing will lend more pressure than direct pressure from a hand. However, this is not true and the additional pressure from the hand over the pressure dressing until the bleeding is stopped is important.
- After applying a pressure bandage, be sure to check distal function and pulse often.

☐ When a limb is affected dress the wound as previously described and consider elevating the extremity if you are able, although this has never been proven to be effective.

☐ In the past, this was the point when "pressure points" would be used over inflowing arteries with the concept of diminishing the flow into the area of injury, which would allow the wound to clot.
- This is <u>no longer recommended</u>.
- There is no evidence to show that pressure points are effective for stopping bleeding.
- There is a risk of limb injury / ischemia from inhibiting the blood flow into the whole limb.
- The bleeding may actually worsen the bleeding due to compression of the out flowing vein and back pressure into the venous system.

■ Third line of action: Tourniquet

☐ If the first two methods do not control the bleeding and if the victim is in danger of bleeding significantly, then use a tourniquet.

☐ Tourniquets are to be used only if the wound is on a limb.

☐ A tourniquet may be the first line of control necessary in a life-threatening hemorrhagic wound as described in the "**M**" of massive hemorrhage in MARCH.

☐ It is reasonable to place a tourniquet initially in order to staunch massive hemorrhage in your primary assessment of the patient. Once the patient is stabilized, then you may go back and better assess the wound / injury and determine whether you can control the bleeding with the initial two steps previously described and then to loosen the tourniquet.

☐ You can use a commercially available tourniquet or you may improvise a tourniquet out of a strip of cloth at least two inches wide and a stick or some other rigid item to act as your windlass.

☐ Never use wire, twine, cord, or any other thin material that will not apply a wide enough area of pressure but may cut the skin.

■ **How to place a tourniquet**
  ☐ Place the tourniquet over the smoothed sleeve or trouser leg if possible.
  ☐ Place the tourniquet around the limb two to four inches above the wound.
  ☐ Do not place the tourniquet on a joint or directly over a wound or a fracture.
  ☐ If the wound is just below a joint then place the tourniquet as close to the joint as possible but not on the joint.
  ☐ Once the tourniquet is in place, it should be tightened so that all bleeding stops.
  ☐ If you are using an improvised cloth strip, then tie a half-knot and place the windlass on the knot. Then tie a second half-knot on the windlass and then tighten than by twisting it until the bleeding stops.
  ☐ Secure the windlass so that it does not unwind.
  ☐ Mark the time that you placed the tourniquet on the patient's forehead so it is rapidly visible to other personnel when the care for the victim.

■ Sometimes you may initially apply a tourniquet and treat a bleeding wound with a pressure dressing and potentially control the bleeding.
  ☐ In these cases, it is appropriate to fully dress the wound with the pressure and/or hemostatic dressing while the tourniquet is tightened and then to loosen the tourniquet to see if the bleeding has been controlled with the dressing.
    ● If bleeding continues, then the tourniquet must be tightened again.
    ● If the bleeding is controlled then you should loosen the tourniquet but leave it in place in case the bleeding recurs.
    ● There is no indication to intermittently loosen a tourniquet for "perfusion" of an extremity.

Anesthesia

Topical anesthesia
■ Topical anesthesia is somewhat effective for skin lacerations and can be appropriate for wilderness medicine, if somebody carries it with them.
■ The common formulation is a combination of lidocaine, epinephrine, and tetracaine (LET).
  ☐ The solution is soaked into sterile gauze and placed directly over the wound for 20-30 minutes.
  ☐ An area of blanching at the site of administration indicates adequate anesthesia.

Local anesthesia
■ Local anesthesia using an injection of 1% lidocaine (without epinephrine) is the standard method for achieving soft tissue anesthesia for closing a wound.
■ Use of local lidocaine requires additional supplies (syringes, needles, etc.) and precautions, such as sharp disposal and protection of the lidocaine from extreme temperatures. However, syringes and needles themselves have multiple uses in wilderness medicine.

If one is not prepared with the above supplies, the wound may require treatment without the benefit of anesthesia, which may diminish the ability to effectively clean and treat a wound.

Irrigation

High-pressure irrigation is the most important intervention to prevent infection.

Irrigate the wound with a solid stream of disinfected water or saline.

If available, use a syringe with a catheter tip (ideally, an 18 or 19 gauge needle or catheter) to create a high-pressure stream of water.

If a syringe is not available, fill a plastic bag or hydration system with the cleanest fluid available (tap water has been shown to be as effective as sterile saline). Poke a small hole in a corner of the bag, and then close the top of the bag to create a seal in order to force a stream of high-pressured water from the bag.

A plastic water bottle with an adjustable top may also be improvised and used.

Gently separate the wound edges and irrigate while holding the syringe or bag over the wound.

Rinse the wound forcefully with the water, protecting your skin and eyes from fluid splashes. If a splash shield is not available, a 4x4 gauze pad can be taped at the opening of the irrigation system.

A generally accepted principle is to irrigate with at least 60 mL of fluid per centimeter of injury, with a minimum total volume of 200 mL.

Debridement

It is important to remove visible foreign matter from the wound to minimize infection, inflammation, discomfort, and skin tattooing.

If possible, also remove any clearly devitalized tissue, which may serve as a culture medium for any remaining bacteria.

Debridement should be followed with another round of high-pressure irrigation and reexamination.

Abrasions

Abrasions should be irrigated as described above. If anesthesia is required, topical anesthesia may be used, as it is usually difficult to infiltrate the entire area of an abrasion.

Debridement is extremely important to prevent against permanent scarring due to retained foreign bodies.

Blisters

If a small blister or hot spot forms, place a donut-shaped dressing of moleskin over the affected area, with the donut hole matching the actual size of the blister or hot spot.

- ☐ The moleskin may be anchored by tincture of benzoin or a similar product and secured with tape.
- ☐ Several layers of moleskin may be used.
- ☐ Avoid opening or puncturing small, intact blisters.
- What size and when a blister should be intentionally ruptured are controversial. In general, if the blister is 2 cm in diameter or larger, then it is likely to spontaneously rupture and may be amenable to initial treatment by intentionally rupturing it. However, the reality is that there is no best answer for this issue.
- In those cases where it is large enough or already ruptured, wash the area and puncture the base of the blister with a sterile needle or sterilized safety pin. Debride the external flap of skin from the blister, apply an antibiotic ointment and cover the blister with a sterile dressing. This can be protected with moleskin or mole foam.
- Hydrocolloid dressings have increased in popularity, also providing protection and comfort.
- Hot spots and blisters should be inspected daily. If an intact blister becomes infected, drain and débride it and seek medical attention.

Puncture Wounds

- Although the surface of a puncture wound should be cleaned to facilitate examination, puncture wounds themselves should generally NOT be irrigated, as this may further push in contamination. The wound should be dressed without closure. Puncture wounds should be evaluated more frequently than simple lacerations, as they are associated with a high risk of infection.

General Laceration Wound Closure

In the wilderness, it is difficult to achieve adequate wound care as outlined above. If the provider is well prepared and resources are available, closure techniques may mirror those of a clinic and sutures may be used. However, in many situations this protocol may not be feasible or appropriate.

- The decision is broken down to three potential courses of action
  - ☐ Primary closure with suture, staples, tape or tissue adhesive
    - Advantage = rapid treatment with potentially earlier mobility and less pain
    - Disadvantage = higher risk of infection
  - ☐ Delayed primary closure (DPC): This means irrigating and debriding the wound and then packing it. Remove the packing at 48 – 72 hours and irrigate the wound and then close it using one of the described closure methods.
    - Advantage = less risk of infection with similar cosmetic outcome to primary closure
    - Disadvantage = potentially more pain and loss of functionality of that area which could be problematic in the wilderness.

☐ Heal by secondary intention which means irrigating and debriding the wound and then packing it with at least daily dressing changes and allowing the wound to heal on its own without any closure techniques.

- Advantage = lowest risk of infection
- Disadvantage = largest scarring and potentially more pain and loss of functionality of that area which could be more problematic in the wilderness.

Interestingly, there is no improved outcome (in terms of cosmetic appearance) of primary closure versus delayed primary closure.

Closure may be achieved most simply by using micropore tape.

Remove a wound closure strip from its backing and tape the wound together. The tape should close the wound so the edges of the wound touch but are not mashed together.

If necessary, trim the hair around the edges of the wound so the tape will adhere better.

Make sure the tape overlaps at least 1 inch on each side of the wound. Use as much tape as needed, with each strip placed several millimeters apart.

If micropore tape is not readily available, duct tape with perforations made with a safety pin may suffice. The holes should be made from the sticky side pushed out towards the non-sticky side so that it will allow better drainage of fluid from the wound.

Sutures and staples can both be used effectively if continued cleanliness of the wound can be assured, and are more appropriate for large wounds and those in high-tension areas.

Staples can be used anywhere except the face. Some believe that micropore tape and staples will adequately close the majority of skin wounds in the wilderness. However, personal preference and packing limitations will dictate what closure material one decides to bring.

Tissue adhesives may be used for closing small and uncomplicated lacerations.

The chemical is applied on top of the wound and serves as a bandage to close the wound.

They are as effective as sutures for low-tension areas.

They also produce an impenetrable barrier that requires a thoroughly cleansed wound.

Tissue adhesives are easy to transport, but are moderately expensive and sensitive to cold temperatures and prolonged exposure to direct light.

If applying a tissue adhesive, do NOT use topical antimicrobials, as these petroleum-based products will dissolve the glue.

Dressing

Wound dressing is important for protection from the environment and prevention of infection and can be accomplished in a number of ways.

If a commercial non-adhesive/stick pad or dressing is not available, improvise using a 4 x 4 pad covered in an antibiotic ointment. Cover this dressing with an absorbent gauze dressing, then secure with tape.

If the injury is on a flexible part of the body – an elbow or finger, for example – immobilize the joint with a splint to prevent the wound from reopening.

Antibiotics

Topical antibiotics are appropriate for all skin wounds, unless a skin adhesive is used.

Bacitracin or mupirocin are reasonable choices. Neomycin is less ideal because it is associated with allergic reactions.

Another ideal topical antimicrobial is honey. The osmolarity and bacteriostatic compounds in unprocessed honey make it an extremely effective, inexpensive and readily available alternative for topical application.

Systemic antibiotic administration for lacerations is still a debated subject. Adequate cleansing and protection from the environment are much more important factors in prevention of infection. As stated above, multiple factors must be considered when determining whether or not to administer systemic antimicrobials prophylactically.

Indications for systemic antimicrobials generally mirror those in the clinical setting:

- ☐ Complex or mutilating wounds
- ☐ Grossly contaminated with penetrating debris
- ☐ Extensive lacerations of the ear and cartilage
- ☐ Penetration of bone, joint, or tendon
- ☐ Animal bites
- ☐ Open wounds in patients with valvular heart disease, diabetes, or immunosuppression

Additionally, wounds that cannot be adequately protected from the environment may benefit from prophylactic antibiotics.

Any wounds with signs of infection should receive antibiotics. These signs include:

- ☐ Pain
- ☐ Redness
- ☐ Swelling
- ☐ Purulent discharge
- ☐ Fever

Antimicrobial prophylaxis should be generally administered for 3 to 5 days. A longer course provides no added protection against infection and increases the risk of resistance. Current acceptable choices for prophylaxis include a first-generation cephalosporin, amoxicillin-clavulanate, or clindamycin. Suspicion of MRSA may require different antibiotic coverage such as trimethoprim/sulfamethoxazole, clindamycin, or doxycycline.

Treatment for active infection should be administered for 7-10 days and should be tailored to suspected organism and local resistance patterns.

Dressing changes and wound checks should be performed at least once daily in the backcountry.

Most infections begin within 48 hours, but aggressive and gas-forming infections may begin within hours.

Special Lacerations

Scalp

The extent and severity of scalp lacerations are often initially obscured by surrounding hair that is matted with blood. Copious irrigation is often necessary to visualize the laceration. Hair may be trimmed if necessary, but this should be limited to the immediate area of the laceration, since the surrounding hair can later be twisted into strands and used to approximate the wound edges. Once the margins of the scalp laceration have been defined, local or topical anesthetics may be applied.

Physical examination of a scalp laceration should assess the integrity of the galea aponeurotica tissue layer that overlies the skull. A significant galeal laceration, or the presence of a de-gloving injury, mandates evacuation. This is especially true in victims with mental status changes who may have an underlying skull fracture.

Minor scalp lacerations can be effectively treated in the wilderness setting. After the application of analgesia and wound exploration, mechanical high-pressure irrigation should be employed. Surgical debridement of scalp wounds should be kept to an absolute minimum, because it may be difficult to mobilize wound edges to cover the resulting soft tissue defect.

Staples are effective in closing scalp lacerations.

For small lacerations, the "hair tie" technique may be effective. For this you roll several strands of hair together on each side of the wound, then you cross those over the wound and roll those together in one big roll and then secure that roll with tissue adhesive, super glue or possibly tape. This is only effective for wounds 1 – 2 cm in length.

Face

Superficial lacerations to the face may be managed in the wilderness.

However, if there are injuries to any of the following the victim should be evacuated for definitive management: facial nerve, parotid gland, lacrimal ducts, eyelids, ear or nose cartilage.

Anesthesia for lacerations to the face can be achieved using topical, local or regional blocks, depending on available resources and expertise. As with other lacerations, high-pressure irrigation is the method of choice for mechanical cleaning, and surgical debridement should be limited to obvious areas of necrotic tissue. The face has an excellent blood supply; consequently, wound closure using micropore tape or a skin glue can be effective and produce satisfying cosmetic results.

Torso

Torso lacerations require evaluation for fascial penetration. If the anterior fascial layer is penetrated, the injury should not be considered a skin injury, but rather an injury to the underlying region. Specifically, if the fascial layer of the chest or abdomen is penetrated, the patient should be immediately evacuated.

Distal Extremity

Management of extremity lacerations in the wilderness requires careful judgment because of the potential involvement of underlying structures.

This is especially true with the hand, where critical structures lie close to the surface.

A detailed neurovascular evaluation of all extremity lacerations should be performed as well as an inspection of the wound throughout the range of motion as tendon injuries may easily be missed.

Any evidence of neurovascular functional compromise with a hand wound mandates evacuation.

Animal Bites

Animal bites should be cleaned, débrided and dressed as described.

Antibiotics should be strongly considered.

Definitive wound closure is rarely appropriate because of the high risk for infection. Specific treatment is discussed in the animal bites chapter.

Superficial Burns

Treat with aloe-vera gel.

For comfort, cool the area with damp wet cloths.

Avoid further exposure to heat and sunlight.

Partial and Full Thickness Burns

Gently clean the burn with cool water to remove loose skin and debris.

Trim away all loose skin.

Apply a thin layer of antibacterial ointment to the burn and cover with a non-adhesive, sterile dressing. Inspect the wound and change the dressing at least once a day.

Do not apply ice directly to burns for more than 15 minutes, as this may cause more tissue damage due to a decreased blood supply to the area.

Burns that compromise blood flow or respiratory drive

A severe full-thickness burn across the chest or an extremity may produce an eschar, which can result in respiratory or circulatory embarrassment.

If the patient with a burn over the chest wall develops respiratory distress, or if a circumferential extremity burn develops circulatory compromise during evacuation, an incision through the subcutaneous tissue in the proper planes can save life or limb.

One should be familiar with these techniques of escharotomy before attempting to utilize them.

PREVENTION

As skin injuries are among the most common injuries in the wilderness, simple preventative measures can be taken to decrease the risk of and from them.

Improper knife handling and care are also responsible for an excessive number of skin injuries.

Adequate lighting should be used in the wilderness as much as possible to avoid falls and other injuries.

■ Tetanus is a life-threatening infection, and many wounds in the wilderness are considered tetanus-prone. ALL individuals should have their tetanus immunization updated before participating in wilderness activities. If they have not and sustained a wound, they should have their tetanus updated as soon as they return from the wilderness.

EVACUATION GUIDELINES

Evacuation of patients with wounds should occur when necessary to preserve life, limb, function, and when an infection cannot be controlled.

An individual with even a minimally infected friction blister of the foot could require evacuation, whereas a forearm abscess with surrounding cellulitis may be monitored if the proper tools and antibiotics are available.

■ Burn evacuation guidelines mirror those that require treatment in a burn center:
- □ Partial thickness burns greater than 10% TBSA
- □ Full thickness burns greater than 1% TBSA
- □ Partial or full thickness burns involving the face, hands, feet, or genitals
- □ Electric burns
- □ Burns complicated by smoke inhalation (The victim's airway may become obstructed from severe swelling in the throat.)
- □ Burn victims who are medically ill

QUESTIONS

1. **Which type of wound is least likely to become infected, and thus would be the best candidate for backcountry closure?**
   a. A cut from a knife leading to a 2 cm forearm laceration
   b. A crush injury caused when mountain biker strikes the ground with his lower leg
   c. A puncture wound through the plantar surface of the foot caused by a piece of broken glass at a campground
   d. A stab wound to the abdomen inflicted by a pocket knife

2. **All of these would be acceptable topical antimicrobials except**
   a. Bacitracin
   b. Mupirocin
   c. LET (lidocaine, epinephrine, tetracaine)
   d. Silvadene

3. **Which burn does NOT require evacuation?**
   a. A camper wakes up when his tent has caught on fire because he didn't properly put out his campfire. He is able to evacuate from the tent, but he is coughing frequently and has singed nose-hairs
   b. A patient with burns on the forearm after attempting to treat a snakebite by placing jumper cables adjacent to the area and starting the car
   c. A patient with 4 centimeters of erythema only which is located on the dorsum of the forearm after brushing against hot firewood
   d. A patient with diabetic neuropathy and blistering of the plantar surface of the foot after stepping on hot coals

4. **Which is necessary to evaluate when examining a wound in the wilderness?**
   a. Location, extent, and depth of the wound
   b. Presence or absence of foreign body
   c. Bone, tendon, or joint involvement
   d. All of the above

5. **Which wound requires evacuation?**
    a. A 2 day old puncture wound of the foot that has developed surrounding erythema and is extremely painful to walk on, despite the administration of prophylactic antibiotics
    b. A 3 day old 2 cm arm laceration that has developed some purulent drainage in an afebrile patient who can be started on antibiotics
    c. A 4 cm leg laceration that has been irrigated, has no foreign body, bone, tendon, joint involvement, and is secured with duct tape
    d. A 6 cm laceration of the head closed with staples

6. **Which is the best way to treat a simple friction blister?**
    a. Clean the area, cut a ring of moleskin, adhere with benzoin and cover with athletic tape and lamb's wool if necessary
    b. Cut a ring of moleskin, adhere with benzoin, cover with tape and place on prophylactic antibiotics
    c. Evacuate all friction blisters
    d. Ignore it; most blisters pop or stop hurting sooner or later

7. **For which wound should a tourniquet be used as the primary method of hemostasis?**
    a. An amputation of the little finger at the level of the distal phalanx
    b. An amputation of the leg at the level of the knee, sustained in a high-speed 4-wheeler collision
    c. A rapidly bleeding scalp laceration
    d. A radial artery laceration

8. **Which wound would be the best candidate for antibiotics?**
    a. A 1 cm facial laceration that occurred 12 hours ago
    b. A 1 cm laceration over the index finger metacarpal-phalangeal joint, obtained in a fight the night before
    c. A 2 cm laceration of the palm due to a clean pocket knife 4 hours ago
    d. A 3 cm scalp laceration that occurred 6 hours ago

9. **Which best describes a superficial partial-thickness burn?**
   a. A burn that includes the dermis and epidermis with a central painless white area
   b. A large burn with exposed muscle and bone
   c. A painful area of erythema without blistering or tissue loss
   d. A painful area of erythema with blistering

Answers:

1. a
2. c
3. c
4. d
5. a
6. a
7. b
8. b
9. d

CHAPTER 3

Musculoskeletal Injuries

This chapter describes how to recognize and treat musculoskeletal injuries in the wilderness.

Objectives:

- Be able to identify and treat life-threatening musculoskeletal injuries
- Describe methods to help identify fractures and dislocations
- Discuss when to reduce and splint fractures in the wilderness
- Describe various methods to properly manage dislocations, strains, and sprains in the wilderness
- Be familiar with musculoskeletal injuries associated with some common wilderness activities

CASE 1

You are biking on a single-track trail with a friend. You come around a bend and hear a call of distress. You slow your bike to a halt as you look to your right where the edge of the trail turns into a downward slope. Lying on his right side, amongst a pile of scattered boulders, is a middle-aged man. His bike is about seven feet uphill from him. As you go through your initial assessment, you notice that he is favoring his left shoulder. The patient is very sensitive to movement of his left shoulder and complains of severe pain. The left shoulder appears to be dislocated. Further examination shows that he is neuro-vascularly intact over the left arm and hand.

1. What is your approach to this injury?
2. What is the more common direction of dislocation of the shoulder?
3. Would you reduce this man's shoulder in this case?
4. When would you consider doing a reduction in the field?
5. What other important assessments do you need to make?

CASE 2

At the tail end of an intense day of hiking on day five of your eight-day backpacking trip, one of your group members abruptly stops and grabs the front of her left knee. You remove her pack and have her sit in a comfortable position. She explains that she was jumping off a three-foot ledge and twisted her knee because the lateral side of her left foot landed unsteadily on a small rock. She heard a "popping" sound when the injury occurred. You begin your exam and notice that her left knee appears to be swollen when compared to her uninjured right knee.

1. What tests will you perform to assess the patient?
2. How would you determine if she requires evacuation?
3. How will you stabilize this injury?

CASE 3

You are heading on a day trip to do some rock climbing and have with you your basic first-aid kit, some food, a knife, flashlight, and change of clothes that you carry with you on all day trips. You come across a male frantically searching for help, screaming that his buddy has fallen and has a significant leg injury that will not allow him to walk. As he leads you towards the patient, he tells you they were scrambling around on some rocks over a cliff. His friend had tried to complete a five-foot jump from one cliff edge to another, slipped and fell about 30 feet. You smell alcohol on the breath of this individual, and he admits they had "one or two beers." You approach the scene and see a male in his mid-twenties lying near some rocks at the bottom of a 10-foot wide canyon enclosed by two 30-foot cliff faces. You approach the patient.

1. How do you proceed with the assessment?
2. Can you clear his cervical spine or will he need cervical immobilization?
3. Which fracture(s) may be placed in traction in the field?
4. What are the contraindications to traction?

GENERAL

- Management of orthopedic injuries begins only after massive hemorrhage as well as the patient's airway, pulmonary, and cardiovascular status have been stabilized.
- Initial evaluation of the musculoskeletal system should include careful attention to stabilization of the spine.
  - ☐ The cervical, thoracic, and lumbar spine should be inspected closely and palpated for signs of fracture or instability.
  - ☐ Once the spine is stabilized or cleared, attention is focused on the pelvis and extremities.
- An open pelvic fracture with associated GI and/or GU injuries carries a 50 percent mortality rate.
- The shoulder is the most commonly *dislocated* major joint.
  - ☐ Anterior dislocation of the shoulder is the most common type of shoulder dislocation, occurring in over 90% of shoulder dislocations.
  - ☐ While uncommon, posterior shoulder dislocations occur most often with a direct blow to the anterior shoulder after a seizure or electrical / lightning injury.
- A posterior hip dislocation occurs in about 85 percent of hip dislocations.
- The ankle is the most commonly *sprained* major joint.

BASIC FRACTURE MANAGEMENT

Assessing for Fracture in the Wilderness

- In the wilderness, you must rely on your physical examination to best determine whether a bone is fractured.
- Always compare the injured side to the uninjured side.

History elicited from the patient should include: Time and mechanism of injury, sound or sensation consistent with fracture, subsequent ability to use the injured area, and numbness or weakness of the extremity.

Pain and tenderness that is consistent with a fracture includes:

- ☐ Pain and point tenderness to palpation over a specific area of the bone
- ☐ Reproduction of pain with axial compression along a long bone or with torque on the bone

Deformity: An unusual or abnormal shape, position, or movement of the bone or joint.

Inability to use the extremity: If the patient cannot move the limb or joint, or is unable to bear weight on it, a fracture should be suspected.

Swelling and bruising: rapid swelling with ecchymosis at the fracture site.

Crepitus: the grinding of bones that can sometimes be heard or felt when touching or moving a fractured bone.

Percussion: percussion over the bone proximal to the fracture site while placing a stethoscope more distally may aid in detection of a fracture. This should be done on both the injured and uninjured side. The side with the fracture will not transmit the percussion as loudly.

Ultrasound: handheld ultrasound may assist as a diagnostic tool, if available and practical. As ultrasound becomes more portable and visualization improves, this technology is becoming more frequently utilized out of the hospital setting.

Management of an Open Fracture

An open fracture is one where the bone is actually visible penetrating through the skin or when there is a wound through the skin at or near the fracture site. The bone penetrating through the skin is obvious to recognize. However, it is more difficult, especially in the field, to determine if a wound near a fracture actually communicates with the fracture. The reason that a small puncture or laceration near a fracture is considered an open fracture is that the fractured bone may have penetrated the skin as the fracture occurred and then retracted back under the skin. The best approach is to assume that a break in the skin near a fracture is an open fracture.

Open fractures should be evacuated as soon as possible, because they are at very high risk for infection and typically require intraoperative irrigation.

Wilderness management of open fractures depends a great deal on the amount of time that you have to evacuate the patient.

In general, management is as follows:

- ☐ Administer the best possible pain control.
- ☐ Irrigate or clean the wound and the protruding bone if present.
  - ● Remove gross debris initially.
  - ● Irrigate with clean and disinfected water in order to try to minimize the wound contamination.

- Depending on the severity of injury, this may be a painful process and the ability to provide proper care may depend on the degree of achievable pain control.

☐ Reduce the fracture if the bone is still penetrating through the skin. If you are uncomfortable or unable to reduce the fracture, then the next best option is to dress the protruding bone with a clean and preferably sterile bandage after irrigation and cleaning of the bone and wound.

☐ Reduction is performed by providing traction, reproducing the mechanism of the fracture, and then attempting to realign the fracture pieces.

☐ Administer antibiotics that have good coverage against skin bacteria plus anaerobes that may contaminate from the soil. Reasonable choices include cephalexin, amoxicillin plus clavulanate, levofloxacin, or cefazolin 1g plus gentamicin 5mg/kg.

☐ Splint the extremity.

☐ Prior to attempted reduction, a neurovascular exam must be performed distal to the injury. If neurovascular compromise is noted, emergent reduction should be attempted.

☐ Cover the wound with a sterile or clean dressing.

☐ While continuing to hold the reduced limb in alignment, apply a splint to reduce further motion.

Management of a Closed Fracture

Management of closed fractures depends on the fracture site, neurovascular status, the patient's ability to function, proximity to evacuation, and ability to control pain. Management of specific fractures is discussed below.

In general, it is not necessary to reduce a fractured limb unless circulation or neurological status distal to the site of injury is diminished, pressure of the fragment against the skin is significant, or gross deformity makes it difficult to splint and transport.

Reduction is easier if it is done soon after the injury before swelling, pain, and muscle spasm make it more difficult.

When reducing, straighten the limb by reproducing the direction of the initial fracture, then pulling axial traction on the fracture fragment. This should be done while an assistant holds traction above the fracture.

Once reduced, maintain the desired position while applying a splint to prevent further motion.

Reevaluate the circulation to ensure it has been restored or improved and has not been worsened by the manipulation.

Splinting

Splints reduce pain and help to minimize bleeding by preventing movement of the fracture ends and nearby joints.

Improperly loose splints can allow the fracture ends to shear or compress nearby vessels and nerves.

A splint applied too tightly can lead to circulation and neurological compromise at or distal to the splint.

The splint should immobilize at least one joint above and one joint below the fracture site.

Remove all jewelry and accessories such as watches, bracelets, and rings before applying the splint.

Fashion the splint on the *uninjured* body part first and then transfer it to the injured area to minimize discomfort.

The key elements of a splint include rigidity for stabilization and padding for comfort.

Multiple materials may be used as splint:

- ☐ Prefabricated splints (such as the SAM® splint) are very effective, pliable, and reusable.
- ☐ In the wilderness sticks, boards, skis, paddles, heavy cardboard or rolled-up magazines or newspapers may be effective.
- ☐ Pad the splint with soft material, such as clothing. Use plenty of padding over bony protrusions such as elbows, knees, and ankles.
- ☐ If no other objects are readily available, the patient's body works very effectively as a splint.
  - Upper extremity fractures can be immobilized with the shoulder adducted, the elbow flexed to 90 degrees, and the forearm placed across the abdomen. The bottom of the patient's shirt can be folded up over the upper extremity and then secured with safety pins or tape.
  - Lower extremity injuries can be splinted by securing the injured limb to the non-injured lower extremity.

Secure the splint in place with straps, tape, belts, and strips of cloth, webbing, or rope. Tie firmly, but not tightly enough to cause discomfort. Secure the splint in several places, both above and below the fracture. Do not tie directly over the injured area.

Once the splint is placed, the patient should be instructed to identify and notify medical personnel for changes in sensation or level of pain.

Check circulation often. Swelling within the confines of a splint can cut off circulation to the limb. If this occurs, loosen or reposition the splint to allow blood flow.

After splinting, elevate the injured body part to minimize swelling.

The splint should immobilize the fractured limb in its functional position.

- ☐ In general, the upper extremity should be splinted so that the shoulder is adducted, the elbow is flexed to 90 degrees, the wrist is splinted in 30 degrees of extension, and the fingers slightly flexed as if holding a 12-ounce bottle or can.
- ☐ The lower extremity should be splinted with the hips in neutral, the knees slightly flexed, and the foot at 90 degrees flexion (except an Achilles tendon rupture, which should be splinted in passive equinus).

Compartment Syndrome

In the extremities, most of the muscles and bones are contained within soft tissue sections called compartments. These compartments are enclosed by fascia that does not allow for much swelling.

A compartment syndrome occurs when there is an injury within that compartment – typically a fracture – and there is a great deal of swelling and bleeding that is contained within the compartment. Because of the tight fascia, the pressure within the compartment rises, which may then compromise flow to the muscles at the capillary level and smaller. When this occurs, it leads to ischemia of the muscles and nerves within that compartment, which can culminate with necrosis of those muscles and nerves.

Compartment syndrome is most common in the lower leg, but it can occur in any extremity.

Consider a compartment syndrome any time that the soft issue of an injured extremity/fracture becomes increasingly tense and painful or the patient has increasing pain with movement of that injured area.

Compartment syndrome typically occurs from internal pressure rising within that compartment, but it can also occur from an external compression such as splints or dressings that are too tight.

Compartment syndromes are commonly identified with the 5 Ps:

☐ Pain with passive stretch of the muscle distal to the fracture (this is the earliest sign)

☐ Pressure (increased tenseness of the area around the fracture)

☐ Paresthesias (numbness or tingling distal to the injury). This is due to ischemia of the nerves that travel within or through that compartment.

☐ Pallor (decreased color in the extremity), which is a late sign.

☐ Pulselessness (loss of pulses is a late and very serious sign). When this sign occurs, the pressure within that compartment is very high and the patient has probably already had significant damage to the muscles and nerves within that compartment. Do NOT wait for this sign to make the decision that the patient may have a compartment syndrome.

If these signs appear, loosen any restricting dressings, splints or clothing. Do NOT elevate the limb (keep at the level of the heart), and emergently evacuate the patient.

If the patient is complaining of severely worsening pain or is developing the early signs (pain with passive stretch, paresthesias) then he or she should be evacuated emergently.

LIFE-THREATENING FRACTURES

Spinal Fractures

Any accident that places excessive pressure or force on the head, neck, or back can result in fractured or dislocated vertebrae.

Care must be taken in the wilderness when treating back and neck injuries. Further twisting or jolting of the spinal column may further damage the spinal cord.

Because of the association of head and cervical spine injuries, patients with significant head injuries should be assumed to have cervical spine injuries, especially if the patient is unconscious.

If a spinal injury is suspected, the physical exam should include determination of motor strength, sensory response to light touch and pinprick, and documentation of Babinski reflex.

Thoracolumbar spine fractures occur most frequently at the thoracolumbar junction. In the wilderness, falls from significant heights or high-velocity impact are the most common causes of these fractures.

Signs and Symptoms

The patient has bony tenderness in the neck or back.

The patient is unconscious or has an altered level of consciousness in association with trauma.

There are significant cuts and bruises along the spine.

There is weakness, numbness or tingling in the patient's extremities.

There is another extremely painful injury, such as a fractured femur or dislocated shoulder, which might distract him or her from noticing the spinal pain.

The patient is under the influence of alcohol and/or drugs that may alter his or her perception of pain.

Ruling Out Cervical Spine Fractures

You may use clinical criteria to rule out potential cervical spine fractures using validated methods such as the Canadian C-spine or NEXUS (National Emergency X-ray Utilization Study) algorithms.

☐ No posterior midline spinal tenderness to palpation

☐ No altered level of consciousness due to drug or alcohol intoxication

☐ No painful distracting injury – a distracting injury is defined as what "you as the provider" consider painful enough to cause a patient to not realize (e.g. distract the patient) that they have neck pain

☐ No neurological deficits

☐ Some algorithms will use mechanism of injury as an additional screening tool to determine which patients need cervical spine stabilization. In addition to the above, consider stabilizing the cervical spine following injury sustained through the following mechanisms:

● Fall from greater than 3 meters

● Axial load to cervical spine (fall directly on head)

- High speed motor vehicle collision
- Rollover or ejection from motorized vehicle

☐ In situations where unnecessary immobilization may have the potential to add further injury to the patient or rescuers (combat, remote and dangerous environment) a more aggressive algorithm may be required. The **Wilderness Medical Society (WMS) practice guidelines for spine immobilization in the austere environment** offers the following recommendations for decision making:

- No immobilization with penetrating trauma
- Following blunt trauma with a mechanism of injury suspicious for spine trauma, immobilization should be performed when any of the following are present:
  - Severely injured patient
  - Altered mental status (GCS<15, evidence of intoxication)
  - Presence of neurologic deficit
  - Thoracic or other *significant* distracting injury
  - Significant spine pain or tenderness (≥7/10)
  - Patient unable to voluntarily flex, extend, or rotate the spine (cervical or thoracolumbar) 30° in each plane, regardless of pain.

Treatment

■ Immobilize the patient's head, neck, and back. If the patient is not breathing or is having trouble breathing, straighten the injured area only enough to open an airway.

■ If the patient is found in a position other than supine or if the neck is bent at an angle, the rescuer can attempt to straighten it with gentle in-line traction in order to stabilize it in a neutral position.

☐ Once the rescuer begins to manipulate the injured cervical spine, he/she must hold manual stabilization until it can be more definitively secured.

☐ If there is more than expected resistance to movement of the spine, if movement causes increased pain or an increase in neurologic symptoms, the spine should not be rotated and should be secured in the position in which it lies.

☐ High cervical spine fractures (occipitoatlantal or atlantoaxial) may be made worse by excessive traction, so only the amount of force necessary to control movement and position of the neck should be used to move the spine.

■ Malleable splints, such as the SAM splint, may be very effective to help stabilize the cervical spine.

■ Place rolled-up clothing, life jackets, blankets, or plastic bags filled with sand or dirt around the patient's head, the sides of the neck, the shoulders, and from the armpits down alongside the trunk to prevent movement.

☐ Secure the head to these supports with tape or straps.

☐ Secure the rest of the body to a flat board.

☐ If an unstable cervical spine fracture is suspected, manual stabilization should be utilized throughout the evacuation in addition to the above methods, as even the most rigid collar will not fully stabilize a cervical spine fracture.

Treat for shock and evacuate the patient as soon as possible.

Pelvis Fractures

Pelvic fractures are often associated with significant life-threatening hemorrhage due to the numerous vessels that course through the pelvic region.

There is also a risk of injuries to the intestines, bladder, uterus, and the sacral spinal nerve roots.

An open pelvic fracture with associated GI and/or GU injuries carries a 50% mortality rate.

Signs and Symptoms

Suspect a pelvis fracture if there is pain in the pelvis, hip, or lower back.

The patient may present the following symptoms:

- Unable to bear weight and will be very sensitive with pain around the waistline or hips
- Pain and tenderness with palpation and compression of the pelvis
- Abnormal motion or crepitus on palpation and compression of the pelvis
  - If an unstable pelvic fracture is suspected, or any crepitus is felt on exam, do NOT repeat exams, as any movement can shear vessels, increasing bleeding
- Bruising over the pelvic area to include the perineum
- Neurologic deficit over one or both of the legs
- Hematuria or inability to urinate
- Bleeding from the urethra, rectum, or unexpected vaginal bleeding

Treatment

If an unstable fracture is suspected, pelvic splinting is important to prohibit motion, minimize bleeding, and control pain.

- There are multiple effective commercial products available to splint and immobilize the pelvis.
  - Alternatively, one may use a wide belt, sheet, or piece of clothing that is wrapped around the pelvis and tied tightly to immobilize the pelvis and to hold the pelvic ring together. Care should be used to ensure that the compression occurs at the level of greater trochanters of the hips and pubic symphysis, and not over the lower abdomen or superior iliac crests.
  - When transporting the patient, place padding between the legs, then strap the legs together. This, too will work do decrease movement at the level of the pelvis.

Treat for shock, but do not elevate the legs.

Femoral Fractures

A fractured femur can produce one to two liters of blood loss into the thigh, leading to shock.

Midshaft femur fractures may be placed in traction prior to evacuation. Theoretical advantages of traction splinting:

☐ Decreases amount of bleeding into the thigh

☐ Improves pain control

☐ Inhibits further vascular damage by fracture fragments

☐ Prevents converting a closed fracture into an open fracture

There have been conflicting studies regarding the utilization of traction splints. A small minority of fractures is amenable to traction.

Traction is acceptable if there will be prolonged evacuation. If the injury occurs in close proximity to a higher level of care, evacuation should not be prolonged to fashion a traction splint. In this case, the femur may be splinted in place.

Traction should NOT be performed if:

☐ A pelvic fracture is suspected

☐ Ankle or foot fracture is suspected, due to pressure from the ankle harness

Treatment

There are multiple commercial traction devices acceptable for wilderness travel. Depending on the expedition, the medical officer in charge should determine the efficiency of carrying commercial traction splints.

Improvised traction may also be effective, but the method should be practiced prior to the event. Before placing an improvised traction splint on the patient, it should be tested on the patient's uninjured leg. Once tested, place the splint on the injured side.

■ Improvising a traction splint:

☐ There are many ways to improvise a traction splint in the wilderness but the following components should be available:

- Ankle attachment (use webbing or a band of cloth)
- Upper thigh (crotch) attachment
- Strong support that is one foot longer than the leg
- Method to fix the two attachments to the support
- Method to pull traction
- Padding

In general, about 10% of the patient's body weight should be applied in traction. If pain is significantly relieved, this, too, can be an adequate endpoint.

Padding should be placed behind the knee so that it is in slight flexion.

■ If unable to fashion a traction splint, splint the injured leg in place, then secure the two legs together with straps after padding between the two legs.

■ Treat for shock, checking the patient's circulation by palpating distal pulses and observing capillary refill periodically.

UPPER EXTREMITY FRACTURES

Clavicle and Shoulder Girdle

Fractures are usually stable and require minimal treatment other than a simple sling and swath. Figure-eight slings are not necessary and are no longer recommended.

Humeral Shaft

Non-displaced proximal fractures require sling and swath.

Displaced fractures or fractures associated with pain despite sling and swath should be treated with a posterior or sugar tong splint with the elbow flexed at 90 degrees.

Distal Humerus and Forearm

Splint elbow at 90 degrees of flexion.

Splint should generally immobilize elbow and wrist, which should be in a functional position at 30 degrees of extension.

Wrist and Metacarpal

Splint the hand in position, as if the patient was holding a baseball or 12-ounce can, by placing an object of similar size (for example, a rolled up sock or rolled SAM splint) in the hand. In general, the wrist should be splinted at 30 degrees of extension, the metacarpo-phalangeal (MCP) joint at 70 degrees of flexion, and the intraphalangeal (IP) joints at 15-20 degrees of flexion.

Phalanx

If possible, the provider may reduce fractures of the hand and fingers along with their commonly associated dislocations. Immobilize a fractured digit by buddy taping the digit to the adjacent one. A piece of gauze or cloth should be placed between taped digits to reduce friction and absorb moisture.

MCP joints should be splinted at 70 degrees of flexion and IP joints at 15-20 degrees of flexion.

LOWER EXTREMITY FRACTURES

Knee

A fracture to the knee should be suspected if (Pittsburgh knee rules):

☐ The patient has suffered blunt trauma or fall as a mechanism of injury plus either of the following:

- Age younger than 12 years or older than 50 years
- Inability to walk four weight-bearing steps on examination

- ☐ This is 99 percent sensitive for a fracture, but only 60 percent specific as ligamentous and other injuries may cause significant pain and inability to bear weight.
- ☐ If a fracture is suspected, the patient should be splinted with knee in slight flexion and non-weight bearing.
- A direct blow to the knee may result in patella fracture, which can be difficult to differentiate from contusion, as there may not be obvious deformity. Treat as indicated above.

Tibia/Fibula

- Incorporate the joint above (knee) and below (ankle) in a splint for any fractures.

Ankle

- Suspect a fracture if the patient has (Ottawa ankle rules):
  - ☐ Bone tenderness along the distal 6cm of the posterior edge of the tibia or tip of the medial malleolus
  - ☐ Bone tenderness along the distal 6cm of the posterior edge of the fibula or tip of the lateral malleolus
  - ☐ Inability to bear weight for four steps immediately and on your exam
- Use a bulky compression dressing and devise a U-shaped splint, L-shaped splint, or the combination of the U and L-shaped splints that wrap around the ankle.

Tarsal Bones

- Calcaneus or talus fractures usually occur during falls from significant heights.
- Suspect a calcaneus fracture when the patient has heel pain and tenderness, typically with deformity and crepitus.
- Talus fracture may mimic ankle fracture, with majority of tenderness distal to the malleoli.
- Due to the forces required to cause these fractures, injuries elsewhere should be suspected. Calcaneus fractures in particular are associated with compression fractures of the lumbar vertebrae.
- Suspect a fracture of the midfoot if the patient has:
  - ☐ Bone tenderness at the base of the fifth metatarsal
  - ☐ Bone tenderness at the navicular bone
  - ☐ Inability to bear weight for four steps immediately and on your exam
- Use a bulky compression dressing and devise a U-shaped splint that wraps around the ankle and can be secured on both sides of the leg. Patients should not bear weight and should be evacuated.

Metatarsal fractures

- Treat with posterior splint and non-weight bearing.

Phalanx

- Displaced fractures may be amenable to reduction.
- Suspected fractures of second through fifth toes are treated with buddy taping to adjacent toes and stiff-soled boots or shoes.
- Suspected fractures of the great toe should be splinted and may require evacuation due to the pain produced by the force of the toe-off part of the gait.

DISLOCATIONS

General

- A dislocation occurs when enough force is placed across a joint to separate the bone from its articulation.
- Dislocations are most common in the fingers, shoulder, elbow, and patella.
- Dislocations can damage blood vessels, nerves, muscle, and ligaments.
- In general, dislocations should be reduced as soon as possible because muscle spasm increases as time from injury lengthens.
  - □ This also reduces pain, risk of circulatory or neurological damage, and can make patient transport and evacuation much safer.
  - □ If you are unable to reduce the dislocation, splint the extremity in the position in which it is found in order to decrease pain.
- Pain should be significantly relieved after reduction. If significant pain persists, fracture or persistent dislocation should be suspected.
- If reduction is unsuccessful after three attempts, if uncomfortable performing the reduction, or if unsure about associated fractures, it is best to splint the extremity in position and evacuate the patient.
- If you do not have access to sedatives, local intra-articular injection of lidocaine or bupivacaine, in addition to narcotic pain medication (if available), may allow reduction without sedation. This should only be performed if you are comfortable with this procedure.

Mandible

- Frequently occurs without trauma (for example, yawning), especially in patients with prior dislocations.
- Patient is unable to close mouth.
- If associated with trauma then suspect fracture of the condyle and avoid attempts at reduction.
- It is reduced by provider placing thumbs on lower posterior molars and pressing down, then posteriorly.
- Significant muscle spasm may be present, requiring sedation.

After reduction, the patient should be instructed not to open mouth more than 2 cm. A hand should be placed under the chin when yawning, generally for at least one week.

Upper extremity

Shoulder (glenohumeral joint)

An anterior dislocation of the humerus is one of the most common dislocations that can occur.

It is usually caused by direct force to the arm when abducted and externally rotated.

The shoulder typically has a squared-off appearance on the affected side.

As with all dislocations, the ability to reduce the glenohumeral joint without sedation decreases quickly as muscle spasm sets in.

Reduction is obtained when the patient can move the arm towards the opposite shoulder. There are many methods to reduce a shoulder dislocation.

☐ One of the most commonly used methods is traction or counter traction. With the patient lying on his back (supine), place a piece of cloth around his torso, with the closed end of the loop on the side of the dislocation. If you have an assistant, he/she should hold the ends of the cloth on the other side of the patient. Alternatively, wrap these around a secure object, such as a tree. Pull traction along the axial line of the extremity while externally rotating the arm. Reduction may occur at this point. If reduction has not occurred, once the arm is maximally externally rotated, begin abducting the arm. Along this arc, reduction should occur.

☐ Other effective methods include:

- Slowly abducting the patient's shoulder to the overhead position of full abduction (Milch technique), then externally rotating the shoulder as if "picking an apple from a tree." This method must be performed slowly with a pause any time the patient complains of worsening pain.

- Slowly and externally rotating the patient's shoulder fully (external rotation technique), then abducting his/her shoulder. This is a very slow maneuver, similar to the Milch technique.

- Allowing the patient to lie prone with the injured arm dangling free. Traction or weights may be slowly added to assist in relocation.

- Scapular manipulation (pushing the tip of the scapula medially and upward) is frequently used in addition to the prone position and may help improve the success of this, or any of the methods of reduction.

After reduction, the patient's arm should be placed in a sling and a swath.

Elbow

Elbow dislocations are usually posterior and are caused by hyperextension with a fall on an outstretched hand.

There will be a bony posterior deformity and shortened forearm.

Method for reduction is as follows:

- [ ] Have an assistant hold counter-traction on the upper arm
- [ ] Apply traction downward on the proximal forearm by placing one hand inside the elbow on the forearm, and away from the patient's elbow, by placing another hand at the patient's wrist
- [ ] Reduction is usually apparent; if unsure, when the patient can fully flex the elbow, reduction has been obtained
- [ ] Splint with the elbow at 90 degrees and place in a sling and swath

Fractures, especially supracondylar fractures in children, may mimic elbow dislocations. If unsure, if unable to achieve reduction, or if nerve injury is suspected, splint the arm in position and evacuate the patient.

Finger

DIP dislocations can be reduced with traction while pushing the dislocated base of the finger back into place.

Dislocations of the MCP or PIP joints should be reduced manually without traction. Traction can convert the injury to a complex dislocation requiring surgery.

After reduction or if unable to reduce finger or wrist dislocations, buddy tape and splint the hand in the position of holding a baseball or can.

Lower extremity

Hip

The dislocated hip, which is a posterior dislocation, will typically cause the leg to be rotated internally, shortened and adducted.

A fracture of the neck of the femur must be suspected in a leg that is rotated externally, shortened, and *abducted*. If there is concern that there is a fracture, then do not attempt reduction as it could cause displacement of a non-displaced hip fracture, which would significantly worsen the outcome.

Given the significant force and relaxation required to overcome muscle spasm and soft tissue interposition, it may not be possible to relocate in the wilderness without significant sedation. Dislocations of total hip replacements often can be reduced with less effort and less need for sedation.

The most common technique for reduction is as follows:

- [ ] With the patient lying supine, the assistant applies counter-traction to the pelvis.
- [ ] The provider flexes the patient's hip and knee to 90 degrees, and straddles the patient.
- [ ] The provider then pulls traction on the thigh, in an axis perpendicular to the supine patient, ideally pulling the hip into place. Gentle internal and external rotation of the hip during reduction may facilitate success.
- [ ] The hip must be immobilized to the other extremity regardless of whether or not reduction was accomplished, and the patient must be evacuated. An exception would be successful reduction of a dislocated total hip, particularly in a patient who has experienced previous dislocations. In this scenario, satisfactory reduction does not require immobilization or evacuation.

Patella

- The patella most frequently dislocates laterally.
- If the patella is displaced superiorly, a patellar tendon rupture should be suspected. The knee should be immobilized and splinted, and the patient should be evacuated.
- A dislocation can be easily reduced, frequently without sedation, by flexing the hip, then placing medial pressure on the patella with both thumbs, while extending the knee. After reduction, place a knee splint with the joint in extension.
- The patient may be able to walk with the aid of a crutch after reduction is accomplished.

Ankle

- Dislocations are usually associated with fracture and significant force.
- Neurovascular compromise or significant skin tenting are frequently associated with ankle dislocation, which has the potential to result in necrosis, making an attempt at reduction necessary in the field.
- With the knee bent, grasp the posterior heel and apply traction, attempting to realign as closely as possible.
- Place a posterior splint for stability and evacuate the patient.

Toe

- These are easily reduced with traction.
- After reduction, buddy tape the injured toe to the adjacent toe for one to three weeks.

SPRAINS

- A sprain is the stretching or tearing of a ligament caused by twisting, wrenching, or stretching movements beyond the ligament's normal range of motion.
- Sprains are most common in the finger, ankle, wrist and knee.
- Symptoms include pain, swelling, and discoloration.

Treatment

- Assess for neurovascular compromise.
- General treatment for sprains is summarized by the acronym RICES:
    - ☐ **R**est the joint from activity and stress.
    - ☐ **I**ce: Apply ice at least 3 times per day for 15 to 20 minutes if it is available in your wilderness setting.

- ☐ **C**ompression: Follow the ice with a compression wrap. Cover the sprained joint with a sock, cloth, or other light material and then wrap tightly. The wrap should compress the joint, but not so tightly that it restricts circulation or causes pain.
  - ☐ **E**levation: Elevate the injured area above the level of the patient's heart to minimize swelling.
  - ☐ **S**tabilization: Tape or splint the injured joint for transport.
- Ligament ruptures leading to joint instability may require orthopedic intervention. These should generally be splinted in position of function until definitive evaluation can be arranged.
- Follow the RICES treatment protocol for the first 72 hours after the injury.
- Evacuation may be necessary if the patient cannot safely mobilize or if the patient's pace creates a dangerous situation for the rest of the group.

INJURIES RELATED TO SELECTED WILDERNESS ACTIVITIES

Skiing

- Knee injuries are extremely common in skiing. It is most common to tear the major ligaments of the knee. If a patient presents with severe swelling due to a twisting fall, it is best to immobilize and treat with RICES. A full assessment may be difficult until swelling diminishes (usually after a couple of days).
- Finger fractures and thumb injuries (including ulnar collateral ligament rupture; gamekeeper's thumb) are also common in skiing. Treat using the above principles.

Snowboarding

- Wrist sprains or fractures are the most common upper extremity injury among snowboarders.
- In the lower extremity, ankle injuries are common, although knee injuries are more common in those wearing stiffer boots.
- A fracture of the talus is called "snowboarder's fracture" and can occur when the snowboarder falls forward with his or her front foot everted or their back foot inverted. If this is suspected, splint the ankle in place.
- All snowboarders should wear helmets. Due to the force of falls from snowboards, concussions may be significant.

Mountain Biking

- Abrasions are extremely common in mountain biking. Proper wound care should be applied.
- Shoulder dislocations are common due to falls. Shoulder dislocations are more commonly anterior, but in mountain biking, it is common to posteriorly dislocate the shoulder. Reduction of either may be achieved by methods described above.
- Concussions and head injuries are very common in mountain biking. Therefore, the primary assessment, need for stabilization of the spine with a collar, and full neurological exam are very important. Other common mountain biking injuries include wrist and forearm fractures from a fall on an outstretched hand (FOOSH). Reduce and splint these as previously directed.

Climbing

- Severe climbing injuries are rare, but a fall from height can result in serious injuries. Always assess to stabilize the most severe injuries first and prepare for evacuation even if the injuries are apparently minor in a fall from height.
- Maintain a high suspicion for internal bleeding from various injuries not obvious on initial assessment.

QUESTIONS

1. **Which of the following statements regarding the wilderness approach to reduction of dislocations is most accurate?**
   a. Dislocated joints should not be reduced without access to radiography and sedative medications
   b. If performed promptly by a provider familiar with reduction techniques, up to three attempts as soon as possible after dislocation are generally recommended
   c. The longer one waits to reduce, the better, as the muscles will eventually fatigue
   d. Traction-countertraction is the only recommended method for reduction of shoulder dislocations in the wilderness

2. **Which one of the following dislocations is unlikely to be relocated in the wilderness setting?**
   a. Ankle
   b. Finger
   c. Hip
   d. Shoulder

3. **Which one of the following is important to perform when splinting a potential fractured forearm?**
   a. The splint should flex the wrist into a 30-degree position
   b. The splint should immobilize the elbow and wrist
   c. The splint should immobilize the elbow, wrist and shoulder
   d. The splint should immobilize the wrist only

4. **Which one of the following is a concern when managing a patient with a potential pelvic fracture in the wilderness setting?**
   a. Fracture fragments tearing the femoral artery at the time of fracture
   b. Internal hemorrhage due to bleeding vessels in the pelvis
   c. Splinting it will cause movement of the pelvic bones, which will cause more damage
   d. Spinal fracture is a commonly associated injury with pelvis fracture

5. Which one of the following is not part of the acute therapy for the management of a patient who has an ankle sprain?

    a. Active motion with full weight bearing

    b. Elevation above the heart

    c. Rest when possible

    d. Stabilization with a splint or tape

Answers:

1. b

2. c

3. b

4. b

5. a

CHAPTER 4

Altitude Medicine

This chapter describes how to recognize, prevent and treat health conditions caused by high altitude.

Objectives:

- Recognize the signs and symptoms of acute mountain sickness, high altitude cerebral edema and high altitude pulmonary edema
- Understand that gradual ascent is the key to preventing altitude illness
- Understand that descent is the most important treatment for altitude illness
- Describe pharmacologic methods of treating altitude illness; including the use of acetazolamide, dexamethasone and nifedipine
- Identify additional methods for preventing and mitigating altitude illnesses

CASE 1

A 38-year-old male from New York City takes a ski trip to Colorado. He flies to Denver and then rents a car and drives directly to his accommodations at a ski resort. That night he sleeps poorly and awakes with a splitting headache. Attributing his headache to his restless night, he takes some acetaminophen, drinks coffee, and heads to the rental shop to get set up for a day of skiing. On his way to the rental shop, he becomes very nauseated. He then decides that he must have eaten something wrong the night before and decides to head to the resort's medical clinic, where he meets you.

1. What is your recommendation for treating this victim?
2. Is there anything you would recommend to him for preventing these symptoms on future trips?
3. Does he need to return to New York or can he stay and wait through his illness?

CASE 2

You are based at a medical aid station at a base camp in Denali National Park when a 26-year-old climber is brought to your tent. He is breathing at a rate of 40 breaths per minute and coughing up pink frothy sputum. He is tachycardic to a rate of 140 beats per minute and has diffuse crackles bilaterally. Your pulse oximeter is reading 48%.

1. What are your initial steps in managing him?
2. Should he be evacuated or can he be "tuned up" at the aid station?
3. If evacuation is not possible due to weather, what can you do to help him until evacuation is possible?
4. If this person recovers, is he at risk for long-term complications?

BACKGROUND

- High altitude is defined as starting at a terrestrial elevation of 1500 meters (4,950 ft)
- Very high altitude is defined as 3500 – 5500 meters (11,500 – 18,000 ft)
- Extreme altitude is above 5500 meters
- High-altitude syndromes are usually seen at altitudes in excess of 2500 meters (8250 ft) and are caused by hypobaric hypoxia.

- Acute mountain sickness (AMS), high altitude cerebral edema (HACE) and high altitude pulmonary edema (HAPE) are the three major syndromes of altitude illness and are considered a failure of acclimatization.
- Graded ascent is the safest method to facilitate acclimatization and prevent altitude sickness.
- Hyperventilation and dyspnea on exertion are normal responses at altitude.
- Increased urination is also a normal physiologic response to altitude.
- Hyperpnea followed by brief periods (3-10 seconds) of apnea is common while sleeping at altitude.
- Alcohol consumption increases susceptibility to altitude illness.
- Age, gender, and fitness level do NOT play a role in susceptibility to altitude illness.
- Acute mountain sickness occurs hours to days after ascent to an altitude above 2000 meters.
- Acute mountain sickness is the beginning of the continuum of illness with HACE representing end-stage AMS.
- HAPE is a pulmonary form of altitude illness that can occur with or without AMS or HACE.
- HAPE and HACE are both medical emergencies and delays in treatment can be fatal.
- HAPE is the most common cause of death related to the high-altitude syndromes.

PATHOPHYSIOLOGY

General

- Compared to sea level, barometric pressure drops by one-half at 5500 m (18,000 feet) and two-thirds at 8800 m (29,000 feet).
- This drop in barometric pressure and, therefore, the partial pressure of oxygen results in hypobaric hypoxia.
- Acclimatization is a set of physiological responses that occurs over time in response to this hypobaric hypoxia.
  - ☐ The primary benefit of these responses is improved delivery of oxygen to the tissues.
  - ☐ Successful acclimatization protects against altitude illness and improves aerobic exercise ability at altitude.
  - ☐ On exposure to altitude, the carotid body senses hypoxia and signals the medulla to increase the ventilatory rate.
  - ☐ 80% of ventilatory compensation to altitude takes place over the first 4 days.
  - ☐ In response to hyperventilation, the kidneys secrete bicarbonate, which induces a metabolic acidosis that allows hyperventilation to continue.
  - ☐ Increased catecholamine release stimulates an increase in heart rate, blood pressure, and cardiac output.
  - ☐ Over days to weeks, there are increases in hematocrit and capillary density, as well as increased mitochondrial density at the cellular level.

Mechanism of Injury

Acute Mountain Sickness (AMS)

AMS is characterized by relative hypoventilation, fluid retention and redistribution, impaired gas exchange, increased intracranial pressure and possibly endothelial cell dysfunction.

High Altitude Cerebral Edema (HACE)

HACE is characterized by severe brain edema in addition to hemorrhage and thrombosis that are likely secondary events.

HACE is a vasogenic edema of the white matter, and thus a leaky vasculature problem, not a fluid overload problem.

Rising intracranial pressure results in decreased cerebral blood flow and a cycle of worsening ischemia and increased pressure leading eventually to coma and death.

High Altitude Pulmonary Edema (HAPE)

HAPE is a form of permeability edema associated with high pulmonary artery pressures.

The most likely mechanism is that hypoxia results in pulmonary hypertension and uneven pulmonary vasoconstriction.

This combination may result in over-perfusion and "stress failure" of the capillary membrane in selected areas of the vascular bed.

Autopsies have shown diffuse alveolar damage and neutrophil-laden alveolitis with HAPE.

Alveolar hemorrhage is a late common feature.

HAPE also likely results from alterations in the sodium-driven clearance of alveolar fluid.

HAPE is a leaky vessel and pulmonary artery pressure problem but not a fluid overload problem, which makes it different from the pulmonary edema seen with congestive heart failure. Therefore, the treatment of HAPE is different from treating a cardiac patient with pulmonary edema.

CLINICAL PRESENTATION

Acute Mountain Sickness

History is the key to diagnosing AMS because there are no specific physical exam findings.

A key to the history is the ascent profile looking at both total elevation gain and the rate of gain.

AMS is a common illness that may occur in 10% – 70% of individuals, depending primarily on the rate of ascent.

Headache is a not a necessary symptom in order to diagnose AMS, but is almost always present.

- The Lake Louis Consensus criteria is a standardized international symptom set that allows one to diagnose AMS.
- AMS is diagnosed in the setting of a recent gain in altitude with the presence of a headache and at least one of the following symptoms:
  - ☐ Dizziness or lightheadedness
  - ☐ Fatigue or weakness
  - ☐ Nausea/vomiting/anorexia
  - ☐ Insomnia
- Risk factors for AMS
  - ☐ Prior history of AMS
  - ☐ Fast or high ascents
  - ☐ Obesity
  - ☐ Men and women and children are equally susceptible.

High Altitude Cerebral Edema

- HACE represents a progression of AMS to the point of life-threatening end-organ damage.
- HACE is defined as severe AMS symptoms with additional obvious neurologic dysfunction:
  - ☐ Ataxia: this is the most common presenting sign of HACE
  - ☐ Altered level of consciousness
  - ☐ Severe lassitude
- While the boundary between AMS and HACE can be blurry, HACE almost never occurs without antecedent AMS symptoms as a harbinger.
- The progression of AMS to coma typically occurs over 1 – 3 days.
- HACE and HAPE are often present simultaneously. (up to 70% of the time in one series)

High Altitude Pulmonary Edema

- HAPE usually evolves over 2 – 4 days after ascent to altitude.
- The Lake Louis consensus criteria for HAPE diagnosis are:
  - ☐ Symptoms: at least two of:
    - Dyspnea at rest
    - Cough
    - Weakness or deceased exercise performance
    - Chest tightness or congestion
  - ☐ Signs: at least two of:
    - Crackles or wheezing in at least one lung field
    - Central cyanosis

- Tachypnea
- Tachycardia

The primary symptoms are dyspnea at rest, cough and exercise intolerance.

The initial symptom will often be a marked decrease in exercise tolerance in an individual as compared to prior days.

Occasionally, a pink frothy sputum is produced, but this is usually later in the illness.

Neurological symptoms may be seen with concomitant HACE.

Physical examination findings include tachycardia, tachypnea, fever, rales/crackles and central cyanosis.

Hypoxemia and respiratory alkalosis are universally present.

Radiologic findings are consistent with increased permeability pulmonary edema.

Mild cases may resolve within hours after descent. In contrast, severe cases may progress to death within 24 hours, particularly if descent is delayed.

There are HAPE susceptible individuals who genetically are at high risk of developing HAPE with every ascent.

PREVENTION

Graded ascent is the safest method to facilitate acclimatization and to prevent altitude illness.

Current recommendations for climbers without experience at high altitude are to spend two to three nights at 2500 – 3000 meters before further ascent.

- ☐ Increases of greater than 600 meters in sleeping altitude should be avoided.
- ☐ One should consider an extra night of acclimatization for every 300 – 900 meters of altitude gain.

Acetazolamide 125 mg PO BID starting 1 – 2 days before ascending is effective for AMS prophylaxis.

Mixed evidence suggests that gingko biloba (120 mg PO BID starting five days prior to ascent) may be helpful in preventing acute mountain sickness. However, it cannot reliably be counted on to be of benefit and thus is no longer recommended

Ibuprofen has been shown to effectively treat and prevent high altitude headache. It remains unclear if it actually has effect on preventing AMS.

Prophylaxis against HAPE should be reserved only for those with previous episodes of HAPE.

- ☐ Nifedipine slow release 20 mg PO Q 8 hours has been shown to be effective for prophylaxis in these individuals.
- ☐ Salmeterol has also shown to be effective in reducing the risk of HAPE in those known to be susceptible to recurrent episodes. 125 mcg inhaled BID is the dose.
- ☐ Phospodiesterase inhibitors tadalafil and sildenafil have also been shown to be effective in decreasing the risk of HAPE in those at risk, though Nifedipine remains the gold standard.
- ☐ HAPE susceptible individuals should limit ascent rate to no more than 350 meters (1155ft) a day

TREATMENT

Acute Mountain Sickness

- Discontinue ascent and rest.
- Acetazolamide 250 mg PO Q 12 hours until symptom free.
- Acetazolamide is the treatment of choice for AMS as it facilitates acclimatization.
- Dexamethasone can be used as a monotherapy in sulfa allergic individuals or in addition to acetazolamide in severe AMS. For AMS treatment, it is given as 4 mg PO Q 6 hours for two doses. The patient must then not continue ascent until 18 hours after last dose AND must be symptom free.
- Supplemental oxygen can improve symptoms rapidly.
- Descent is the definitive treatment.

Acetazolamide

- The gold standard for prevention and treatment of AMS
- A carbonic anhydrase inhibitor, it causes the kidney to secrete bicarbonate resulting in diuresis and a metabolic acidosis with compensatory hyperventilation
- Sulfa based so it should not be given to those with a history of anaphylaxis to sulfa
- More recent literature questions the cross-reactivity between acetazolamide and sulfa antibiotics, but one should use caution in its use in those with allergies to sulfa medications.
- Side effect of parasthesias is common and dose dependent
- Decreases exercise tolerance at sea level and may do so at altitude in some cases

High Altitude Cerebral Edema

- IMMEDIATE descent (almost always with assistance) is imperative and should not be delayed unless descent poses a greater danger to the parties involved (i.e. weather, terrain). Even modest elevation losses can be helpful.
- In addition to descent, administering dexamethasone 8 mg IM/PO as a loading dose followed by 4 mg IM/PO Q 6 hours should be given immediately.
- Acetazolamide 125 mg PO TID should be given if the victim is able to tolerate oral medications.
- Oxygen supplementation should be given when available.
- If descent is not possible, place the victim in a portable hyperbaric chamber for 4 to 6 hours.
- Recovery with prolonged sequelae, especially ataxia, lasting up to weeks is common.
- Most who survive eventually fully recover neurologically.

High Altitude Pulmonary Edema

- IMMEDIATE descent is imperative (likely with assistance as exertion will worsen symptoms). All that may be required is 500 to 1000 meters of descent before improvement is observed.
- Supplemental oxygen, if available, should be administered.
- Rest after descent.
- Nifedipine 20 mg PO followed by 10 mg PO Q 8 hours. If the victim is unable to tolerate oral medications, then empty the capsule sublingually.
- If descent is not possible, then place the victim in a portable hyperbaric chamber.
- Neither supplemental oxygen, hyperbaric therapy, nor any other intervention should delay an opportunity to descend.
- Acetazolamide can be modestly helpful in improving oxygenation.
- Furosemide has been utilized in the past, but it has fallen out of favor. This is because HAPE victims are not fluid overloaded and there is an increased mortality in animal studies.
- There have been excellent initial study results with the use of sildenafil (Viagra) and tadalafil (Cialis) in the prevention of HAPE; there will likely be more work on this in the future.

EVACUATION GUIDELINES

- With all altitude-related illness, the definitive treatment is always descent. However, descent is not the same as evacuation. In select circumstances, victims with altitude-related illness can descend for a period of time while their bodies acclimatize before re-ascending.
- Victims with AMS do not necessarily need to be evacuated:
  - ☐ Rest at the current altitude, and medical interventions, such as acetazolamide and dexamethasone, may be sufficient for complete recovery within 24 to 48 hours.
  - ☐ Extreme caution should be used if the victim is to continue to ascend, because symptoms can progress to HACE.
  - ☐ Victims should be symptom free for at least 24 hours after steroid use before once again proceeding to ascend.
- Victims with HACE should be evacuated after descent:
  - ☐ While full neurologic recovery is likely if they survive, sequelae such as ataxia can persist for weeks.
  - ☐ For this reason, victims with HACE are not safe to attempt re-ascent on the current expedition.
- Victims with HAPE should be evacuated:
  - ☐ Death from HAPE can proceed rapidly, so descent followed by evacuation should not be delayed.

☐ Some climbers with mild HAPE (characterized by dry cough, mild tachypnea at rest) may be reluctant to abort an expedition, as these trips usually represent thousands of dollars of investment. As a medical provider, in extremely mild cases, you can advise them to descend until symptom free and then wait for a symptom free period of at least three days for further acclimatization. However, if symptoms return upon re-ascent, after a second period of acclimatization, that person should be evacuated.

QUESTIONS

1. **Which one of the following is the factor that most predisposes to altitude illness?**
    a. Alcohol intake
    b. Current altitude
    c. Fitness level
    d. Rate of ascent

2. **Which of the following is not considered appropriate treatment options for acute mountain sickness?**
    a. Acetazolamide 250 mg PO BID
    b. Descent
    c. Dexamethasone 4 mg PO Q 6 hours for 48 hours
    d. Rest and discontinuation of ascent

3. **What is the proper sequence of interventions for the victim with high altitude pulmonary edema?**
    a. Descent, oxygen, nifedipine, rest
    b. Descent, oxygen, rest, nifedipine
    c. Nifedipine, oxygen, rest, descent
    d. Oxygen, descent, rest, nifedipine

4. **Which of the following is <u>not</u> a clinical feature of high altitude pulmonary edema?**
    a. Ataxia
    b. Cyanosis
    c. Tachycardia
    d. Tachypnea

5. **High altitude cerebral edema differs from acute mountain sickness in which one of the following ways?**
    a. Altered mental status or ataxia are hallmarks of HACE
    b. Ataxia is commonly seen in AMS
    c. Headache is only seen in AMS
    d. Vomiting is only seen in HACE

Answers:

1. **d**
2. **c**
3. **b**
4. **a**
5. **a**

CHAPTER 5
Avalanche

This chapter discusses the fundamentals of avalanche safety, rescue, treatment and survival

Objectives:

- Be able to describe and recognize factors that predispose to avalanche occurring
- Be able to understand the utility of avalanche safety and survival tools
- Recognize that the time to recovery is the most significant factor for victim survival
- Be able to describe the most appropriate way to organize a rescue
- Understand the types of injuries causes by avalanche burial
- Be able to understand treatment options based on burial time

CASE 1

Just prior to a ski resort's season opening, you and a group of three friends decide to take advantage of recent snowfall by hiking up the mountain with your skis and snowboards to get some "fresh tracks." While all of you are experienced, you are the only person familiar with the local terrain.

1. What preparations need to be made before departure to improve the safety of your trip?
2. What are the essential tools you need to carry?
3. Describe the type of route you wish to select to safely lead your friends up the mountain.
4. When is it time to descend the mountain, and what safety measures will be taken?

CASE 2

After getting to the summit and enjoying lunch, you and your friends are prepared to descend the mountain. One member of your party decides to hike a few hundred feet farther along the ridgeline so that he can ski down the center of the bowl. When he is skiing within the bowl, the snow starts to move with him and then suddenly collapses under him. He is swept down the mountain in the ensuing avalanche. You try to keep sight of your friend as long as possible as he tumbles down the mountain, but as the snow settles and stops, you are only able to identify a ski pole and a mitten on top of the debris.

1. What are some of the greatest threats to your friend's survival?
2. Describe how you and your remaining friends will organize yourselves to try to rescue him.
3. What risks do you need to be mindful of while attempting to rescue the victim?
4. Describe how you would use various avalanche safety and survival tools to improve the victim's chance of survival.

CASE 3

Thankfully your friend had prepared for avalanche terrain and was wearing an avalanche beacon. However, it takes you over 35 minutes to finally find him buried 3 feet deep in the debris snow. He doesn't seem to be moving or response to your voice commands.

1. What are some of the major factors regarding your medical treatment plan?

2. Did any of you pack equipment to access vital signs, core temperature, establish an airway, splint a fracture or call for help?
3. Describe how you and your two remaining friends will continue medical treatment given the current situation.

BACKGROUND

Facts

- Human factors contribute to nearly all avalanche accidents.
- The most important factor in avalanche survival is the amount of time buried in the snow.
- Depth of burial is the second most important factor in avalanche survival.
- Fully buried avalanche victims have a greater than 90 percent chance of survival if extricated within 18 minutes.
- Injury and death due to avalanches have dramatically increased over the past two decades.
- Asphyxiation is the predominant mechanism of death among avalanche victims.
- As many as one-third of avalanche victims sustain significant blunt trauma.
- Hypothermia is a rare cause of death among avalanche victims.
- Avalanches can be predicted by snow conditions and terrain.
- Avalanches can reach speeds of up to 100 mph in less than 10 seconds.
- Snowmobiler's account for the largest group of backcountry users who are killed in avalanches in the United States.
- Noise does not trigger avalanches.
- Avalanches are caused by four main factors: slope angle, snow pack, a weak layer in the snow pack, and a trigger.
- In the vast majority of avalanche burials, the victim or someone in the victim's party triggered the avalanche.

Factors That Predispose to Avalanches Occurring

Decision Making in Avalanche Terrain

- Human factors contribute to nearly all avalanche accidents.
- Human factors encompass all those factors that can influence people and their behavior.
- When it comes to risk management, people behave and think differently.
- Minimizing risk by traveling wisely with good techniques and avoiding high-risk terrain.
- Choosing the right terrain should be a consensus decision made by a cohesive group.
- Working as a cohesive group is done through planning, observation and communication.

Weather Factors

- Snow falls to the ground as crystals that go through metamorphic changes based on rain, sun, and temperature changes.
- These metamorphic changes bond snow pack together into strong or weak layers.
- Weather affects snow pack differently in each climate zone (i.e. coastal, interior, continental).
- Long cold dry spells can cause weaker "faceted" layers into the snow pack, where as deep compact snow exposed to consistently warmer air can cause stronger "rounding" snow pack.
- Strong winds carry windward snow and redistribute dense unstable layers on leeward slopes.
- These thick snow deposits on leeward slopes can shear off and cause a slab (wind) avalanche.
- Extended periods of snow melting are more likely to cause a slab avalanche.
- Any recent heavy snowfalls, particularly when the snow falls on old snow that has gone through freeze/thaw cycles, can also increase the risk of avalanches.

Terrain

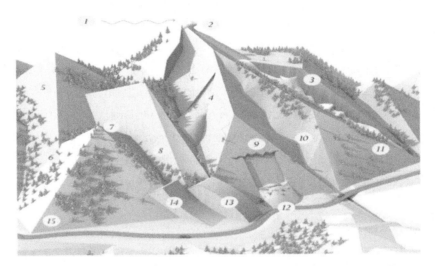

Created by Sam Moulton & Molly Loomis

1. **Windward** - wind-eroded slopes are usually fairly safe. **Leeward - wind-loaded slopes** can be very dangerous.
2. **Cornices** are obvious indicators of the prevailing wind direction and more prone to slides.
3. Traveling above a **cliff band** is never a good idea, especially if the slope is avalanche prone.
4. **Loose-snow avalanches**, often called **point releases**, usually start from a single source.
5. **Slope aspect**—snowpack can vary dramatically depending on how much sun it gets.
6. **Surface hoar** is a layer of feathery crystals from exposed snow on cold, clear, calm nights. These snow crystals don't bond well and are notorious for causing weak layers in snow pack.
7. **Safe zones** are places where members of your group can watch one another from a secure location, such as a ridgeline or a tight cluster of trees on a low-angle slope.

8. The **prime avalanche angle** for a slope is 38 degrees, with most slides occurring between 35 and 45 degrees. Less the 25 degrees and steeper than 60 degrees have a lower incidences.

9. **Slab avalanches** are the result of **a weak layer, a bed surface, terrain steep enough to slide, and a trigger. Slabs** can propagate farther down the slope and create larger dangerous slides.

10. **Terrain traps** like streambeds or gullies allow avalanche debris to pile up, making a deep burial more likely while increasing your odds of getting caught in an avalanche.

11. Exposed slopes with few young, widely dispersed trees are red-flag warnings of **frequent slide path** and more prone to avalanche.

12. Avalanche paths that spill over roads cause a **depression zone**, making it harder to rescue.

13. **Convex slope** or rollover pull snow downhill due lower compression strength (gravity) —making it more prone to sliding and more dangerous.

14. A **concave slope** naturally compresses snow—gravity adds strength to the snowpack.

15. Chose an established route, like a **skin track** or a boot-path, through trees keeps you out of the path of avalanche slides. Try to always choose the route with the least exposure.

Avalanche Types

Slab Avalanches

Most avalanche accidents occur from slab avalanche and are commonly triggered during or just after a snowstorm.

These are also referred to as wind, wet or storm slab avalanches.

Slab avalanches occur when two layers of snow, such as granular snow on smooth snow, do not adhere to one another.

It starts as a cohesive unit (slab) of snow, which fractures from surrounding snow.

Slab avalanches need a relatively strong layer of snow over a relatively weaker layer. Because these two layers are well beneath the snow surface, the danger is often invisible.

Clues such as sinking, cracking, or collapsing snow should alarm you of snow layer instability.

Loose Wet Snow / Dry Snow Avalanches

Wet snow (cement) avalanches occur anytime that there are prolonged periods of elevated temperatures that warm up the snow surface. This is more common in the spring.

They primarily occur in the afternoon, after the sun has had time to melt the top several centimeters of the snow surface. They are slower moving but more difficult to escape.

Dry snow (powder) avalanches start as a single point and grow into a fan shape as they progress down the mountain.

These are typically smaller and less destructive when compared to a slab avalanche.

Dry snow (sluffs) slides are common to skiers /snowboarders after freshly fallen new snow.

However, high density and heavy slides can drag victims over rock formations and cliffs, even if the slide is small.

When large and fast enough, avalanches can send shock waves in advance of their descent, increasing the amount of destruction in the path of the avalanche.

PATHOPHYSIOLOGY

General

The pathophysiology of death by avalanche follows the sequence of trauma, acute airway obstruction, early asphyxia, late asphyxia and hypothermia.

Trauma

Approximately one-fourth of avalanche victims have massive trauma as the primary cause of death.

Multiple injuries, such as spinal and long bone fractures, blunt abdominal trauma and closed head injuries are sustained as the avalanche victim is dragged over rocks and through trees.

Primary protection from brain trauma through the use of helmets in the wilderness is highly recommended.

Acute Airway Obstruction

Inhalation of snow by the avalanche victim results in rapid asphyxiation if the victim is unable to clear his or her airway. This more difficult as the slide slows and comes to stop.

Acute airway obstruction or acute asphyxiation is responsible for the immediate drop in survival observed after 19 to 35 minutes of burial.

If a victim can be rescued within 18 minutes, the survival rate is greater than 91%. The survival rate drops to 34% in burials between 19 and 35 minutes.

Early and Late Asphyxia

If chest movement is not restricted to the point of compromising breathing mechanics, survival depends on the size of the air space created near the victim's face as the snow flows down to a stop.

All air pockets will ultimately fail for two reasons:

☐ Heat from the expired air causes an ice lens to form on the air-snow interface, preventing continuous gas exchange.

☐ Re-breathing expired air with increased carbon dioxide (3% to 5%) and decreased oxygen (16%) content results in hypercapnia, hypoxemia and eventually death from asphyxiation.

Hypothermia

- Avalanche victims die from trauma or asphyxiation far sooner than they die from hypothermia.
- While hypothermia can significantly increase the morbidity of the victim, it is the primary cause of death in 1% of avalanche victims.
- The rate of core cooling is unlikely to cause life-threatening hypothermia before 90 minutes of burial.
- After one hour, only 1 in 3 victims buried in an avalanche is found alive.

AVALANCHE SAFETY AND SURVIVAL

Safety

- Education is the key to avalanche avoidance. Specific field instruction with avalanche professionals is encouraged.
- Planning, observation and communication is the key to good decision making in avalanche terrain.
- Alternatively, travel with a guide who is knowledgeable in avalanche safety and who can recognize dangerous terrain.
- When traveling, never travel directly above any member of your party.
- Avoid terrain traps like cliffs, bodies of water, crevasses, roads where debris pile up or valley bases within a known avalanche slide path.
- Avoid gullies and narrow valleys. These serve as run-out zones where avalanches far up the mountain can funnel through, burying everything on the bottom of the gully.
- Travel on ridgelines above start zones. In dense forest or well away from damaged vegetation.
- Travel from one safe zone to another one person at a time. If an exposed area needs to be crossed, never expose more than one person at a time. Keep the rest of the party in a safe area so that they can perform a rescue if an avalanche does occur.
- Be on the lookout for "red flags," such as collapsing, cracking snow or sinking into wet snow.
- Start on low angle slopes, which are less than 30°, before venturing to steeper slopes. This gives you the opportunity to better assess snow stability before traveling on more risky slopes.
- When traveling through avalanche-prone terrain, always send one person at a time and follow the same tracks.
- If forced to move in an avalanche zone, keep close to the sides or flanks of the zone.
- Use releasable bindings so that if caught in an avalanche your skis do not trap you at the bottom of the debris (the "anchor" effect).
- Let someone at home know where you have gone and when he or she can expect you back.
- Always call the Forest Service or Avalanche Forecast Center for a report of the current snow conditions.

- Always carry avalanche rescue equipment, including at a minimum, an electronic avalanche rescue transceiver (beacon), a shovel and probe, and practice using them.
- The RECCO reflector is a passive electronic reflector that can be detected by those equipped with its notebook-sized detector.
- Always wear a helmet.

Survival

- If an avalanche starts, attempt to escape to the side.
- If caught in an avalanche, attempts should be made to remove all ski equipment including skis and poles.
- Lightweight backpacks may be left on as they may provide some measure of spine protection.
- Heavy mountaineering packs should be jettisoned as they hinder "swimming" in the avalanche.
- Once caught, the most important thing to do is to get a hand or both hands in front of the face to create and protect an air pocket.
  - ☐ If caught, attempting to "swim" to the surface of the debris is no longer the most important thing to do – maintaining an air pocket is.
- Human-triggered avalanches stop suddenly, so you may not have an opportunity at that time to create an air pocket.
- Creating an air pocket is the most important key to survival.
- Snowmobilers caught in an avalanche should try to remain on the vehicle, as those thrown off are twice as likely to be buried.

AVALANCHE VICTIM RESCUE

- If an avalanche is witnessed, the survivors should make every effort to maintain sight of the victim as he/she is pushed down the slope.
- Once the survivors lose sight of the victim, a mental note should be made of the area where the victim was last seen using fixed landmarks such as rocks and trees.
- As more than one avalanche is possible in the same area, extreme caution should be used by the rescuers to avoid getting caught in a second avalanche. One member of the rescue party should be designated as the team leader and should stand at a safe distance away from the debris and other rescuers and look out for potential danger.
- Transceivers (beacons), shovels, and probes constitute the basis of avalanche survival and rescue equipment.
- Transceivers work on the assumption that an avalanche victim can be found within the "golden fifteen minutes" after burial (after 15 minutes, the chances of survival dramatically decrease).

If a member of a party is buried in an avalanche, rescuers should switch their transceivers from the "send" to the "receive" mode. This will allow rescuers to pick up the signal transmitted by the victim's beacon. Using a systematic pattern, rescuers can hone in on the victim's signal with their receiving transceivers.

- ☐ A rule of thumb is to start at the place where the victim was last seen and work "downstream," making wider and wider switchbacks as you travel down the avalanche path.

- ☐ Leave surface clues such as gloves and ski poles in place where you found them so that other rescuers can probe around them or walk around them with a transceiver to see if a signal is picked up in the area around the articles.

- ☐ Once the maximal signal is obtained on the lowest sensitivity setting, then the transceiver is placed on the snow where the signal is strongest and rescuers start to probe in a grid-like fashion around the signal.

- ☐ Once a body is felt with the probe, leave the probe in place and dig the snow out around the probe, using caution as to not further injure the victim with the shovel.

- ☐ If multiple victims are involved, turn off the victim's transceiver once he/she is extricated so as to not interfere with the signal of another victim's transceiver.

TREATMENT

Hypoxia and hypercarbia are major threats to life in avalanche victims.

As with any victim, primary attention should first be given to MARCH protocol.

- ☐ If the victim is not breathing spontaneously, clear all snow and debris that may be obstructing the airway and listen for breath sounds.

- ☐ If the victim is still not breathing spontaneously, then initiate rescue breathing. If resistance is met, reassess for airway obstruction.

- ☐ Continue the primary assessment and treat as discussed in the Patient Assessment chapter.

Because major trauma frequently accompanies avalanche burial, cervical spine precautions should be used when extricating the victim.

If lethal injuries are present at the time of extrication, then attempts at resuscitation are not recommended.

Resuscitative efforts should continue on an asystolic victim buried more than 45 minutes if an obvious air space is identified at extrication.

Continue with the secondary assessment as previously discussed.

Keep in mind the patient's exposure to the environment. Snow can be insulating. Once the victim is extracted from the snow and exposed to wind, core body cooling can accelerate if the body is not

properly insulated against the environment.

EVACUATION GUIDELINES

■ Any avalanche burial victim should be evacuated immediately.

■ The entire party should turn around and discontinue the trip if there is any concern for potential additional avalanches.

■ If on a multi-day tour or if caught in a storm such that evacuation poses as much risk as proceeding on the trip, then the involved parties should stop and make every reasonable effort to find shelter in a safe area (such as digging a snow cave in a heavily wooded area) until the storm clears and a safe route can be navigated.

International (IKAR) Standard for Avalanche Rescucitation

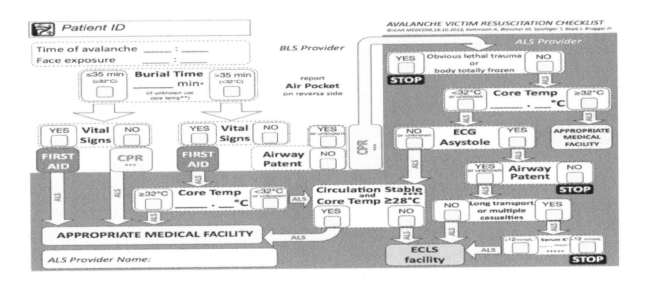

QUESTIONS

1. **Which one of the following is the most important determinant of avalanche victim survival?**
    a. The ability of the victim to create an air pocket around his or her face
    b. The fitness level of the buried victim
    c. The length of time which the victim is buried
    d. Type of avalanche in which the victim is caught

2. **When traveling over snow in the wilderness, which one of the following guidelines should be observed?**
    a. Exposed areas are frequently safest as there is less risk of being injured against a tree
    b. Gullies and narrow valleys are generally safe places to travel
    c. Talk in low, hushed voices so as to not disrupt an avalanche
    d. Travel one person at a time when crossing hazardous areas

3. **When performing a rescue for an avalanche victim, which one of the following is TRUE?**
    a. Rescuers should turn their transceivers from "receive" to "send" mode
    b. More than one avalanche in the same area is rare
    c. Cervical spine precautions should be observed when extricating avalanche victims
    d. Hypothermia is the biggest concern with avalanche victims before rescue

4. **If caught in an avalanche, which of the following should be attempted?**
    a. Create an air pocket around the mouth and face
    b. "Swim" to the surface
    c. Ski to the side of the slide
    d. All of the above

Answers:
1. c
2. d
3. c
4. d

CHAPTER 6
Heat-Related Illness

This chapter describes how to recognize and treat health conditions caused by excessive heat and how to help prevent these injuries.

Objectives:

- List risk factors for heat-related illness
- Discuss the body's four primary mechanisms of heat regulation
- Discuss the body's general response to heat stress
- Describe the etiology and management of patients with heat cramps and heat syncope
- Know the similarities and differences between heat exhaustion and heat stroke
- Discuss methods to help prevent heat-related illness
- Know which methods of cooling are most effective in treating heat-related illness, and when to stop active cooling
- List evacuation guidelines for victims with heat-related illness

CASE

During a long distance running event, three people present to your first aid station.

Patient #1: A 27-year-old female who "passed out" while standing at a hydration table where she had stopped to drink some fluids. She regained consciousness shortly after falling to the ground. She is alert and oriented to person, place, time and event. Her blood pressure is 110/70 mmHg and her pulse is 120 bpm. She denies dizziness, nausea or weakness and asks you if she can continue running.

Patient #2: A 42-year-old male complains of severe spasms in his right calf muscle. His blood pressure is 130/85 mmHg and his pulse is 95 bpm. He is in severe pain. He has been drinking large amounts of water throughout the day.

Patient #3: A 35-year-old male is brought to the aid station by bystanders who state the man was moving erratically and was "just not acting right." The victim's blood pressure is 150/90 mmHg, his pulse is 140 bpm, his rectal temperature is 40.5° C, and respirations are 34 breaths/min. He is oriented only to his name. On exam, he is covered in sweat, is agitated, and is warm to the touch.

1. What other information would be helpful in diagnosing and treating each person?
2. What is the etiology of each victim's illness?
3. What is the next step in management for each person?
4. Can any of these people continue the race?
5. Who, if anyone, needs to be evacuated immediately?

BACKGROUND

Heat-related illnesses are a common cause of weather related death in the United States.

Between 2006 and 2010, a total of 3,006 deaths in the USA resulted from heat-related illness (annual mean: 601). This is 31% of all weather related causes of death during this period.

Mortality rates associated with heat stroke range from 10 to 75 percent. Mortality increases in situations where the patient has significant comorbidities and initial treatment is delayed by more than two hours.

The classic definition of a "heat wave" is defined as three or more consecutive days with environmental temperatures above 90° F (32.2°C). However, a more rational definition is dependent on the region and the normal conditions for that region.

Risk Factors for Heat-Related Illness

Medical Conditions
- ☐ Heart disease
- ☐ Skin diseases (scleroderma, ectodermal hyperplasia)
- ☐ Extensive burns
- ☐ Dehydration
- ☐ Vomiting
- ☐ Diarrhea
- ☐ Endocrine disorders (hyperthyroidism, diabetes)
- ☐ Neurologic diseases (autonomic neuropathies, Parkinsonism, dystonias)
- ☐ Delirium tremens
- ☐ Fever

Environmental
- ☐ Exercise in a hot environment
- ☐ Lack of air conditioning or proper ventilation
- ☐ Inappropriate clothing (occlusive, heavy, or vapor-impermeable)
- ☐ Lack of acclimatization
- ☐ Decreased fluid intake
- ☐ Hot environments (inside of tents or autos in the sun, hot tubs, saunas)

Drugs and Toxins
- ☐ Beta-blockers
- ☐ Anticholinergics
- ☐ Diuretics

- ☐ Ethanol
- ☐ Antihistamines
- ☐ Cyclic antidepressants
- ☐ Sympathomimetics (cocaine, amphetamines)
- ☐ Phenothiazines
- ☐ Lithium
- ☐ Salicylates

■ Other Risk Factors
- ☐ Salt/water depletion
- ☐ Obesity

PATHOPHYSIOLOGY

Four Mechanisms for Heat Regulation:

Evaporation

- Evaporation is the most efficient method
- Thirty percent of body cooling at average temperatures is due to evaporation.
- As external temperatures reach 95° F, evaporation becomes the major mechanism for heat dissipation.
- Evaporation is most effective in a dry environment. As the humidity approaches 100 percent, the body loses its ability to dissipate heat.

Radiation

- Radiation is the transfer of heat between the body and the environment via electromagnetic waves.
- It does not require an intervening medium.
- Radiation accounts for over 50 percent of cooling, as long as ambient air temperature is lower than body temperature.

Conduction

- Conduction is the direct transfer of heat between two objects in direct contact.
- Because conduction requires direct contact between two objects, heat loss from the body is minimal except in certain circumstances, such as when lying on cold ground or when immersed in water.

Convection

- Convection is heat transfer between the body and a moving gas or liquid – typically air and water.
- The rate at which heat is transferred depends upon how fast the air or water is moving as well as the temperature of each substance.

Physiological Response to Heat Stress

Vasodilation

- This especially occurs in the skin, which can increase blood flow from 0.2 L/min to 8 L/min.
- Simultaneously, the renal and splanchnic vasculatures vasoconstrict to shunt heat away from the core.
- The heart responds to massive vasodilation and decreased peripheral vascular resistance by increasing heart rate and cardiac output.
- The net effect is increased blood flow to the skin, which facilitates heat transfer to the environment.

Increased Catecholamines

This results in activation of an increased number of sweat glands.

This stimulates active glands to become more active.

Sweating increases the amount of evaporative heat loss.

Inhibition of Metabolic Heat Production

This is controlled by the hypothalamus.

Less metabolic heat production decreases the amount of heat that the body has to regulate.

The body's physiological responses eventually deteriorate as cardiac output reaches its limits. In conjunction with the limits of the cardiovascular response, progressive electrolyte and water depletion further contribute to heat injury.

Stages of Heat-Related Injury

Heat-related injury can be divided into three progressive stages: acute, enzymatic and late

Acute phase

Activation of inflammatory mediators from endothelial cells, leukocytes and epithelial cells

Hypoperfusion of the GI tract, leading to migration of bacterial products into the bloodstream

Respiratory alkalosis from hyperventilation accompanied by metabolic acidosis from increased glycolysis and hyperlactemia

Enzymatic phase

Disturbance of coagulation cascade, which results in elevated coagulation and fibrinolysis

Endothelial injury and diffuse microvascular thrombosis

Multiple effects culminate in disseminated intravascular coagulation (DIC)

Late phase

Hepatic dysfunction secondary to DIC. Cholestasis and hepatocellular necrosis, with elevation of AST, ALT, and serum bilirubin levels, usually within 12 to 24 hours

Renal failure from dehydration, vasodilatation, and hypotension

Central nervous system injury leading to cerebral edema, petechial hemorrhages in the brain, and neuronal degradation

Cardiovascular dysfunction leads to hypotension and compensatory vasoconstriction

The consequence of these final steps in heat injury is shock and eventual death.

CLINICAL MANIFESTATIONS OF HEAT INJURY

Heat injury presentations occur on a spectrum of severity, ranging from minor to life threatening.

Heat Cramps

Background
- Heat cramps occur when significant salt and water losses are replaced with a hypotonic solution, such as water.
- This creates a relative hyponatremia, which lowers the threshold for skeletal muscle cell depolarization.
- This eventually leads to sustained involuntary contraction of skeletal muscle.

Clinical Presentation
- Heat cramps are brief, intermittent and involuntary contractions of skeletal muscle.
- They most commonly involve the calves, but may occur in any voluntary skeletal muscle.
- They usually occur unilaterally and are quite painful.
- The patient with heat cramps classically offers a history of the following:
  - ☐ Prolonged activity in a hot environment
  - ☐ Good hydration, typically with a hypotonic solution such as water
  - ☐ Poor salt/electrolyte intake

Treatment
- Mild cases
  - ☐ Oral salt replacement with a 0.1% to 0.2% saline solution.
  - ☐ This can be easily made with ¼ to ½ teaspoon of table salt added to a quart of water.
- Severe cases
  - ☐ IV normal saline (0.9% NaCl)
  - ☐ Begin with a one-liter bolus; repeat if necessary.

Heat Edema

Background
- Dependent extremity swelling due to interstitial fluid pooling as a result of hydrostatic pressure, vascular leak, and cutaneous vasodilatation
  - ☐ High temperature leads to vasodilatation, which results in dependent edema.

Clinical Presentation
- Dependent extremity swelling in hands and/or feet

Treatment

- Benign, self-limited condition; elevation and/or frequent voluntary contraction of muscles will redistributed edema
- May use compression stockings for ongoing edema

Heat Syncope

Background

Heat syncope is a form of orthostatic hypotension that results from volume depletion, peripheral vasodilatation and decreased vasomotor tone.

Patients are typically not profoundly dehydrated or hyperthermic.

Heat syncope typically affects two populations: the non-acclimatized and geriatric individuals.

Heat syncope usually afflicts standing, stationary individuals.

- ☐ By standing upright, blood pools in the lower extremities because of gravity.
- ☐ Additionally, peripheral blood vessels are dilated to facilitate heat transfer to the environment.
- ☐ Increased vagal tone may also occur, which may cause bradycardia.
- ☐ The combined effect of these factors leads to decreased cardiac output and poor cerebral perfusion. The flow of oxygen to the brain may descend below the threshold where unconsciousness occurs.

Clinical Presentation

Prodromal symptoms of heat syncope include:

- ☐ Lightheadedness
- ☐ Vertigo
- ☐ Restlessness
- ☐ Nausea
- ☐ Yawning

If cerebral perfusion is compromised, loss of consciousness or syncope will occur.

Syncope typically resolves once the patient is horizontal, as this facilitates redistribution of blood from the lower extremities back into central and cerebral circulations.

There may be tonic jerking associated with syncope, but generalized seizure activity should not occur.

Treatment

The actual loss of consciousness of heat syncope should be brief and resolves once venous return to the brain improves.

Treatment to improve central and cerebral blood flow should be instituted:

- ☐ Lie the patient flat
- ☐ Elevate the feet
- ☐ Remove from direct sunlight
- ☐ Move to a cool area if possible

Heat Exhaustion

Clinical Presentation

Heat exhaustion is a form of heat illness that represents significant heat stress, leading to intravascular volume and sodium depletion.

Symptoms of heat exhaustion include:

☐ Weakness

☐ Lightheadedness

☐ Fatigue

☐ Nausea with or without vomiting

☐ Headache

☐ Thirst

Signs of heat exhaustion include:

☐ Tachycardia

☐ Tachypnea

☐ Profuse diaphoresis (may be absent)

☐ Orthostatic hypotension

☐ Hyperthermia may or may not be present, but body temperature should be < 40°C (104° F)

☐ Absence of altered mental status

Heat exhaustion is part of the continuum of heat illness that progresses to heat stroke.

Treatment

Heat exhaustion is treated with liberal volume and electrolyte replacement after cessation of all immediate activities.

Specific treatment includes:

☐ Removal from the direct sunlight into a cool, shaded area

☐ Restrictive clothing should be loosened

☐ Aggressive oral hydration

☐ If the patient is hyperthermic (> 38°C), active cooling measures should be initiated.

- One very effective way to cool a hyperthermic patient is to make the patient "sopping wet" with tepid (comfortable room temperature) water and fan the patient with anything that increases air movement and thus evaporation of the water.

- Ambient temperature water lessens the shivering reaction and helps to keep the skin vessels dilated, which increases heat transfer.

- Shivering will increase core body temperature and should be avoided.

Oral hydration should adhere to the following guidelines:

☐ Cold water or sports beverage

☐ Beverage should not exceed 6% carbohydrate content. Increased carbohydrate content inhibits gastric emptying and fluid absorption.

- ☐ A general rule is that every pound lost to sweat should be replenished with 500 mL or 2 cups of fluid.
- ☐ The treatment goal for mild heat exhaustion should be 1 – 2 liters over 2 – 4 hours.

Heat Stroke

Clinical Presentation

Heat stroke is a true medical emergency and is classically defined as

- ☐ Severe hyperthermia (core temperature > 40° C [104° F])
- ☐ Central nervous system (CNS) disturbances
- ☐ Anhidrosis (absence of sweating) *although this may be absent.*

Experience has shown that following these three symptoms as strict criteria for the diagnosis of heat stroke is too conservative and may delay critical treatment.

CNS abnormalities are the hallmark of heat stroke and thus the most sensitive indicators of significant heat injury.

Central nervous system disturbances include:

- ☐ Ataxia
- ☐ Irritability
- ☐ Confusion
- ☐ Combativeness
- ☐ Bizarre behavior
- ☐ Seizures
- ☐ Hallucinations
- ☐ Syncope
- ☐ Decorticate and decerebrate posturing
- ☐ Hemiplegia
- ☐ Coma (very late finding)

One of the earlier neurological manifestations of heat stroke is ataxia because the cerebellum is very sensitive to heat stress.

Mild elevation in temperature does not preclude the diagnosis of heat stroke. A rectal or other core thermometer should always be utilized in the evaluation of a heat-related injury patient as non-core temperature determinations may be misleading and delay treatment.

Anhidrosis is classically associated with heat stroke. However, it is usually a very late finding and can-not be relied upon to make an accurate diagnosis. Typically, heat stroke patients are profusely dia-phoretic until the very late stages of the illness.

The key to treatment and prevention is in understanding that heat exhaustion and heat stroke are not separate entities but are a continuum of the same illness. The onset of central nervous system abnormalities should alert providers that a patient is suffering from significant heat illness.

Treatment

■ The initial resuscitative effort should include:

☐ Assess airway, respirations, circulation and intervening where necessary

☐ High flow oxygen via face mask, if available

☐ Intravenous access; two lines if possible

☐ Cardiac monitoring, if available

☐ IV infusion of normal saline or lactated Ringer's solution should be started. Ideally 1 to 2 liters cooled to 4° C should be given within the first hour. Monitor breath sounds for the development of pulmonary edema.

☐ Continuous vital signs monitoring

☐ Monitor core temperature by placing a rectal probe, if possible

■ Active Cooling:

☐ Remove all restrictive clothing

☐ Cold-water immersion (CWI); if available, whether in the field or the hospital

● CWI has been shown to reduce core temperature twice as fast as evaporative cooling and has been demonstrated to be safe in young, healthy heat stroke victims.

● CWI is now a class IA recommendation for field and hospital treatment by the Wilderness Medical Society.

● Remove all of the victim's clothes and submerse their trunk and extremities in a cold-water bath or another readily available body of water.

● There should always be someone managing the head to ensure that it stays above the water.

● If a source for CWI is not available, repeated dousing of the victim with cold water or snow is also an option.

☐ Evaporative and convective cooling (Class IC recommendation)

● If cold-water immersion is unavailable, not tolerated, or in classic heat stroke patients or those with multiple medical problems where ice-water cooling may be inadvisable.

● The victim's skin should be kept "sopping wet" with tepid (comfortable room temperature) water if available, and continuously fanned to promote evaporation.

● The tepid water allows for skin vasodilation as well as decreasing the chance of shivering.

● If tepid water is not available, then cold water is perfectly fine

● If available, ice packs and cold compresses may be placed in area where large arteries run, such as the groin, axilla and neck.

☐ The initial treatment goal is to drop the body core temperature to below 40°C (104° F) as rapidly as possible

☐ The secondary treatment goal is 39°C (102°F). At this temperature all active cooling should be discontinued to avoid overshoot hypothermia.

■ Antipyretics such as acetaminophen, aspirin and NSAIDs are not effective and should not be used.

EVACUATION GUIDELINES

■ A patient who has had a syncopal episode that is thought to be heat-related should only have brief loss of consciousness and should recover quickly. Any patient who has prolonged loss of consciousness, persistent pre-syncope signs and symptoms, more than one episode of syncope or signs of heat stroke should be evacuated.

■ A patient with severe heat cramps that do not respond to oral salt solutions, or someone who has multiple cramps should also be considered for evacuation, depending on the situation.

■ Heat exhaustion victims *may not* need to be evacuated:

☐ As long as the patient can adequately be protected from the environment.

☐ In mild cases, close observation in the field for development of heat stroke, as well cessation of heat-generating physical activities for 24 to 48 hours is recommended.

☐ If the patient develops behavioral changes, a temperature above 39°C (102.2°F), or has a syncopal episode while under observation, he or she should be considered a potential heat stroke victim and be evacuated immediately.

■ Heat stroke is a serious medical emergency and any patient with signs or symptoms of heat stroke should be evacuated as soon as possible.

PREVENTION

■ The three main categories of prevention include hydration, heat dissipation and acclimatization.

■ General hydration guidelines include:

☐ Drink 4 to 8 ounces of water or sports beverage every 15 to 20 minutes during mild to moderate exertion.

☐ Hydrate with a goal of clear urine instead of a set amount of intake.

☐ Consume salt-containing foods or add salt to water if exposed to heat for time periods greater than 2 to 3 hours, especially if using only water for hydration.

☐ To make a palatable salt solution, add ¼ to ½ teaspoon of salt to a liter of fluid. Flavored drinks that are cold are more palatable.

☐ Most commercially available sports drinks may be diluted by 50% for ideal electrolyte and carbohydrate concentrations.

■ To help dissipate heat:

☐ Wear loose fitting clothing that allows air circulation and sufficient evaporation.

☐ Avoid direct sunlight when possible and wear light-colored clothing.

☐ Frequently douse exposed skin with cool fluids or cool misting spray.

■ Acclimatization to heat has been proven to decrease the incidence of heat injuries and improve performance in hot environments. General guidelines for acclimatization are as follows:

- ☐ Adults should gradually increase the time and intensity of activity over 7 to 10 days.
- ☐ Children and elderly require 10 to 14 days to maximize acclimatization.
- ☐ Persons who are from temperate or cold climates and will be travelling into a hot environment can acclimatize by going into a sauna or steam room for increasing amounts of time 7 to 10 days before making the trip.
- ☐ The process of acclimatization will activate the renin-angiotensin-aldosterone axis, which will increase sodium conservation, maximize sweat production, expand plasma volume, and aid the cardiovascular system in adapting to the new environment.
- ☐ De-acclimatization usually occurs within 1 to 2 weeks of being removed from the hot environment.

■ Finally:

- ☐ Minimize use of medications that would limit the thermoregulatory response
- ☐ Consider previous history of heat injury as a risk factor for recurrence (for at least months after the initial event).

QUESTIONS

1. **All of the following increase the risk of heat illness except:**
   a. Alcoholism
   b. Cardiac medications, such as beta-blockers and calcium channel blockers
   c. Diarrhea
   d. History of heat injury
   e. All of the above increase the risk of heat injury

2. **Which is the most efficient of the four primary methods of heat regulation in the body?**
   a. Conduction
   b. Convection
   c. Evaporation
   d. Radiation

3. **Heat cramps are most likely to occur in which patient?**
   a. A runner on a hot day drinking water alternating with a sports drink
   b. A runner on a hot day drinking 6 to 8 oz of water per hour for 2 hours
   c. A runner on a hot day drinking 6 to 8 oz of water per hour for several hours
   d. A runner on a hot day not rehydrating with anything

4. **The major difference between heat stroke and heat exhaustion is which one?**
   a. Core body temperature
   b. Neurologic findings, including altered mental status
   c. The presence or absence of sweating
   d. The presence of vomiting

5. **Which one of the following is the most effective way to cool a patient with heat stroke?**
   a. Cold water evaporative cooling
   b. Cold water immersion in a safe body of water
   c. Ice packs to the axilla/groin
   d. Tepid water evaporative cooling

6. **Acclimatization to a hot environment should take how long for the average adult?**
   a. 1 to 3 days
   b. 4 to 6 days
   c. 8 to 10 days
   d. 11 to 14 days

7. **At what core temperature should active cooling be stopped to help prevent the development of overshoot hypothermia?**
   a. 37° C (98.6° F)
   b. 38° C (100.4° F)
   c. 39° C (102.2° F)
   d. 41° C (105.8° F)

Answers:

1.	e	5.	b
2.	c	6.	c
3.	c	7.	c
4.	b		

CHAPTER 7

Cold-Induced Injuries and Illness

This chapter describes how to recognize and treat health conditions caused by cold and how to help prevent these injuries.

Objectives:

- Understand the mechanisms by which the body loses heat
- Review the pathophysiology of hypothermia, frostbite, and other cold-related injuries
- Recognize and treat hypothermia and frostbite in the wilderness with limited resources
- Understand the evacuation criteria for frostbite and hypothermia
- Be able to describe methods to prevent cold injury

CASE 1

After spending several weeks acclimating to high altitude conditions, Scott Fisher, an experienced climber and founder of the adventure company Mountain Madness, led his team towards the summit of Mt. Everest. After climbing through the night, Fisher's team finally reached the peak early on the afternoon of May 10, 1996. Conditions at Everest's summit were extreme, with raging winds and temperatures averaging negative 25°C. The team descended into 75 mph winds and near-whiteout conditions. They lost their bearings and decided to huddle together in an attempt to wait out the storm, hunkering down a mere 400 meters from high camp. The team was eventually rescued by Anatoli Boukreev, one of the guides who had managed to make it back ahead of the storm. All members of the expedition were saved except for Fisher, who had lagged behind to assist the weaker climbers in the group. Boukreev made several attempts to reach Fisher but was unsuccessful and forced to turn back because of the severe weather conditions. Fisher had been climbing with Lopsang Sherpa, a long-time friend and climbing partner, when he collapsed an hour outside of camp. Lopsang was eventually forced to leave Fisher in an attempt to go for help when it was clear that Fisher would not be able to continue. Unfortunately, this help would not arrive until the following day, when Fisher was found dead from hypothermia. Interestingly, his body was discovered with mittens off and down suit unzipped in an apparent attempt to undress. Fisher was one of eight people who perished on one of the deadliest days in Everest's history.

1. What are the mechanisms by which the body loses heat?
2. What are the stages of hypothermia?
3. Why have multiple victims of hypothermia been found attempting to undress despite freezing temperatures?
4. If medical care was available, what interventions could have been pursued to save Scott Fisher's life?

CASE 2

After saving money for a over a year, Mike, an experienced rock and ice climber, set off with his climbing partner on a dream vacation to climb Mt. McKinley in Alaska. Being a seasoned outdoorsman and knowing the extremes of temperatures that exist at McKinley's summit, Mike left California well prepared to do battle with the elements. Included in his gear was a new, top-of-the-line pair of mountaineering boots to protect his feet from cold-related injuries.

Three weeks into the expedition, Mike and his climbing partner made camp a few hours from the summit when a storm front moved in with blinding snow and subzero temperatures, forcing them to remain in camp for an extra two days. Somehow over the course of this period, Mike was separated from his boots but decided to continue on with a pair of standard ski boots rather than risk a hazardous descent through avalanche terrain to retrieve his gear. On the third day, as the snow died down, Mike and his partner decided to attempt a summit push.

A couple of hours into their journey, Mike began to experience pain and numbness in his feet. As they continued on, his symptoms began to grow worse with increasing stiffness in his toes. Mike was well aware that his symptoms were consistent with the early stages of frostbite and was forced to decide between returning to camp and pressing on for the summit.

1. What are the initial signs and symptoms of frostbite?
2. What is the treatment of frostbite?
3. What are complications Mike could expect if he continued his push for the summit?
4. What conditions should be distinguished from frostbite?

CASE 3

Anna Bagenholm was a 29 year-old Orthopedic surgery resident and expert skier in Norway who liked to ski in the mountains surrounding her town after work. On one particular momentous occasion, the day her mentor was to celebrate his retirement, she and two of her colleagues set out to take a few runs prior to the nights festivities. As she descended a route she knew very well, she lost control of her skis and fell backwards, head first onto an ice covered stream. The ice opened and swallowed her head and torso. She was trapped under 7 inches of ice.

Her colleagues arrived immediately, but were unable to free her from the ice. They called for help from a cell phone. Anna struggled as her companions held fast to her skis, finding an air pocket under the ice. She struggled for more than a half an hour, eventually becoming lifeless. The initial rescue team could not free her from the ice and after more than an hour, the second rescue team was able to cut her free from the ice.

After extricating her from the ice, she was lifeless, pulseless, not breathing with fixed and dilated pupils.

1. What is your initial assessment of this patient?
2. How would you address her cardiopulmonary status in the field
3. What interventions to address her status can be expected and prepared for in the hospital?
4. When is it appropriate to presume a patient 'cold and dead'?

HYPOTHERMIA

Although extreme cases, one can learn from the stories of Scott Fisher and Anna Bagenholm that even the most experienced and prepared individuals can succumb to hypothermia.

Between 2006 and 2010, a total of 6,652 deaths in the USA resulted from cold-related illness (annual mean: 1330). This is 63% of all weather related causes of death during this period.

Most think of hypothermia as a condition associated with prolonged cold exposure, but it can also result from immersion accidents, may occur in any season, and in either tropical or temperate climates.

Hypothermia occurs more frequently in the urban homeless, intoxicated, or patients with comorbidities.

The lowest known core temperature from which a patient with accidental hypothermia has been successfully resuscitated is 13.7°C (57°F)

Physiology

The healthy body maintains a core temperature of 37°C +/- .5°C.

Humans have a limited physiologic means to avoid development of hypothermia.

Shivering is our primary method of heat production, increasing the metabolic rate.

The body conserves heat through vasoconstriction of skin and extremities.

Pathophysiology

A core body temperature of 35°C or less defines hypothermia.

The primary mechanisms by the body loses heat include radiation, conduction, convection, and evaporation. These mechanisms are all discussed in the Heat-Related Illness chapter.

Poor insulation, wet clothing, and vasodilators such as alcohol all accelerate heat loss.

Trauma and severe illness may also compromise temperature regulation.

Perception of temperature is closely linked to skin temperature rather than core temperature; for example, shivering may begin when core temperature is 37 degrees Celsius.

Hypothermia compromises cardiac function, leading to decreased output and fatal arrhythmias

The body must expend energy in order to shiver and to vasoconstrict peripherally.

☐ Depletion of energy stores leads to a loss of temperature homeostasis and vasodilatation.

☐ When this occurs, blood rushes back to the skin and the individual feels warm.

☐ This may lead to the phenomenon known as "paradoxical undressing," whereby hypothermic individuals take off their clothes despite being cold.

☐ This paradoxical undressing precipitates a further drop in core temperature as blood returns to cold extremities and is subsequently circulated back to the core.

After-drop refers to a decrease in the core temperature as the extremities are rewarmed.

☐ As the periphery vasodilates during rewarming, blood volume increases to these areas.

- ☐ Cooled blood returns to the core, decreasing overall body temperature.
- ☐ In cases of severe hypothermia, cardiac arrest may result from even a small (5 degree Celsius) subsequent drop in core temperature

Clinical Presentation

A core thermometer (rectal or esophageal) is ideal for diagnosing hypothermia as temperature measurement may be grossly inaccurate using peripheral methods.

- ☐ It is important to note that most commercial thermometers can only register temperatures down to 34.5°C.
- ☐ Since most people faced with hypothermia in the wilderness do not have thermometers, this is an impractical means of diagnosing this condition.

Individuals must therefore rely on clinical symptoms to make the diagnosis.

Classification

A number of guidelines grade severity of hypothermia. Most of these use temperature as a means of classification. However, as mentioned above, accurate core temperature measurement in austere environments is often impractical.

The standard classification system is detailed below.

Mild Hypothermia

A core temperature ranging from 32° to 35°C defines mild hypothermia.

At this level, the cold temperature defense mechanisms are still working and will cause pallor and sensation of cold, secondary to maximal peripheral and cutaneous vasoconstriction.

The victim may manifest uncontrollable shivering.

Mental status may become impaired with varying degrees of confusion, ataxia, and disorientation.

Urinary frequency is common, due to increased renal perfusion caused by elevated cardiac output and peripheral vasoconstriction increasing blood flow to the kidneys.

The victim may have an elevation in vital signs, including tachycardia, tachypnea, and hypertension.

Moderate Hypothermia

A core temperature ranging from 28° to 32°C defines moderate hypothermia.

Blood pressure, heart rate, and respiratory rate are all decreased.

Individuals exhibit confusion as well as dilated pupils and muscle rigidity.

Thermoregulation is less effective (shivering) and exogenous rewarming is required.

☐ Shivering ceases at and below a core temperature of 30°C (86°F)

☐ Cardiac dysrhythmias are common and unless rewarming is possible, the victim will eventually cool to ambient temperature and die.

Severe Hypothermia

☐ A core temperature between 24°C and 28°C defines severe hypothermia.

☐ At this temperature, the victim will go into a deep coma with dilated pupils and muscular rigidity.

☐ Blood pressure will be barely palpable and the pulse may be as low as 10 to 20 beats per minute.

☐ Life-threatening dysrhythmias, such as ventricular fibrillation, are easily induced in these victims with even with the slightest of movements. Chemical or electrical conversion of such rhythms is nearly impossible without core rewarming.

Profound Hypothermia

☐ Core temperature below 24°C

☐ Significantly low rate of survival

☐ High likelihood of cardiac arrest

Swiss Staging System

☐ The Swiss Staging System was developed for use in a wilderness setting by rescue personnel and focuses on clinical findings as opposed to temperature.

☐ The system is simple, easy to recall and interpret and meant to correspond to the standard temperature ranges.

☐ Limitations of the system pertain to variability of clinical response to particular temperatures potentially leading to an under appreciation of severity of hypothermia.

☐ The modification below substitutes the Swiss numbering with stages with which most providers are familiar.

TABLE 1: Hypothermia Classification

	Temperature	Clinical Picture
Mild hypothermia	32 to 35°C (92 to 95°F)	Hypertension Tachypnea Tachycardia Skin pale and cold Uncontrollable shivering Urinary frequency Impaired judgment
Moderate hypothermia	28 to 32°C (82 to 90°F)	Hypotension Bradycardia Bradypnea Stop shivering Dilated pupils Slurred speech Decreased level of consciousness Dysrhythmias
Severe hypothermia	24°C to 28°C (77 to 82°F)	Apnea Profound hypotension Severe bradycardia Nonreactive pupils Muscle rigidity Pulmonary edema Life-threatening dysrhythmias Death
Profound hypothermia	< 24°C (75°F)	Life-threatening dysrhythmias likely Signs of life may be absent

TABLE 2: "Modified" Swiss Staging System

Stage	Clinical Symptoms	Typical Core Temperature
Mild	Conscious, shivering	32-35
Moderate	Impaired consciousness, not shivering	28-<32
Severe	Unconscious, not shivering, vital signs present	24-<28
Profound	No vital signs	<24

Treatment

General

- Ensure scene safety prior to any attempts at resuscitation
- Treatment should be guided by these important factors:
  - ☐ Level of consciousness
  - ☐ Intensity of shivering
  - ☐ Cardiovascular stability
- The most important consideration in treating hypothermia in the field is preventing further heat loss.
  - ☐ Accomplish this by removing the victim from the situation that caused him or her to become hypothermic, transporting the patient to a shelter, removing wet clothing and providing an insulating barrier around the patient.
  - ☐ Prevent conductive heat loss with the use of insulating materials including clothes, blankets, sleeping bags, sleeping pads, etc.
  - ☐ Evaporative heat loss is addressed through application of a vapor barrier; such as bubble wrap or a tarp.
- Anything that can be done to help rewarm the victim will be helpful, such as sitting by a fire, and carbohydrate-rich food or beverages. Importantly, avoid alcoholic beverages, which may actually exacerbate hypothermia by causing a peripheral vasodilatation.
- Handle the patient gently, as excessive physical stimulation may precipitate fatal arrhythmias.
- In a rescue situation, it is important to remember the premise that "no one is dead until they are warm and dead." (And consider the exceptions to this premise).
  - ☐ The caveat to the above "rule" is that an individual in the wilderness may have died from a non-hypothermia related condition such as trauma or a medical illness. In this case, rewarming would obviously be of no use and would therefore not warrant risking the safety of rescuers to evacuate the individual's body.
  - ☐ Without obvious signs or a history of such insults, measures to resuscitate and rewarm the patient should be initiated.
- As mentioned above, vital signs may be markedly abnormal in hypothermic patients and should be checked over a 60 second span to assure accuracy.
- As discussed in the previous section, people suffering from severe hypothermia may be severely comatose, though alive and salvageable with proper medical care. Hypothermia decreases basal metabolic rate and lowers oxygen requirements, which may in turn allow victims to survive for a prolonged period without a detectable perfusing rhythm.
- The following are specific recommendations for treatment of the different levels of hypothermia in the field. However, keep in mind that field treatment of hypothermia is notoriously difficult, and arrangements should begin for evacuation as soon as it is determined that the victim cannot actively rewarm himself or herself.

Mild Hypothermia

Remove the victim from the elements and shelter them to avoid further heat loss.

The individual should completely undress, then dress in dry clothes and be wrapped in blankets, taking special care to cover the head and neck to avoid heat loss from radiation.

Carbohydrate-rich beverages and foods may be helpful in both rewarming and meeting increased caloric requirement for shivering, taking care to avoid alcohol.

Limited exercise may generate some heat, however this is not advised in moderate and severe hypothermia.

☐ A shivering patient who may be hypothermic should be kept as warm as possible, and observed for at least 30 minutes before exercising.

☐ If the patient is alert and can stand without difficulty, begin with low intensity exercise and increase gradually as tolerated.

Do not use baths or water immersion to treat even mild hypothermia. This intervention may increase the likelihood of after-drop, exacerbate hypotension and cause cardiovascular collapse. However, placing the distal extremities (hands and arms up to the elbows as well as feet and legs up to the knees) in warm (42 – 45°C) water has been shown to effectively rewarm patients with mild hypothermia.

Body-to-body rewarming may improve comfort of the mildly hypothermic patient as a result of decreased shivering, but should not be done at the expense of delayed evacuation.

☐ WMS recommends body-to-body rewarming in mild hypothermia to increase patient thermal comfort if enough personnel are available and if it does not delay evacuation to definitive care (1B).

Generally speaking, those suffering from mild hypothermia will have a favorable outcome as long as the cooling process is halted.

Moderate Hypothermia

In moderate hypothermia, the individual has exhausted their capacity to achieve rewarming by shivering and more aggressive treatment must be pursued.

Active rewarming must be performed in order to get their body temperature to a near-normal level.

Attempt rewarming in the field with items such as large electric heat pads or blankets, warm water bottles, Norwegian charcoal-burning heat pack, the U.S. military Hypothermia Prevention Management Kit (HPMK), etc.

Areas of the human body with the highest potential for conductive heat loss include the axillae, chest and back. Concentrating external rewarming measures in this area yield the greatest effect. Of note, the upper torso is safer than the extremities when utilizing external rewarming measures.

If conditions prohibit the use of a fire to warm fluids, one may use chemical heaters such as those found in military "meals ready to eat" for this purpose. Warm beverages may be somewhat effective to actively rewarm victims. The rescuer must first assess level of consciousness to avoid risk of aspiration. Do NOT place those chemical heaters on the skin to warm the patient as it creates a risk of thermal burn.

Severe/Profound Hypothermia

Severe hypothermia is a true medical emergency that requires aggressive treatment and prompt medical management with evacuation for initiation of active core rewarming. These victims have no ability to reheat themselves at this stage.

It is important to consider that victims suffering from this condition may exhibit altered mental status if they are still conscious. Therefore it is vital to ignore pleas of "Leave me alone, I'm okay" because these individuals are in serious trouble.

■ The classic teaching of no patient is dead until he or she is warm and dead is a useful guideline. However, contraindications to resuscitation in the field include obvious fatal trauma and inability to perform chest compressions because of stiff chest wall.

Care must be taken in handling victims suffering from this condition as extremely cold core temperatures can cause cardiac irritability.

  ☐ Even the slightest jolt may cause these individuals to degenerate into life-threatening dysrhythmia such as ventricular fibrillation.

  ☐ This becomes extremely important in determining when CPR needs to be initiated. As discussed earlier, victims with severe hypothermia may have faint pulses, severe bradycardia, and appear to be dead. Thus, we recommend assessing vital signs over a minimum of 60 seconds.

  ☐ Initiation of CPR in a patient with pulses may precipitate an arrhythmia due to the preexisting cardiac irritability.

If available, administer warmed intravenous fluid, as this may also be helpful in the treatment of severe hypothermia. As little as 500 cc of a normal saline bolus can stabilize cardiac conduction and prevent life-threatening dysrhythmias.

  ☐ Extreme vasoconstriction may prohibit or make challenging the initiation of an intravenous line. In this situation it has been shown that saline infusion through an intraosseous line, if available, is just as effective.

Above all else, it is crucial to closely monitor individuals suffering from this condition. Remember that severe hypothermia may mimic other medical conditions and may mimic death as well. Because the victim has lost his or her ability to thermoregulate, evacuation with active core rewarming at a medical facility must be the ultimate disposition.

■ Hospital management of severe hypothermia is an evolving science, however, it is important to keep in mind that prompt recognition, evaluation and intervention in this process can lead to positive outcomes.

CPR

There are many cases of full neurologic recover of hypothermic patients even after extended periods of cardiac arrest.

Prolonged cardiac arrest in severely hypothermic patients does not necessarily cause brain injury as it does in normothermic patients.

If the patient has vital signs, even if very slow, CPR should not be performed as it may cause the victim to go into a nonperfusing rhythm.

After determining that the patient has no vital signs, CPR (including breathing) should be initiated.

If the patient is severely or profoundly hypothermic, CPR can be delayed and given intermittently during evacuation if the situation does not allow for CPR to be performed continuously due to safety factors or if it is not technically possible.

Evacuation Guidelines

All victims with moderate and severe hypothermia must be evacuated from the wilderness. They have lost the capacity to rewarm themselves and it is extremely difficult to actively rewarm these victims in the wilderness setting.

Victims with mild hypothermia may not require evacuation as long as they are able to warm themselves and they do not develop any sequelae from the episode.

Patients with severe hypothermia who are hemodynamically unstable or who have a core temperature less than 28°C should be transferred to a hospital capable of providing critical care and extra corporeal membrane oxygenation (ECMO) or cardiopulmonary bypass (CPB) if possible.

☐ Consider bypassing closer facility if critical care facility is less than one hour further.

When transporting hypothermic patients:

☐ Handle the individual very gently to prevent degeneration into a fatal rhythm

☐ Keep him or her horizontal to prevent exacerbating potential hypotension.

Prevention

The single most important aspect in hypothermia prevention is adequate preparation:
- ☐ Maintain awareness of weather conditions
- ☐ Pack sufficient gear
- ☐ Design a contingency plan in case the worst should occur

The weather does not need to be sub-zero in order for hypothermia to set in, as evidenced by the fact that several cases are reported every year in areas that traditionally have warmer climates.

It has been said that hypothermia is the "killer of the unprepared," but even experienced and prepared outdoors people have succumbed to this ailment.

Should the unexpected occur and you are faced with this situation, the following is a list of things that can be done to prevent hypothermia:
- ☐ Find or create a shelter
- ☐ Cover exposed areas of the body
- ☐ Wear several loosely fitting layers of clothing
- ☐ Conserve, share, and create warmth
- ☐ Share body heat
- ☐ Increase heat production through voluntary muscle movement
- ☐ Drink and eat warmed beverages and food
- ☐ Build a fire
- ☐ Monitor for signs and symptoms of hypothermia

FROSTBITE

Background

Frostbite occurs when skin is exposed to temperatures that are below freezing.

While the incidence of frostbite is unknown, it occurs most often in the extremities, with a slightly higher incidence in feet than in hands.

Frostbite can occur in any area of the body.

It more commonly affects exposed areas, but in severe conditions can arise on parts of the body that are covered.

Pathophysiology

The pathophysiology of frostbite can be divided into four phases (**Table 3**): pre-freeze, freeze-thaw, vascular stasis and ischemic.

- In general, it involves the cooling and eventual freezing of body parts by heat loss through the mechanisms discussed previously.
- The end result is the formation of ice crystals in the extra cellular space, intracellularly or both.
  - ☐ Extracellular ice formation leads to cell death due to cellular dehydration even if there is no formation of ice crystals inside the cell.
  - ☐ The extracellular ice crystals bind up free extracellular water, which leads to higher osmolarity outside of the cell than intracellularly. This leads to a net movement of water from intracellular to extracellular space to equilibrate the osmotic difference, leading to cell death.
- However, this is only the beginning of the problem. The ensuing inflammatory response, primarily mediated through thromboxane and prostaglandin pathways, leads to a great deal of secondary damage.

TABLE 3: Phases of Frostbite

Phase	Changes
Pre-freeze	Vasoconstriction with diminished tissue temperature Paresthesias or hyperesthesias from neuronal cooling and ischemia Cell membrane instability Endothelial plasma leakage
Freeze-thaw	Tissue temperature drops below freezing Formation of ice crystals extracellular and intracellular fluid shift across cell membrane Cellular shrinkage/dehydration
Vascular stasis	Fluctuating vasoconstriction and dilation Vascular shunting Plasma leakage Small vessel thrombosis
Ischemic	Thrombosis AV shunting Ischemia Autonomic dysfunction Gangrene

Clinical Presentation

- Frostbite is the freezing of the skin and may involve deeper tissues.
- Frostbite is classified by 2 methods: first – fourth degree and superficial / deep.
- First and second degrees are considered to be superficial and typically heal well with minor sequelae.
- Third and fourth degrees are deeper and associated with very significant permanent damage and tissue loss.
- On initial evaluation one may be unable to differentiate the exact degree of frostbite because it is based on findings after thawing. However, the treatment for all degrees of frostbite is the same, so defining an exact degree early on is unimportant.
- A simplified two-tiered classification after rewarming but prior to imaging is as follows:
  - ☐ Superficial (first and second degree and no or minimal anticipated tissue loss)
  - ☐ Deep (third and fourth degree and anticipated tissue loss)

Superficial Frostbite

First Degree

- Involves the superficial layers of skin
- The skin appears pale or yellowish-white with a raised plaque and surrounding erythema of the affected area. Edema and numbness over the same area is common.
- There is no tissue ischemia, but mild sloughing may occur.
- With rewarming, there will be pain and redness of the involved area.
- After rewarming, the area may be swollen and continue to be red for a period of hours.

Second Degree

- Involves deeper layers of the skin
- The skin appears pale or yellowish-white with a raised plaque and surrounding erythema of the affected area. Edema and numbness over the area is common.
- With rewarming, there will be pain and redness of the involved area.
- After rewarming, the area will be swollen and continue to be red for a period of hours.
- In addition to the redness, the skin will develop blisters over the area of involvement. These blisters will be filled with clear-to-white fluid.

Deep Frostbite

Third Degree

- Complete freezing of the skin and tissue layers under the skin

The skin appears pale or yellowish-white with a raised plaque and surrounding erythema of the affected area. Edema and numbness over the same area is common.

With rewarming, there will be pain, redness, and swelling of the involved area.

After rewarming, the area will be swollen and continue to be red for a period of hours to days.

In addition to the redness, the skin will develop blisters over the area of involvement. These blisters will be filled with hemorrhagic fluid.

Fourth Degree

Involves the skin and deeper tissues to include the muscle, tendon, and bone

The area of involvement appears pale and white while frozen.

Numb to the touch, it has a "chunk of wood" type of consistency

With rewarming there may be significant pain, redness, and swelling of the involved area, excepting areas of dead tissue.

After rewarming, the area will be swollen and continue to be red for a period of hours to days.

In addition to the redness, the skin will develop blisters over the area of involvement. These blisters will be filled with hemorrhagic fluid.

Mottled skin with bluish discoloration forms a deep, dry, black-crusted lesion.

Treatment

Frostbite may associated with hypothermia. If the patient suffers from mild hypothermia, institute treatment for mild hypothermia while concomitantly treating frostbite. However, if the patient suffers from moderate to severe hypothermia, treatment for frostbite should be delayed until the patient is stabilized.

Protect the affected area from further damage; i.e.: remove all wet clothing and replace with dry clothing, remove any tight or constrictive clothing and rings, etc.

Adequately hydrate the patient to prevent dehydration and further risk of ischemia.

Thawing of a frozen body part is a very painful process that usually requires opioid analgesics in addition to NSAIDs. NSAIDs work as an analgesic but more importantly, they inhibit the development of the inflammatory cascade that leads to vasoconstriction, shunting and sludging, all of which lead to worsening ischemia and necrosis.

☐ Administer ibuprofen 400 - 600 mg (6mg/kg) every 12 hours; this dose inhibits prostaglandin formation and is safer for the intestinal tract than higher doses.

An inappropriate or poorly performed thawing process will cause the victim more harm than benefit.

☐ If the frozen part is thawed too slowly the inflammatory response is accentuated, which causes the secondary damage after the freezing injury.

☐ If the temperature is too high, the victim may sustain a burn due to the anesthesia from the injury, which will also worsen the injury.

☐ Refreezing confers significantly greater morbidity than initial freezing, even for extended periods of time.

In general, if there is a chance that a body part may be subjected to a second case of frostbite soon after rewarming, then it should not be thawed initially.

☐ For example, a victim has a frostbitten foot, and he or she must walk out of the area. If there is a chance that the foot may become frostbitten again, it is better to have him or her walk on the frostbitten foot than to thaw it.

Two treatment modalities are employed to address frostbite: active (rapid) and passive rewarming.

Active (Rapid) Rewarming

The primary treatment is rapid rewarming in a controlled manner.

This should only occur when there is no chance of the person refreezing the area of involvement.

The optimal method of rewarming is to place the affected body part into gently circulated water that has been warmed to 37° to 39°C (98.6° to 102.2°F).

This should be done for at least 15 to 30 minutes or until skin regains pliability and returns to its normal color or appears red or purplish.

The temperature must be closely monitored with a thermometer. If it is too hot, it will burn the skin. If it is too cool, it will delay thawing.

Without a thermometer, as monitoring the water temperature is more difficult, a good rule of thumb is to heat the water until it approximates the temperature of a hot tub. If the water is so hot that you are not able to keep your hand in it for an extended period of time (30 seconds), then it is probably too hot.

Do not rub the area as it is rewarming although the victim may gently move that frostbitten area.

Upon sufficient rewarming, the affected area should be allowed to air dry in a warm environment.

Passive Rewarming

Most frostbite will thaw spontaneously when the above measures are accomplished.

Rapid rewarming is superior to passive rewarming. However, without the proper equipment, a reasonable time to definitive care (generally accepted limit of 2 hours) and consideration of environmental challenges, the risk of refreezing rises. If any one of these is not accounted for, passive rewarming is the safest option.

Techniques for passive rewarming include relocating to a warm environment, utilizing body heat from a rescuer as well as the general measures listed above and those described in the prevention section below.

Other Measures

Apply topical aloe vera ointment every 6 hours to superficially frostbitten areas to prevent thromboxane and prostaglandin production.

Dressings have not proven to decrease overall amount of tissue loss and should only be instituted in a practical manner so as not to interfere with extrication. Wrap the affected area with gauze or some other clean, absorbent material. If the hands or feet are involved, separate the fingers with gauze while wrapping.

Generally speaking, frozen parts should not be used for walking, climbing or other activities until definitive care is reached.

☐ However, if the extremity must be utilized for extrication, splint the extremity to minimize motion, padding all joints with extra padding.

☐ Elevate the extremity.

Administration of prophylactic antibiotics for frostbite is not supported by evidence. Administer systemic antibiotics only if there is significant trauma or signs of infection.

Ensure that the frostbite victim is up-to-date on his or her tetanus immunization. Frostbite is considered a tetanus prone wound.

"DO NOTS" OF FROSTBITE TREATMENT

Do NOT attempt thawing by heating with dry heat such as a fire, space heater or oven. The fact that the temperature is not controlled may lead to delay in thawing, but may also burn the tissues because the area is numb and pain is not appreciated.

Do NOT thaw the area if there is any chance that the area will refreeze. If a body part undergoes freezing again soon after being rewarmed the extent of the injury is a multitude more than if there was just a delay in the thawing.

Do NOT rub or massage the area when it is frozen or thawing as this will worsen the injury. The victim may move that area while undergoing thawing, but that should be the extent of the motion.

Do NOT rub the area with snow.

Do NOT debride blisters. Hemorrhagic blisters should not be debrided in the field and are best addressed at the point of definitive care by utilizing guidelines pertinent to risk of infection of rupture. Generally, do not debride clear blisters; however, some are of large enough size to prevent effective extrication (those that are tense or interfere with range of motion). In this case, they may be aspirated.

Prevention

As with hypothermia, the most important aspect of frostbite prevention is adequate preparation.

Keep in mind that maximal prevention technique will include not only protection from environmental threats, but underlying medical conditions as well. Ultimately, one must have adequate perfusion and minimal heat loss to prevent frostbite.

Techniques to maintaining adequate perfusion include:

☐ Maintaining adequate core temperature and body hydration.

☐ Minimize effects of medical problems and avoid substances known to decrease perfusion; i.e.: drugs, alcohol, nicotine, etc.

- Covering susceptible areas of skin with properly fitting dry clothing and footgear is essential during prolonged exposure to cold weather.
- Minimizing restriction in blood flow; i.e.: tight fitting clothing, prolonged rest, etc. Continuous movement, including frequent contraction and relaxation of extremities, may also be helpful in creating transient vasodilation and increased blood flow.
- Maintain a good diet and ensure adequate nutrition.

Techniques to protect from the cold include:

Avoid high-risk environments; i.e.: temperatures below -15 degrees Celsius.

- Protect the skin from wind and cold and avoid excessive perspiration and wet extremities.
- Carry extra gloves, socks, and underwear in a dry waterproof container.
- Appropriately utilize hand and foot warmers.
- In extreme situations, putting one's hand or feet in his or his partner's armpits may provide some added warmth.

FROSTNIP

Frostnip is a cold injury to the skin, without actual tissue freezing as that which occurs in frostbite.

It is the result of prolonged skin exposure to cold temperatures.

Frostnip can be a precursor to frostbite and should therefore be taken seriously.

Signs of frostnip include:

- The affected area will be red and swollen, but the skin will stay soft and pliable.
- Numbness and tingling are possible but should resolve after rewarming.
- Frostnip has only mild pain when rewarming.
- Pain and skin cracking are possible in areas that are repeatedly frost-nipped, potentially leading to infection.
- Areas that are most commonly affected include fingers, toes, ears, and cheeks.

Treatment

Rewarm the injured area using warm water or another heat source.

Take care not to rub frost-nipped areas as this may promote tissue damage.

Unlike frostbite, these injuries should always be rewarmed even if still exposed to a cold environment since the tissue has not yet been damaged and will only become damaged if the process is allowed to continue.

CHILBLAINS

Chilblains occur at temperatures from 0 to 15°C (32 to 59°F) and result from an abnormal reaction of the body to the cold.

Several different conditions have been linked to the formation of chilblains including the following:

☐ Poor circulation
☐ Rapid rewarming
☐ Damp living conditions
☐ Sudden exposure to cold water

Common places where chilblains occur include the backs and sides of fingers and toes, lower extremities, heels, nose, and ears.

Signs of chilblains include:

☐ Itchy, red or purple bumps on the skin that emerge over the course of several hours and can become very painful
☐ Blistering, ulceration, and infection are possible, but they generally resolve spontaneously over the course of one to two weeks.

Treatment

Treatment generally consists of elevation, gentle rewarming, and covering the area with a dry bandage.

Diphenhydramine (Benadryl) may be helpful to relieve the itching.

Prevention

Certain groups of people predisposed to chilblains include children, the elderly, and people with poor blood flow to the arms, hands, legs and feet.

Keep legs and feet warm with leg warmers or wool socks.

Avoid smoking, as this causes constriction of the blood vessels.

Wear warm, waterproof gloves if working in wet environments.

Exercise and acclimatize before prolonged exposure to a cold environment.

Soak hands in warm water and then dry to promote dilation of blood vessels.

IMMERSION FOOT

Immersion foot, also known as trench foot, occurs as the result of several days of exposure to water at non-freezing temperatures. Ambient temperatures generally consistent with immersion foot range from 0 to 10°C (32 to 50°F).

Signs and Symptoms

- Redness followed by bluish discoloration and mottling
- Swelling
- Numbness, tingling and pain (can be described as feeling "wooden" in severe cases)
- Shiny appearance
- Blisters, ulcers, and even gangrene are possible (although uncommon)

Treatment

- Most cases of immersion foot resolve spontaneously over the course of several weeks, provided the feet are removed from the offending conditions.
- Acutely, the affected area should be kept warm and dry.

Prevention

- Keep feet warm and dry by changing wet socks and boot/shoes as often as possible.
- Allow feet to air-dry whenever possible.
- Frequently inspect feet for signs and symptoms of this condition.

TABLE 3: Comparison of Local Non-Freezing Injuries

	Ambient Temperature	Pathophysiology	Signs and Symptoms
Frostnip	< 15°C (59°F)	Local vasoconstriction Freezing of moisture on skin	Erythema Edema Numbness Paresthesia Skin remains soft
Chilblains	0 to 15°C (32 to 59°F)	Local vasoconstriction Followed by vasodilatation Leakage blood into tissue	Red/purple bumps Itchy Painful
Immersion Foot	0 to 10°C (32 to 50°F)	Prolonged exposure to water Local vasoconstriction Neurovascular damage	Hyperemia Cyanosis Mottling Delayed cap refill Erythema Edema Numbness Paresthesia

Evacuation Guidelines

■ All victims with frostbite must be evacuated from the field for definitive rewarming and management of their frostbite. The treatment regimen has just begun with the rapid rewarming.

■ Frostnip, chilblains, and immersion foot do not require evacuation.

QUESTIONS

1. **In which degree of hypothermia is uncontrollable shivering a feature?**
   a. Mild hypothermia
   b. Moderate hypothermia
   c. Profound hypothermia
   d. Severe hypothermia

2. **Which one of the following is NOT a step that should be taken to prevent further hypothermia in the victim who is cold?**
   a. Drinking alcohol
   b. Drinking warm beverages
   c. Removing wet clothing
   d. Using body heat

3. **During which stage of frostbite do ice crystals form?**
   a. Freeze-thaw
   b. Ischemic
   c. Pre-freeze
   d. Vascular stasis

4. **Which one of the following is an important medication that you should administer to the victim who has frostbite before he or she undergoes rapid rewarming of the frostbitten body part?**
   a. Epinephrine
   b. Heparin
   c. Ibuprofen
   d. Nitroglycerin

5. **Which degree of frostbite is associated with full-thickness skin involvement in addition to muscle and tendon involvement with hemorrhagic bullae?**
   a. First degree
   b. Fourth degree
   c. Second degree
   d. Third degree

6. When should frostbite NOT be treated in the field with rewarming?

    a. If the area involves the fingers

    b. If the victim is diabetic

    c. If the victim will be promptly evacuated to an appropriate facility

    d. If there is a possibility of refreezing during the evacuation

7. How does frostnip differ from frostbite?

    a. Frostbite has hemorrhagic bullae whereas frostnip has white to clear bullae

    b. Frostnip only involves the surface of the skin and frostbite extends to the muscle

    c. Permanent damage occurs, but it is very minor with frostnip and more severe with first-degree frostbite

    d. There is no ice crystal formation in frostnip

Answers:

1. a   **5. b**

2. a   **6. d**

3. a   **7. d**

4. c

CHAPTER 8

Lightning Injuries and Prevention

This chapter will train you to recognize, treat and avoid injuries caused by a lightning strike.

Objectives:

- Recognize when and where lightning is more likely to strike in relation to a storm
- Describe the six mechanisms by which one may be injured by lightning
- Be able to describe the etiology of cardio-respiratory arrest due to a lightning strike and the appropriate management of it
- Describe common injuries that are caused by lightning for the following organ systems: cardiovascular, CNS, eyes, ears, autonomic nervous system, and skin
- Understand the concept of reverse triage in the management of multiple casualties from a lightning strike
- Understand that all victims of a lightning strike require evacuation
- List methods to minimize the potential of being struck by lightning

CASE 1

A 23-year-old male is leaning against a vehicle with a large whip antenna when the antenna is struck by lightning. He is thrown back from the vehicle and slightly confused as to what actually happened. On your evaluation, he is awake and alert. He remembers a large flash of light, but the next thing he is aware of is being on the ground 10 feet away from the vehicle. He is otherwise healthy and takes no medications and has no allergies. His vital signs are normal. His physical examination is normal with the exception of an unusual rash on his left chest (pictured below).

1. What is the next step in the management of this patient?
2. Are you at risk of electrical injury from a residual electrical charge if you touch him?
3. Does he require evacuation to a hospital or can he stay out in the wilderness?
4. What are some of the organ systems that may be injured that you must specifically look for?

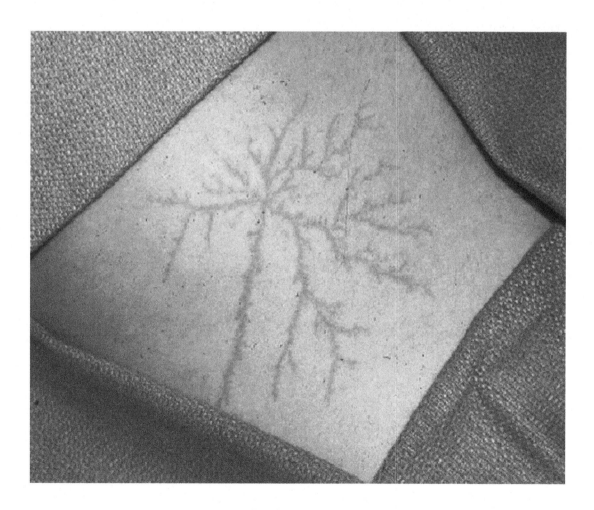

Rash on the left side of the chest of Case 1

CASE 2

You are watching a football team practice when you see lightning and hear thunder approximately five seconds later. The coach sees the lightning as well and calls the team to the center of the practice field to end the practice because of the lightning. As soon as the team breaks to go to the locker room, there is a big flash and boom in the middle of the team formation. You run out onto the field to see several players who are dazed and wandering around as well as eight people on the ground. Three of those individuals are moaning, and three are unconscious but appear to be breathing on their own. One has a large burn wound to his helmet and is pulseless and apneic. The last person is unconscious, apneic, and pulseless with fixed and dilated pupils but does not appear to have any other injuries.

1. What is your next step in the management of this multiple casualty situation?
2. Who is the first person you should attend to?
3. What is the prognosis for the individual with the head burn wound?
4. Is there a risk of lightning striking the same area again?

BACKGROUND

Facts

- Lightning strikes are a common environmental cause of death; with an annual average of 40 in the United States and 24,000 worldwide.
- There are approximately 10 times as many more people struck by lightning who survive.
- The most common time of the day for lightning casualties is in the afternoon.
- The most dangerous times for a severe lightning strike are right before the storm appears overhead and right after it has passed.
- Lightning may travel nearly horizontally as far as 10 miles in front of a thunderstorm and seems to occur out of a "clear blue sky," or at least when it is still sunny.
- Lightning can strike from a storm to the other side of a ridgeline with blue-sky overhead.
- Lightning does strike twice in the same place very commonly.
- A lightning bolt is a massive current pulse up to 30,000 - 110,000 Amps but only for 10 to 100 ms.
- A lightning bolt is typically 2 - 3 cm in diameter, but the ionized sheath is much broader (up to 20 m). The temperature of the sheath is usually about 8,000°C although it has been measured up to 50,000°C.
- For an interesting story of lightning strike and the rescue search "sports illustrated countdown to tragedy" or go to: http://www.si.com/vault/2011/07/18/106089002/countdown-to-tragedy

MECHANISM OF INJURY

Direct Strike

- The patient is hit directly by the bolt of lightning.
- This most commonly occurs to people who are caught in the open.
- The current may flow externally over the body or enter through the orifices and flow through the body internally.
- This is the deadliest type of strike.

Side Splash

- The lightning directly strikes another object such as a tree or building, but the current flow jumps from its original pathway onto the victim.
- This is the most common cause of lightning injury.

These side splashes may also splash indoors from metal objects such as plumbing and telephones.

■ Splashes may occur from person to person when several people are standing close together.

Contact Exposure

Contact exposure occurs when a person is holding on to or touching an object that is either directly hit or splashed by lightning.

The current passes through the object on to the victim.

Ground Current

Ground current is produced when lightning strikes the ground or a nearby object and the current spreads through the ground.

If a person has one foot closer to the strike, then a potential difference may exist between the two feet, and the current will pass up one leg and down the other leg.

This occurs because the body is of lower resistance than the ground.

This is a common mechanism for several people being injured at the same time.

Injury by a Weak Upward Streamer

An electrical streamer heads upward into the sky but does not reach sky lightning and thus does not complete a connection.

The electrical charge passes over and through the involved individual, but it is not nearly as powerful as that of a direct strike that comes from the sky.

Blunt Trauma

Injury occurs due to the impact of the concussive force of the strike itself or from being thrown due to the extreme nature of the muscular contraction from the electrical charge.

It can also be caused by the barotrauma of the strike as the lightning superheats the air surrounding the streamer.

PATHOPHYSIOLOGY

General

Lightning is neither a DC nor an AC current. It is best described as a unidirectional massive current impulse of electrons.

In addition to flowing on the outside of the body (flashover), this current may also enter the body through the cranial orifices (eyes, ears, nose, and mouth) and flow through the body. This may explain why some patients have certain injuries such as ocular and/or ear, and others do not.

Although the current flow occurs over a very short period of time, the amount of current is significant.

Injuries occur from a "short circuiting" of several of the body's electrical systems as well as the more direct trauma and indirect trauma due to muscular contraction and being thrown.

Lightning does not leave a residual charge on a victim of a strike, so there is no need to be concerned about getting shocked or injured by rescuing a person who has been struck by lightning.

Lightning Injury Evaluation by the Organ System

Cardiovascular

The most common cause of death in a lightning strike victim is cardiopulmonary arrest.

After the lightning strike, the heart becomes asystolic. However, due to automaticity, the heart soon begins to contract in an organized manner.

If concomitant respiratory arrest occurs due to a paralysis of the medullary respiratory center, the heart may deteriorate back into asystole secondary to the hypoxia. This respiratory arrest usually lasts longer than the cardiac arrest and is the major reason it is important to provide rescue breathing in lightning strike victims with cardiac arrest.

Other complications include:

- ☐ Direct myocardial damage or necrosis
- ☐ Coronary artery spasm
- ☐ Acute global cardiac dysfunction
- ☐ Atrial and/or ventricular dysrhythmias
- ☐ Pericardial effusion
- ☐ The ECG may show ST segment changes consistent with ischemia or infarction as well as prolongation of the QT intervals

Central Nervous System

When current traverses the brain, there can be coagulation necrosis of the brain, formation of epidural and subdural hematomas, intraventricular hemorrhage and paralysis of the respiratory center.

Those patients who suffer cranial burns are four times more likely to die than those without cranial burns. This is an important consideration in the management of the mass casualty situation.

Direct cellular damage to the respiratory and cardiac centers in the fourth ventricle of the brain may occur, especially if current passes through the orifices of the head.

Seizures may occur secondary to the initial hypoxia from respiratory arrest or due to intracranial damage. These are usually transient, although they may continue for the first few days.

Confusion and anterograde amnesia are very common.

Traumatic brain or spinal injury may occur due to being thrown.

Neuropsychological sequelae are very common.

- Memory impairment
- Difficulty concentrating
- Sleep disturbances
- Personality change with increased lability and aggression

Autonomic Nervous System

Commonly there is instability of the ANS (autonomic nervous system) for several hours after the injury.

More severely injured patients may have lower extremity paralysis (keraunoparalysis) or in some cases upper extremity paralysis.

- In these cases, the involved extremities appear cold, clammy, mottled, insensate and pulseless.
- This is usually the result of autonomic instability and intense vascular spasm, which has been likened to Raynaud's phenomenon in appearance.
- Keraunoparalysis usually occurs due to ground current.
- These findings usually resolve spontaneously after a few hours.

Peripheral Nervous System

Common symptoms include paralysis, pain, and paresthesias.

Symptoms may be delayed by weeks to years.

If present, the prognosis is poor for recovery.

Respiratory System

Acute respiratory arrest due to the loss of respiratory drive.

Pulmonary contusion and hemorrhage can occur.

Skin

Deep burns are unusual after lightning injury. At the most, some deep partial thickness burns may occur.

Often, there are no burns, especially with ground current.

There are four types of skin effects:

- ☐ Ferning (Case 1) – also called feathering or Lichtenberg figures
  - These are not actual burns, but an unusual pattern that occurs due to the electron shower. This skin finding is pathognomonic for lightning injury.
- ☐ Linear burns
  - These are usually superficial and superficial partial thickness burns that occur from steam production from sweat or water on the victim due to the increased temperatures associated with the lightning strike.
- ☐ Punctate burns
  - These are multiple, closely spaced but discrete circular burns that individually range from a few millimeters to a centimeter in thickness. These resemble cigarette burns.
- ☐ Thermal burns
  - These are regular thermal burns that occur when a patient is wearing a metal object, such as a belt buckle or necklace, which heats up due to the electrical current traveling through it.
  - There may also be thermal burns if clothing ignites.

Musculoskeletal System
- ■ Fractures and dislocations may occur due to intense muscular contraction or from being thrown.
- ☐ The significant muscular necrosis and extremity damage seen in electrical injuries is unusual in lightning injuries.

Ocular
- ☐ One-half of all lightning victims will have ocular injuries.
- ☐ Cataracts are the most common ocular injury. These may develop immediately or as late as two years after being struck.
- ☐ Transient bilateral blindness of unknown etiology is not uncommon.
- ☐ Other injuries include corneal lesions, hyphema, retinal detachment, optic nerve atrophy, and vitreous hemorrhage.
- ☐ Dilated and unreactive pupils cannot be used as a sign of death, as this may occur after lightning injury.

Ear
- ☐ Temporary deafness can occur due to the intense noise and shock wave.
- ☐ 30 to 50 percent of victims will sustain rupture to one or both tympanic membranes.
- ☐ Disruption of the ossicles and/or mastoid bone can occur.
- ☐ Facial palsies due to direct nerve damage of the facial nerve as it runs through the auditory canal.

Pregnancy
- ☐ There are only 13 cases reported of lightning strikes to pregnant women.
- ☐ Maternal outcome is generally good. However, there is a reported 50 percent rate of fetal death.

CLINICAL PRESENTATION

Single Victim

The identification of a victim of a lightning strike is easy if the strike was witnessed.

However there may be situations where you will come across a person who is confused, amnestic, disheveled or possibly unconscious. In those situations it will take some time and focus to determine the cause of the individual's symptoms. In the case of the unwitnessed victim, clues that can assist you include the environmental clues such as a recent storm or lightning. Clues that pertain to the victim include confusion and amnesia as well as prominent physical findings such as fixed dilated pupils, ruptured tympanic membranes and the pathognomonic skin finding (ferning).

The patient who is identified as a victim of a lightning strike may present along the spectrum from being unconscious, apneic and pulseless to being awake and alert without any complaint.

The degree to which the patient demonstrates signs and symptoms of lightning strike depends upon the type of strike they received (a direct strike causes the most severe symptoms).

The typical victim is an individual who was witnessed to be struck by lightning and is amnestic to the event and has some of the previously described sequelae of lightning strike.

Multiple Victims

The typical description of a multiple casualty lightning strike is one of a sudden flash of bright light followed closely by a loud boom and then chaos.

There will likely be several people who are ambulatory but confused.

There will be people who are lying on the ground but are at least moving or breathing on their own.

These first two groups of people do not require immediate attention.

The final group of casualties that does require your immediate attention is those who are unconscious, apneic, and pulseless.

The fact that you are treating those who appear dead is called **reverse-triage**. The reason for this reverse triage is due to the fact that those victims who are awake or at least breathing have survived the most immediate and potentially critical injury, which is concomitant cardiac and respiratory arrest. Those patients who are apneic and pulseless require CPR in order to get them to the point where their cardiac pacemakers restart and their intrinsic respiratory drive has started again. These are the patients who may sustain cardio-respiratory arrest and regain their heartbeat but still require assistance with breathing for several minutes before their respiratory drive starts. In attempting to decide on which patients you should start CPR, remember that those with head burns are four times more likely to die from the strike.

TREATMENT

- Perform reverse triage and initiate CPR on those patients who are pulseless and apneic before caring for those who have spontaneous signs of life. Those with no spontaneous breathing or heartbeat may recover their heartbeat and will require assisted breathing until their respiratory drive returns. Breathing for these patients may prevent a secondary cardiac arrest due to hypoxia. If a victim does not regain a pulse within 20 to 30 minutes, then one may discontinue the resuscitation.
- Initial steps follow MARCH: massive hemorrhage, airway, respiration, circulation, and hypothermia/hyperthermia and hike versus hospital.
- Call for evacuation to the closest medical facility.
- Stabilization such as splinting of fractures and spinal precautions should be performed as determined on your secondary assessment.

EVACUATION GUIDELINES

- Any patient who is a victim of a lightning strike should be evacuated as soon as possible.
- Even if the individual does not have any overt evidence of damage, there is a high likelihood of some sort of injury that is not served best by staying in the wilderness.

AVOIDING LIGHTNING INJURY

When you hear thunder

- "When thunder roars go indoors". If you hear thunder, then you should seek shelter. This is based on the fact that the distances that sound travels are well within the distance of a lightning strike. Furthermore, you may miss lightning because the clouds or other terrain hides it. There is no safe place outdoors.

Seek shelter in a substantial building or in an-all metal vehicle

- Small shelters such as golf, bus, and rain shelters may increase a person's risk of being struck due to side splash as the lightning flows over the building.
- All metal vehicles are safe because the metal will diffuse the current around the occupants to the ground.
- A convertible is not a safe alternative.
- It is a myth that the rubber tires provide insulation.

If you are caught in a storm outside without a safe building or vehicle

- Stay away from metal objects and those items that are taller than you.
- Avoid areas near power lines, pipelines, ski lifts, and other large steel objects.
- Do not stand near or under tall isolated trees, hilltops, or at a lookout or other exposed area.
- In a forest, seek a low area under a growth of saplings or small trees. Seeking a clearing free of trees makes a person the tallest object in the clearing.
- If you are completely in the open, stay far away from single trees to avoid lightning splashes and ground current. A good position is to squat down with your knees fully bent and your feet together or to sit cross-legged or kneeling on the ground. Keeping the feet together prevents you from being injured by ground current.
- If you are in a group of people, then spread far apart so that a single lightning strike will not take out the entire group.
- If you are on the water, seek the shore and avoid being the tallest object near a large body of water.

If indoors

- Avoid open doors and windows, fireplaces and metal objects such as sinks and plugged-in electrical appliances.
- Do not talk on the telephone as telephone lines may not be grounded like electrical wires.

When in a group

- The group members should be separated by more than 20 feet to limit the potential for mass casualties due to a strike and the ground current. This allows the individuals to watch others and to rescue them if struck.

QUESTIONS

1. **What is the most dangerous time to be struck by lightning in relation to the storm?**
   a. At the first time you hear thunder
   b. In the middle of the storm when the rain is the hardest
   c. The period of time right before the storm actually hits
   d. You are at the same risk regardless of the storm

2. **In which one of the following situations is somebody least likely to get injured by lightning?**
   a. Crouching near the top of a ridge line
   b. Sitting inside a rain shelter on a golf course that is open on the front
   c. Sitting under a large tree that provides protections from the rain
   d. Sitting in an all-metal automobile with the windows rolled up.

3. **A 30 year-old male is struck by lightning and is pulseless and apneic. Which one of the following is correct in regards to the management of this patient?**
   a. CPR is not necessary as his heart will start beating on its own
   b. CPR is not helpful as his heart likely sustained irreversible damage
   c. CPR should be initiated and continued until he begins breathing on his own, then you may stop
   d. CPR should not be initiated as the patient may have a residual charge from the lightning

4. **Which one of the following is NOT an injury commonly seen with lightning strike?**
   a. Amnesia
   b. Cataracts
   c. Ruptured tympanic membrane
   d. Third-degree skin burns

5. **You observe lightning strike a large group of people with the following casualties:**
   a. Awake, alert and sitting up with obvious dislocated shoulder
   b. Awake, moaning and confused
   c. Unconscious, apneic, pulseless, no evidence of injury
   d. Unconscious, apneic, pulseless, obvious burn to the head and face
   e. Unconscious, breathing on own, palpable pulse

6. **What is the correct order that you should triage and care for these patients?**
    a. A, B, E, D, C
    b. B, E, D, C, A
    c. C, D, E, B, A
    d. D, C, E, B, A

7. **Which one of the following is a method to minimize being struck by lightning if you are caught in an open area?**
    a. If caught in the open squat down with your feet together
    b. Seek shelter under the largest tree in the open, ensuring you are leaning against it
    c. Laying supine if you are caught in the open
    d. Sitting under large electrical towers as they are grounded and protected from lightning

Answers:
1.c 2.d 3.c 4.d 5.c 6. a

CHAPTER 9

Drowning and Water Safety

This chapter will train you to treat conditions caused by accidental drowning and methods to prevent this type of injury, according to the following criteria.

Objectives:

- Be able to define the basic terms of drowning, the drowning process, and survival
- Be able to describe the mechanism of shallow water blackout
- Be able to describe the basic pathophysiology of the drowning process
- Be able to describe the effects of drowning on the pulmonary system
- To demonstrate the initial management of a victim of a drowning in the wilderness setting
- Be able to describe which patients require evacuation to a medical setting
- Be able to describe methods to prevent drowning

CASE 1

An eighteen-year-old male falls out of a raft in a class IV rapid and is repeatedly pulled under the water as he fights his way through the rapids. He is pulled out of the water on the shore and is awake and alert. He is coughing vigorously and complains of shortness of breath and a full sensation in his chest. His past medical history is unremarkable. Vital signs: P = 108, RR = 26.

Physical examination is remarkable for obvious respiratory distress with retractions and rales throughout his lungs. The remainder of his examination is normal.

1. What is the next step in the management of this patient?
2. Are there any other vital signs you would be interested in obtaining for this patient, if possible?
3. Are there any medications you could treat him with that you would normally carry with you?
4. Does he require evacuation to a hospital or can he stay in the backcountry with observation?

CASE 2

You are camping by a lake and hear a cry for help. A father is holding his two-year-old son who is crying. According to the father, he was in the shallow water of the lake with his child and he turned his head away for "just a couple of seconds." When he turned back, he noticed his son was under the water and not moving. He immediately grabbed his son who started crying. There was no color change. The child is alert and crying. Vital signs: P=108, RR=20. Physical exam is normal to include normal respiratory efforts and a normal pulmonary exam.

1. What is your next step in the management of this child?
2. Are there any other vital signs you would be interested in obtaining?
3. Does this child require evacuation to a hospital or can he stay at the campsite with observation?
4. If you elect to observe this child, what is the time interval you should observe him?

BACKGROUND

Terminology

Drowning: A process resulting in primary respiratory impairment from submersion / immersion in a liquid medium. The victim may live or die during or after this process. The outcomes are classified as death, morbidity, and no morbidity.

The Drowning Process: A continuum that begins when the victim's airway lies below the surface of liquid, usually water, preventing the victim from breathing air. A victim may be rescued during the drowning process and may not require intervention or may receive appropriate resuscitative measure. In this case, the drowning process is interrupted. However, if the victim is not ventilated soon enough or does not start to breathe on his own, circulatory arrest will ensue, and in the absence of effective resuscitative efforts, multiple organ dysfunction and death will result.

Drowned: refers to a person who dies from drowning

Near drowning: It is the consensus of the International Liaison Committee on Resuscitation (ILCOR) that the term near drowning no longer be used. The term refers to survival for at least 24 hours after a successful rescue from a submersion episode. This usage has led to uncertainty about the meaning of the term, because it has implied certain recovery in many instances, which is not always the case. Furthermore, when the term is translated from English into other languages, the meaning is confusing and imprecise.

Survival: Indicates that the victim remained alive after the acute event and any acute or subacute sequelae.

Immersion: To be covered in water. For drowning to occur, at least the face and airway are immersed.

Submersion: During submersion, the entire body, including the airway, is under water.

Dry vs. Wet Drowning:

The ILCOR recommends that these terms be abandoned.

The terms wet and dry have been used to classify as those who aspirate liquid into their lungs (wet) and those who do not (dry). Frequently it is not possible to determine at the scene whether or not water was aspirated, particularly when the amount of water is small.

Freshwater vs. Saltwater Drowning

At one time, based on animal studies, it was believed that different pathologic pathways existed between drowning in fresh water and salt water.

Freshwater drowning: It was theorized that with freshwater drowning, the aspirated water would be hypotonic and would rapidly pass through the lungs and go into the intravascular compartment. This would create fluid overload and a dilutional effect on serum electrolytes.

Saltwater aspiration: It was theorized that the hypertonic saltwater would cause fluid to be drawn into the alveoli, thus creating massive pulmonary edema and hypertonic serum.

In reality, patients who survive a drowning incident do not aspirate enough volume to cause hemodilution or electrolyte changes. Based on the animal studies, it required an aspiration of at least 22 ml/kg, whereas the typical human submersion victim aspirates less than 10 ml/kg.

The one exception is the Dead Sea, which is extremely hypertonic. In surviving victims, significant effects on serum calcium and magnesium have been observed.

Shallow Water Blackout

A special cause of drowning that occurs in people who hyperventilate before entering the water for an underwater swim.

Hyperventilation significantly reduces the $PaCO_2$ without increasing oxygen storage.

The vigorous underwater activity uses the available oxygen, causing hypoxemia, but before sufficient CO_2 accumulates to provide a stimulus to return to the surface. The patient loses consciousness due to the hypoxemia and drowns.

Epidemiology

In many areas of the world, drowning is a leading cause of death, especially among young children.

According to the World Health Organization, more than 500,000 deaths each year are due to drowning. Since all cases of fatal drowning are not classified as such even for high-income countries, this number probably underestimates the real figures.

Drowning is second only to motor vehicle accidents as the most common cause of accidental death in the United States

Annually in the U.S., there are an estimated 3,880 fatal drownings.

Drowning mainly kills the young.

- 64 percent of all victims are under age 30
- 26 percent of all victims are under age 5
- There is a bimodal age distribution in the young with large numbers of deaths in children age 4 and younger with the second larger increase in adolescents ages 15 to 24.

Freshwater drowning, especially in pools, is more common than saltwater drowning. This includes coastal areas.

Risk factors:

- ☐ Age
  - Children ages 1 - 4 have the highest drowning rate.
  - Among children ages 1 - 14, drowning is the second leading cause of unintentional injury death behind motor vehicle accidents in the United States.
  - The risk of drowning for males increases at age 15 and remains elevated through age 24 years.
- ☐ Location - Victims of different ages drown in different locations.
  - For children ages 4 and under, home swimming pools, bathtubs, buckets pose the greatest risk.
  - Over half of the fatal and non-fatal drownings in adolescents occur in natural water settings, such as lakes, rivers, and oceans.
- ☐ Gender – Nearly 80% of people who die from drowning are male
- ☐ Drugs - Alcohol, in particular, is involved in half of adolescent and adult deaths associated with water recreation
- ☐ Trauma (secondary to dives, falls, and horseplay)
- ☐ Failure to wear a personal floatation device (PFD) - Most boating deaths are caused by drowning with 88% of the victims not wearing PFDs

PATHOPHYSIOLOGY

General

- ■ The basic pathophysiology of submersion injury is respiratory failure with hypoxemia and resultant cardiac ischemia and neurologic injury.
- ■ Older victims who are not immediately unconscious may initially panic and struggle in the water.
  - ☐ They will hold their breath or hyperventilate and try to stay above the water surface.
  - ☐ Breath holding will occur.
  - ☐ Eventually, a breaking point is reached and the body involuntarily (reflexively) breathes, even if the victim is under water. This point is determined by the both $PaCO_2$ and PaO_2.
  - ☐ At the point of involuntary breathing, aspiration and vomiting occur with an impact on at least the pulmonary system.

Organ System Effects

Pulmonary
- ■ The lung is the primary organ of injury.
- ■ Aspirated water evokes vagally mediated pulmonary vasoconstriction and pulmonary hypertension.

Aspirated water also has a significant effect on lung compliance and recoil due to the washing out and destruction of surfactant. This leads to atelectasis and stiff, noncompliant lungs.

All of these effects lead to significant ventilation-perfusion mismatching as well as a diminished oxygen-diffusing capacity. This may result in relative or significant hypoxemia, depending on the extent of the pulmonary injury.

Clinical signs and symptoms:

- ☐ Shortness of breath
- ☐ Air hunger
- ☐ Cough
- ☐ Rales, rhonchi, and wheezing

Cardiovascular

Cardiac dysrhythmias are common and significant in drowning incidents. However, these are usually secondary to the hypoxemia or acidosis and not primary in etiology.

It is unlikely that the dysrhythmias are caused by electrolyte disturbances.

Central Nervous System

12 to 27 percent of drowning victims sustain neurologic damage.

The best predictor of long-term neurological outcome is a normal or rapidly improving mental status during the first 24 hours after the drowning incident.

Insults to the CNS usually result from the hypoxia and/or trauma to the brain or spinal cord.

If the patient has an altered mental status, appropriate evaluation must look for CNS trauma as a source and one should not just ascribe the symptoms to the hypoxia.

Be concerned for cervical spine injuries when victims have been diving into pools or waters of unknown depth.

Electrolytes and Blood Volume

These are usually generally unaffected by the aspiration.

The one exception is Dead Sea submersion victims, who may develop hypermagnesemia and hypercalcemia.

Cold Water Drowning

Water has a thermal conductivity of 25 - 30 times that of air.

Cold-water submersion results in rapidly induced hypothermia. The body's initial physiologic response to this insult is catecholamine release, tachycardia and hyperventilation. This alone may trigger an arrhythmia and lead to sudden death.

Hypothermia leads to muscle fatigue and poor judgment, decreasing the ability to self-rescue.

Theories of how neuroprotective hypothermia may occur prior to irreversible hypoxia include:

☐ The diving reflex, which includes bradycardia, apnea, and peripheral vasoconstriction after the initial tachycardia and hyperventilation

☐ A combination of external skin exposure, icy water aspiration, and ingestion enabling a rapid core temperature drop.

☐ Through these mechanisms, it is postulated that hypothermia decreases cellular metabolism and may limit reperfusion injuries after resuscitation, especially in children.

However, most hypothermic drowning victims are cold from prolonged exposure and are simply dead.

TREATMENT

Rapid but cautious rescue so that the rescuers do not become victims.

The gold standard is immediate and aggressive initiation of ventilation and oxygenation.

Always consider coexistent trauma and institute spinal protections if there is any concern.

If possible, measure blood oxygenation with a pulse oximeter.

Administer oxygen if available.

CPR should be started on any patient with even a remote possibility of success.

☐ Prompt initiation of rescue breathing or positive pressure ventilation increases survival.

☐ Drowning victims with only respiratory arrest usually respond after a few rescue breaths.

☐ Interestingly, the Europeans Resuscitation Council recommends **five** initial rescue breaths instead of two (as recommended by the American Heart Association) because the initial ventilations can be more difficult to achieve in drowning victims.

☐ If there is no response to the initial rescue breaths, the victims should be assumed to be in cardiac arrest and be taken as quickly as possible to dry land where effective CPR can be initiated.

☐ Victims of cold-water submersion should ideally be warmed to approximately 90°F before the resuscitation is terminated.

☐ Victims of warm water submersion or those who are normothermic and have CPR ongoing for 20 to 30 minutes without success may have CPR terminated.

There are no special drainage procedures to "empty" water out of the lungs or stomach.

If the person in unconscious but breathing, the recovery position (lateral decubitus) should be used.

Bronchospasm may be treated with beta agonists, such as albuterol.

There is no currently no role for prophylactic antibiotics or prophylactic steroids.

The Asymptomatic Patient

- In the wilderness, there will be drowning "events" when there is a question of whether an individual actually aspirated any water or had any significant hypoxia before being rescued.
  - ☐ These patients may have some initial coughing as soon as being brought out of the water but will have no cough or respiratory complaints after the initial few minutes.
  - ☐ They will have a normal respiratory rate and a normal pulmonary exam if you listen with a stethoscope or by placing your ear on their chest.
- These patients can be observed without evacuation for a period of six hours.
- After six hours, if the patient still has no respiratory complaints, no cough, and continues to have a normal pulmonary exam then they can continue on with the trip.
- If they develop any respiratory complaints, develop an abnormal exam or vital signs then they should be evacuated.

PROGNOSIS

- Statistics on survival and the incidence of severe neurological deficits after a drowning event are difficult to interpret.
- Unfavorable prognostic factors:
  - ☐ Age 3 and younger
  - ☐ Estimated submersion/ immersion time longer than five minutes
  - ☐ No resuscitation attempts for at least 10 minutes after rescue
  - ☐ Patient in a coma on ED admission
  - ☐ Arterial blood gas pH 7.1 or less
- With two or less of these factors present, there is a 90 percent chance of recovery.
- The presence of three or more of these factors reduces the chance of survival to less than 5%.

EVACUATION GUIDELINES

- Evacuate the following patients
  - ☐ Those who suffered a loss of consciousness
  - ☐ Any patient who required resuscitation, even if it was just rescue breathing
  - ☐ Those who have any difficulty breathing, persistent cough or complaints of air hunger
  - ☐ Those patients with tachypnea or an abnormal lung examination
  - ☐ Those patients with hypoxemia, if you have a pulse oximeter available

Those patients who are asymptomatic with no respiratory distress may be observed for a period of at least six hours for development of new respiratory symptoms. If they are asymptomatic for this entire period, then they do not require evacuation.

PREVENTION

Prevention is more important than any action one can take after a submersion incident has occurred.

Alcohol should be avoided when participating in or supervising water activities.

Everyone on a boat should always wear approved personal flotation devices that will support the person's head above water, even if the person becomes unconscious.

Camp far enough away from water so that people, especially children, do not accidentally wander into the water.

Anyone who works on or near the water should have swimming, rescue, and life-saving skills.

Young children should always be supervised when around water.

- ☐ A one-minute phone call or other distraction is all it takes for a child to become submerged.
- ☐ Toddlers have drowned in toilets and small buckets of water.
- ☐ Toddlers have drowned in bathtubs when left alone with older siblings to watch them without adult supervision.

Patients with seizure disorders should always be supervised if swimming and should probably bathe in showers.

Swimming pools:

- ☐ These should be completely enclosed by a 5-foot fence with self-closing and self-latching locks.
- ☐ This fence should also separate the pool from the house. This means that the pool should not be directly open to the back door of the house.
- ☐ Appropriate life-saving equipment such as a pole to pull people to the side and personal flotation devices should be near the pool.
- ☐ Owners of swimming pools should be trained in CPR.
- ☐ Children whose families have a pool should take swimming lessons early.

QUESTIONS

1. **Which one of the following is the mechanism behind shallow water blackout?**
   a. Hyperventilation results in an increased blood oxygen level, causing one to lose the drive to surface to breathe
   b. Hyperventilation results in an increased blood carbon dioxide level, causing one to lose the drive to surface to breathe
   c. The lowered carbon dioxide level from hyperventilation causes one to seize and lose consciousness under the water
   d. The oxygen level in the blood drops too low before one has the drive to surface to breathe
   e. Vigorous activity causes the carbon dioxide level to drop while under the water

2. **Which one of the following describes the basic pathophysiology of drowning?**
   a. Cerebral edema due to excessive fluid intake and resultant respiratory arrest
   b. Electrolyte dilution resulting in cardiac dysrhythmia and respiratory arrest
   c. Pulmonary injury resulting in hypoxia and possibly cardiac and neurologic injury
   d. Increased compliance and elasticity of the lungs leading to hypoxia
   e. Respiratory difficulty due to pneumonia caused by bacteria in the aspirated water

3. **A 30-year-old male dives headfirst off a cliff into a lake. He surfaces within 5 seconds but is floating and appears to be unconscious. Which one of the following is the most likely etiology for his symptoms?**
   a. He aspirated a large amount of water when he went into the water and became hypoxic
   b. He hyperventilated before jumping in the water and suffered and arrest due to an increased blood carbon dioxide level
   c. He suffered a cardiac arrest due to the suddenness coldness of the water
   d. He suffered a cardiac arrest due to aspiration of hypotonic water and electrolyte dilution
   e. He suffered a cervical injury with resultant paralysis by striking the bottom of the lake

4. **Which one of the following is not part of the management of the drowning victim in the field setting?**
   a. Heimlich maneuver to increase gastric emptying
   b. Immediate CPR if the patient is not breathing
   c. Scene assessment to ensure the area is safe to rescue the victim
   d. Stabilization of the cervical spine if there is concern of injury
   e. Thorough assessment of the respiratory system if the patient is awake

5. Which one of the following is <u>not</u> a method to help prevent drowning?

    a. All rafters should wear personal flotation devices

    b. Alcohol should be consumed in moderation when around the water

    c. Camp sites should be established far away from water, especially when children are present

    d. Swimming pools should be surrounded by a 5-foot fence

    e. Those working around or on water should have CPR and water rescue skills

Answers:

1. d

2. c

3. e

4. a

5. b

CHAPTER 10

Medical Problems in the Wilderness

This chapter will train you to recognize and treat common and life-threatening medical conditions in the wilderness. It will help you to differentiate serious problems that require evacuation from more minor problems that can be treated in the wilderness.

Remember to consider asking patients themselves as well as other participants for available medications if you are not carrying them yourself.

Objectives:

- How to evaluate and treat chest pain including: angina, myocardial infarction, and CHF
- How to evaluate and treat shortness of breath and pulmonary complaints, including: asthma, COPD, pneumonia, and pulmonary embolism
- How to evaluate and treat strokes and seizures
- Be able to recognize and treat hypoglycemia

- Be able to describe the issues associated with diabetes in the wilderness and ways to help manage diabetics who venture into the wilderness
- Be able to recognize, evaluate and treat allergic reactions, from those that are very minor to anaphylaxis
- Be able to list the common and serious causes of abdominal pain and the methods to recognize and manage these problems

CASE 1

A 56-year-old man is on day four of a seven-day rafting trip. While paddling a raft through a calm stretch of water, he begins to experience chest pain with radiation to his left shoulder. He has mild shortness of breath. The symptoms are relieved by rest. He has never had any symptoms like this before. He does not have a cardiac history, does not smoke, and takes no medications. The pain is sufficiently significant that he has to pull over to shore.

1. What is the first step in the management of this person?
2. What are the most concerning diagnoses that you should consider?
3. Does he require evacuation or can he remain on the trip?
4. What are appropriate medicines to give to this person if he remains pain free?
5. If he develops recurrent or constant pain, what medications should you consider giving him?

CASE 2

A 22-year-old female begins to have difficulty breathing while hiking on a trip in Nepal. She is a known asthmatic. She is familiar with her problem and begins to use an albuterol inhaler. This provides some, but not complete, relief. You are four walking days from the nearest city.

1. What is the first step in the management of this person?
2. Does she require evacuation?
3. What are the different causes of asthma?
4. What other medications could you give her?

CASE 3

While in camp, a 44-year-old female has seizure-like activity on day three of a six-day rafting trip on the Colorado River within the Grand Canyon. She has had seizures in the past, but it has been three years since she has suffered a seizure. She takes phenytoin (Dilantin), an anti-seizure medication. She has been in the backcountry before, but this is the first time she has suffered a seizure in this setting. Evacuation is difficult. She is fine one hour after the event. She did not fall or injure herself.

1. What is the first step in the management of this person?
2. Does she require evacuation?
3. How could you adjust her medication regimen to help keep her safe until you can have her evacuated?

CASE 4

While hiking in the backcountry in West Virginia with a group of scouts, you are called to examine a 14-year-old boy who is becoming unresponsive. He is a known diabetic, as indicated by an alert tag hanging on his neck. It is a cool day and there is no evidence that he has fallen. His lungs are clear to auscultation. It is presumed that his blood sugar is low.

1. What is the first step in the management of this boy?
2. How could you check his blood sugar?
3. What are the reasons that his blood sugar would be so low and how might this have been avoided?
4. Does he require evacuation?
5. Are there other medications that could be given to this victim?

CASE 5

You are mountain biking on a trail in the wilderness when you come upon a 17-year-old girl who is on the ground with a number of people gathered around her. She is sitting upright having significant difficulty breathing. You note red, flushed skin and audible wheezing. By bicycle ride, you are approximately one hour from your car and then another 55 minutes, by automobile, from help.

1. What is the most likely diagnosis?
2. What is the next step in the management of this girl?
3. What medications could you give to this victim?
4. Does she require evacuation?

CASE 6

You are the camp physician for a youth camp in the mountains of Colorado. You are two hours by car from a small clinic in the nearest city and three hours away from a hospital. A young boy comes to you with severe right lower quadrant abdominal pain. He is tender but does not have guarding. The pain began three hours ago. He has not had any surgery in the past, denies trauma, has not had a bowel movement in three days, has no appetite, and does not have a fever.

1. What is the next step in the management of this boy?
2. Should you take him to the clinic?
3. What medications could you give to this boy?
4. What is the differential diagnosis?

CASE 7

You are the camp physician for a group of people who are river running in Cataract Canyon on the Colorado River. You are awakened around 6 a.m. by someone who says her tent-mate has been vomiting all night long. Shortly afterwards, you are called to see another person with similar symptoms. By mid-morning there are five people who have been up all night vomiting and now have diarrhea. It is a cloudless sky; the temperature that day will be in excess of 100°F and the biggest rapids of the entire river lay ahead. The only means of evacuating the patients would be to take them out by boat through the rapids.

1. What is the next step in the management of these patients?
2. What medicines could you give to these patients?
3. What is a list of differential diagnoses for these patients?
4. What was the probable source of the pathogen?
5. Could further problems be prevented?
6. What are the risks of staying in camp versus running the rapids?

CARDIAC PROBLEMS

Evaluating and treating cardiac problems can be difficult in a hospital setting where the full spectrum of diagnostic equipment and treatments are available. Not surprisingly this can be much more difficult in the wilderness. This section will review some of the more common cardiac problems and suggest possible treatment options in a wilderness setting.

Angina

- Angina is the term given to chest pain that is associated with diminished blood flow to a portion of the heart that is reversible and does not cause actual damage to the heart. It is cardiac ischemia but not infarction (death of heart muscle) – the reversibility is in contrast to myocardial infarction, discussed below.
- Angina results from an imbalance between cardiac muscle oxygen demand and oxygen supply. This supply may be restricted due to atherosclerotic disease. There are many reasons for an imbalance in oxygen supply and demand to occur in the wilderness:
  - Increased exertion that causes increased cardiac work
  - Cold temperature, which causes a peripheral vasoconstriction and increases cardiac work.
  - Fear, mental stress, and/or pain, all of which increase the release of catecholamines, which in turn increase both heart rate and blood pressure
  - Decreased partial pressure of oxygen as a person gains altitude; this results in less oxygen being delivered to the heart.

Two Primary Types of Angina
- **Stable Angina**
  - Chest pain due to cardiac ischemia that is well known to the patient for a period of several weeks, months or even years.
  - It is commonly due to stable atherosclerosis in the coronary arteries.
  - The patient knows the symptoms and usually knows what level of activity causes these symptoms.

- **Unstable Angina**
  - New chest pain that is concerning for cardiac ischemia OR a changing pattern in formerly stable angina. Specifically, for a patient with known stable angina, unstable angina is the same pain that occurs more frequently, with less exertion or even at rest.
  - This is commonly attributed to a worsening of atherosclerosis in the coronary arteries or a sudden rupture of an atherosclerotic plaque with formation of a partial clot in a coronary artery.

Symptoms of Angina – Stable and Unstable

- Chest pain or pressure
  - ☐ This is often described as a squeezing or tightness
  - ☐ The pain is usually in the center of the chest, but it may occur unilaterally or even across the entire chest
  - ☐ The pain may radiate to the arms, jaw, neck, or back, typically more towards the left
- Shortness of breath
- Nausea or vomiting
- Light headedness or actual syncope
- Diaphoresis

Treatment

- Steps to reduce oxygen demand of the heart muscle are critical
- Rest is the key to recovery of anginal pain
- Reduce exposure to the cold
- Decrease the elevation when possible and if oxygen is available give it to the patient
- Medications
  - ☐ Nitroglycerin (NTG) 0.4 mg sublingual
    - This may be repeated every 5 to 10 minutes until pain is relieved or until three tablets have been given. After three tablets have been given, you may continue to give the NTG if it is working and it is all that you have, which is usually the situation. However, when going beyond the initial 3 NTG tablets, it should be given with a greater time interval between the tablets. If symptoms do not resolve after 3 NTG tablets, you should assume the patient is having a myocardial infarction and begin immediate evacuation plans.
    - The biggest side effect of NTG is a drop in blood pressure. If the patient has a strong radial pulse, then it is probably safe to give them at least one tablet. You should have the patient lying supine when you give them the NTG.
    - Symptoms suggestive of too much NTG include dizziness (lightheadedness), sweating, paleness, nausea/vomiting and a thready radial pulse.
    - NTG is contraindicated if the patient has taken a phosphodiesterase inhibitor such as sildenafil (Viagra) or tadalafil (Cilalis) within the last 24 hours as this will cause an unsafe drop in blood pressure.
    - NOTE: If there is any concern of dropping the blood pressure too much or if the patient is ill appearing, then it may be prudent to not treat with NTG. This is because the NTG can help the pain, but it will not stop or treat a myocardial infarction.

- [ ] Aspirin 325 mg chewed
  - It is chewed to ensure that it is rapidly absorbed.
  - Aspirin is an anti-platelet agent that may decrease the formation of thrombus in the coronary arteries.
  - It is proven to decrease mortality in myocardial infarction.
- [ ] Clopidogrel (Plavix) 300 - 600 mg for unstable angina
  - This is an anti-platelet agent that works through a different mechanism than aspirin.
  - If you have it, then you should give this in addition to the aspirin.

Evacuation Guidelines

All patients with unstable angina must be evacuated from the wilderness as soon as possible.

Acute Myocardial Infarction (MI)

Acute MI is the term given to chest pain that is associated with absent or diminished blood flow to a portion of the heart that causes myocardial tissue death (infarction).

The most common etiology for an MI is an atherosclerotic plaque in one of the coronary arteries that ruptures, causing the formation of a clot within the artery. This clot obstructs the flow of blood distal to that obstruction. If that clot is not relieved as soon as possible, myocardial cell death will occur within 15 to 60 minutes with larger areas of infarction as time progresses.

Symptoms of MI

An acute MI will present similarly to angina; however, the symptoms are usually more severe in nature and last much longer than angina. Typical angina should be relieved within 15 minutes. If symptoms last longer than 15 minutes, the patient should be assumed to be having an MI.

Patients without a prior history of angina should be assumed to be having an MI and treated as such.

Chest pain or pressure:
- [ ] This is often described as a squeezing or tightness
- [ ] The pain may be in the center of the chest, unilateral, or even cover the entire chest
- [ ] The pain my radiate to the arms, jaw, neck, or back, frequently towards the left side

Shortness of breath

Nausea or vomiting

Light headedness or actual syncope

Diaphoresis

An impending feeling of doom

Features that are not characteristic of MI (though do not fully exclude it) are: pleuritic pain (i.e. sharp pain brought on by respiratory movement or cough), pain that may be localized at the tip of one finger particularly at the costochondral junction, very brief intermittent episodes of pain that last a few seconds, or pain reproduced with movement or palpation of the chest wall or arms

Treatment

■ **Immediate evacuation is the most important priority for the patient with a suspected MI. The fastest way to the hospital is the best way to the hospital. This means that you may be required to put a patient through some exertion in order to get him/her evacuated instead of waiting for evacuation.** All of the following treatments are temporizing measures only, until the patient can get definitive treatment with percutaneous coronary angioplasty (cardiac catheterization with stenting of the blocked vessel) or with fibrinolytic agents such as tPA or TNKase.

■ Steps to reduce oxygen demand of the heart muscle are important.
   □ Rest
   □ Reduce exposure to the cold
   □ Try to minimize anxiety

■ Increase oxygenation by decreasing elevation when at higher altitude and by giving oxygen if available.

■ Medications
   □ Nitroglycerin 0.4 mg sublingual
      ● This may be repeated every 5 to 10 minutes until pain is relieved or until three tablets have been given. After three tablets have been given, one may continue to give the NTG; however, it should be given over a longer period of time, checking the patient's radial pulse each time prior to giving an additional dose.
      ● The biggest side effect of NTG is a drop in blood pressure. If the patient has a strong radial pulse, then it is safe to give them at least one tablet. There is one type of MI, right ventricular infarction, which is very sensitive to preload (venous return) reduction. This means the patient may have a significant drop in blood pressure with even one NTG tablet. Understand that this is a potential complication and ensure that you evaluate the patient's vital signs before each NTG tablet by checking for a strong radial pulse each time.
      ● Symptoms suggestive of too much NTG include dizziness (light-headedness), sweating, paleness, nausea/vomiting and a thready radial pulse.
      ● NTG is much less effective in treating MI (clot) than it is for angina (atherosclerosis), as dilation of the coronaries does not relieve the clot that has occurred in a true MI.
      ● NOTE: If there is any concern of dropping the blood pressure too much or if the patient is ill appearing, then it may be prudent to not treat with NTG. This is because the NTG can help the pain, but it will not stop or treat a myocardial infarction.
   □ Aspirin 325 mg chewed
      ● It is chewed to ensure that it is rapidly absorbed.

- Aspirin is an anti-platelet agent that may decrease the formation of thrombus in the coronary arteries if that is the primary problem.
- It is proven to decrease mortality in myocardial infarction.
☐ Clopidogrel (Plavix) 300-600 mg orally
- This is an anti-platelet agent that works through a different mechanism than aspirin.
- You should give this in addition to the aspirin, if available.

Evacuation Guidelines

All patients with acute MI must be evacuated from the wilderness as soon as possible.

Congestive Heart Failure

Congestive heart failure (CHF) is defined as insufficient cardiac function to supply the body's demand for oxygen. Common etiologies include increased salt in the diet, non-compliance with medications and acute MI.

There are two primary types of heart failure. However, note that many patients with CHF will have a combination of these types of symptoms.
☐ Forward cardiac failure, which results in weakness, fatigue, and low blood pressure.
☐ Backward failure with the accumulation of fluid, which results in shortness of breath with pulmonary edema and peripheral edema.

The onset is usually slow, over several days with the gradual emergence of leg swelling and shortness of breath.

Alternatively, congestive heart failure may occur suddenly with dramatic respiratory distress with signs of wheezing, coughing, inability to lie flat, frothy sometime blood-tinged sputum, and eventually cyanosis and death due to hypoxia and pulmonary edema.

In heart failure, the heart muscle contraction is usually weak with a low stroke volume per beat. There are some cases where patients present with normal cardiac contractile function but have impaired cardiac relaxation. This is called diastolic dysfunction.

Symptoms

- Fatigue and weakness: These are universal symptoms of heart failure.
Shortness of breath: This is present in almost all patients and may occur suddenly and dramatically.
Leg swelling (edema): This occurs slowly, is often only present late in the day, and is often gone in the morning after lying flat. Some patients may also retain fluid in their abdomen and note increased girth and weight gain.
Cough: This is a common complaint due to increased fluid in the lungs. Usually there is clear sputum, but occasionally it may be blood tinged.
Anxiety: If patients are anxious, it is from either hypoxemia or significant difficulty breathing.

Nocturia: Patients reabsorb interstitial fluid when they are resting at night and therefore urinate at night more than usual.

Treatment

- Rest
- Reduce exposure to the cold
- Salt restriction
- Fluid restriction if shortness of breath or leg edema is present. This is important, even if the patient is thirsty.
- Increased oxygenation by either supplemental oxygen or descent to a lower altitude.
- Nitroglycerin may help to relieve the patient's shortness of breath and chest pain. Use dosing similar to that for angina, following the same precautions.
- Inhaled beta agonists, such as albuterol, may help to improve the patient's shortness of breath, particularly if they are wheezing.

Evacuation Guidelines

- All patients with acute CHF exacerbations must be evacuated from the wilderness.

RESPIRATORY EMERGENCIES

- The inability to breathe normally is a very bad feeling that is anxiety provoking.
- Respiratory issues are common in the wilderness due to numerous reasons:
  - ☐ Increased allergens
  - ☐ Smoke from campfires
  - ☐ Relative hypoxia and drier air associated with higher altitudes
  - ☐ Increased exertion
  - ☐ Increased physical and emotional stress

COPD Exacerbation (Chronic Bronchitis and Emphysema)

- Patients with COPD generally do not venture very far into the wilderness.
- Patients with COPD usually know that they have it and are on medication to treat it.

Symptoms

- Patients complain of shortness of breath, similar to episodes that they have had in the past.
- Some patients will complain of tightness in their chest in addition to difficulty breathing. This is difficult to differentiate from angina or MI, especially in the wilderness.

Treatment

- Minimize the patient's activities/exertion.
- Review the patient's medicines and administer them if available and needed.
- Increase oxygen for the patient by descent, supplemental oxygen or both if the opportunity is available.
- *Short-acting* inhaled medicines are most helpful in relieving acute symptoms.
  - ☐ Beta agonists such as albuterol (Proventil) or levalbuterol (Xopenex)
  - ☐ Anticholinergic agents such as ipratropium (Atrovent)
  - ☐ Combination beta agonist and anticholinergic agents such as Combivent (albuterol + ipratropium).
- Consider an infectious process such as pneumonia as the etiology for their symptoms.
- Consider antibiotics presumptively to treat for respiratory pathogens.
- Consider steroids if the patient has a delay in evacuation.

Evacuation Guidelines

- Patients with an exacerbation of COPD should be evacuated from the wilderness.

Asthma

Asthma is a chronic, non-progressive lung disorder characterized by increased airway reactivity to irritants, airway inflammation and reversible airway obstruction.

In the wilderness, asthma can be triggered by a multitude of potential etiologies:

- ☐ Increased strenuous activity
- ☐ Exposure to cold and changes in humidity
- ☐ Exposure to environmental allergens
- ☐ Exposure to camp smoke
- ☐ Medication noncompliance due to running out of medications

Symptoms

Patients who have asthma usually know that they have it and are taking medication.

Patients typically present with shortness of breath, wheezing, dyspnea on exertion or dry cough.

- ☐ Most patients will know when they are having an asthma exacerbation based on their previous episodes.
- ☐ They should also be able to tell you whether their current symptoms are mild, moderate, or severe in comparison to previous episodes.

This is useful in terms of judging their response to treatment and need for evacuation.

The differential diagnosis includes CHF, allergic reactions, pneumonia and pulmonary embolus.

Treatment

Mild to moderate exacerbations (speaking in complete sentences):

- ☐ Short-acting inhaled beta agonists such as albuterol or levalbuterol.
- ☐ *Strongly consider* oral steroids to improve symptoms and to prevent recurrence.
- ☐ Possible evacuation depending on the severity and the response to treatment.

Severe exacerbations (only able to speak a few words at a time):

- ☐ Short-acting inhaled beta agonists in repeated inhalations as much as needed.
- ☐ Ipratropium MDI, giving 4 to 6 inhalations every four hours as needed.
- ☐ Intramuscular epinephrine is a major consideration if the patient is not responding to the inhaled medications or if inhaled medications are unavailable.
- ☐ Corticosteroids such as prednisone or dexamethasone must be given. Oral steroids are just as good as IV/IM steroids.

Evacuation Guidelines

Patients with severe exacerbations of asthma must be evacuated from the wilderness.

Those patients with mild to moderate exacerbations must be monitored closely and should have their activities limited. They do not require evacuation unless their symptoms do not resolve with field treatment.

Pneumonia

In the wilderness, pneumonia is a clinical diagnosis based on the history and exam findings.

Symptoms
Chest pain that may be dull or sharp and may have a pleuritic component

Cough that may be dry or productive of sputum

Shortness of breath and/or dyspnea on exertion

Fever and chills

Increased respiratory rate

Treatment
Start antibiotics, even if unsure it is best to be conservative
- ☐ Fluoroquinolones
- ☐ Macrolide such as azithromycin
- ☐ Other considerations such as doxycycline

Remember to consider medication allergies

Keep the patient well hydrated

Evacuation Guidelines
■ If you suspect pneumonia, then the patient should be started on antibiotics and evacuated.

Pulmonary Embolism (PE)

Traveling a long distance with relative immobilization places someone at risk of developing a deep venous thrombosis (DVT) and/or a PE. This is an important consideration in those who traveled great distances to begin their wilderness adventure.

High-altitude climbers are more susceptible to PE, particularly if they are dehydrated.

Risk factors for PE:
- ☐ Previous history of a blood clot/DVT/PE
- ☐ Factor V Leiden disorder – this is a common heritable disorder of clotting where Factor 5 cannot be inactivated by activated Protein C.
- ☐ Long travel time to get to the destination
- ☐ Leg trauma
- ☐ Being tent bound or sitting on a raft for a long period of time
- ☐ Oral contraceptives, especially in women over age 35 who smoke
- ☐ Family history of blood clot/DVT
- ☐ History of cancer or recent surgery

Symptoms

- Symptoms may look similar to pneumonia
- Sudden onset of chest pain that may be dull or sharp and may have a pleuritic component
- Cough that may be dry or productive of bloody sputum
- Shortness of breath and/or dyspnea on exertion
- Syncope
- Increased respiratory rate
- Fever
- Unilateral leg swelling

Treatment

- There is no specific treatment that can be given in the wilderness that will help these patients.
- Recognition of this potential diagnosis is the most important part of management of these patients.
- Aspirin and clopidogrel are two medications that could theoretically help.
- Descent if at altitude and supplemental oxygen may help those with greater symptoms.

Evacuation Guidelines

- All patients with suspected PE should be evacuated as soon as possible

NEUROLOGIC EMERGENCIES

Cerebral Vascular Accident (CVA)

- The two types of stroke are:
  - ☐ Ischemic: most common type of CVA (stroke). An obstruction of blood flow to a portion of the brain leads to one-sided weakness, paralysis, trouble talking or facial droop. This obstruction is most commonly a small intra-arterial blood clot.
  - ☐ Hemorrhagic: this stroke is due to intra-cerebral bleeding, most often from high blood pressure or a ruptured brain aneurysm. Patients usually have a significant headache and a denser neurologic deficit or complete loss of consciousness
- The signs and symptoms of each are not consistent enough to allow one to discern an ischemic stroke from a hemorrhagic stroke in the wilderness.
- The only true way to tell the difference between ischemic and hemorrhagic strokes is by brain imaging (CT or MRI). This is an issue in the wilderness, as one should not treat a patient with a hemorrhagic stroke with aspirin or clopidogrel as these medications may make bleeding (and symptoms) worse.
- Always consider hypoglycemia as an etiology for stroke-like symptoms.

Symptoms

Signs and symptoms of a CVA vary depending on which part of the brain is affected. It can be a single sign or a combination of any of the following depending on the area and extent of the involvement.

- ☐ Alteration of mental status
  - Confusion
  - Stupor
  - Unconsciousness
- ☐ Difficulty speaking or an inability to speak
- ☐ Ataxia with or without vertigo
- ☐ Weakness to complete paralysis
  - Hemiparesis to hemiplegia
  - Involvement of a single leg, arm or even a hand
  - Unilateral facial involvement
- ☐ Paresthesias to complete numbness with involvement similar to weakness

If symptoms resolve quickly, then it is more likely a transient ischemic attack (TIA), sometimes called a "mini-stroke". However, a TIA is a harbinger of a stroke, so even if the symptoms resolve the patient must be evacuated as soon as possible.

Treatment

Treatment for presumed ischemic CVA or TIA is the same.

Evacuate as soon as possible.

Aspirin is indicated in ischemic CVA but not hemorrhagic CVA.

- ☐ However, ischemic CVA is much more likely than a hemorrhagic CVA.
- ☐ A single aspirin is unlikely to adversely affect a hemorrhagic stroke, but we do not recommend giving aspirin to a patient with a known hemorrhagic stroke.
- ☐ Overall it is a judgment call on whether to give an aspirin to a patient with signs of a stroke.

Clopidogrel (Plavix)

- ☐ This is another potent anti-platelet agent that may help the patient with an ischemic CVA.
- ☐ Same issues in regards to ischemic versus hemorrhagic CVA and giving aspirin apply to clopidogrel.

Evacuation Guidelines

All patients with CVA or TIA should be evacuated from the wilderness as soon as possible.

Seizures

Seizures are an uncommon medical problem in the wilderness because most people with this disorder tend to avoid wilderness activities.

Generally, patients should be seizure-free for approximately six months before attempting to trek into the wilderness for any significant amount of time.

There are numerous reasons for a patient with a known seizure disorder to seize in the wilderness:

- ☐ Fatigue and lack of adequate sleep
- ☐ Diminished absorption of their medications due to dietary changes
- ☐ Missed medication doses due to the rigors of the trek and different schedule than home
- ☐ Increased stress

Note that hypoglycemia is an alternative cause of seizures and should be considered as a diagnosis

Symptoms

There are many forms of seizures including partial and generalized. Generalized seizures involve a loss of consciousness and may involve tonic and clonic phases lasting from one to five minutes with loss of bowel or bladder function followed by a postictal phase of confusion and fatigue.

Seizures lasting longer than 5 minutes, repeat seizure activity for longer than 30 minutes or without regaining normal consciousness in between indicates status epilepticus. Mortality rate is as high as 30 percent and permanent neuronal damage may result within one hour in patients with uncontrolled seizures

Treatment

Consider hypoglycemia as an etiology. (See section on diabetes for further details).

Allow the seizure to run its course. Most will resolve spontaneously within 1 – 5 minutes.

While the patient is seizing you can do things to protect them from harm.

- ☐ Remove the patients from any hazards, such as pulling them out of water or away from a cliff edge.
- ☐ Lay the patient on the ground so that they do not fall and hurt themselves further. Do not restrain them or hold them down.
- ☐ Lying them on their side may help avoid aspiration. Once they have stopped seizing consider the recovery position.
- ☐ Move objects away from the patient so that they do not knock the objects onto themselves.
- ☐ Do NOT try to prevent them from biting their tongue by placing objects in their mouth. They will NOT swallow their tongue. You will do more harm by placing objects in their mouth.

If status epilepticus occurs you may attempt to treat the patient with a benzodiazepine. However, this will be problematic unless you can get an IV in the patient. IM and PR can work, but it is not optimal.

The trip must be stopped until the patient is out of the postictal phase. This may last hours to up to a day and can be characterized by drowsiness, confusion, nausea and headache.

Evacuation Guidelines

Evacuate all of those who have had a new seizure or status epilepticus.

If the patient has a known seizure disorder, it might be possible to increase the patient's anti-seizure medicine and to keep them in the wilderness as long as there are no other risks such as falling from a significant height or drowning. This should only be done in conjunction after a thorough discussion with the patient regarding the risks.

DIABETIC EMERGENCIES

Diabetic patients may venture in the wilderness and have very few limitations.

Fortunately, most who choose to venture into the wilderness know their diabetes well and are usually able to manage it appropriately on their own.

Diabetics should carry a method to measure their serum glucose level on their trips.

- ☐ Colorimetric strips work well in the backcountry if there is any concern of their glucometer not working or breaking. This is an important consideration at altitude and at low temperatures.
- ☐ The diabetic should educate additional personnel on how to use their glucose monitoring equipment in case they are unable to measure it themselves. This is especially important for you to know if you are going to be the medical provider on a wilderness trek.

Some precautions for diabetics venturing into the wilderness:

- ☐ Make sure their diabetes is stable for one year before going to altitude.
- ☐ Ensure that they stay well hydrated.
- ☐ If the person requires insulin they need to ensure that they have a way to maintain the medication at the appropriate temperature, otherwise it may become ineffective.
- ☐ Do they have enough medicine to last for a period of time past the scheduled end of the trip in case it is extended due to unforeseen circumstances?
- ☐ They must monitor their serum glucose closely.
- ☐ Always keep a sugar source nearby to treat low blood glucose if necessary.

Hypoglycemia

Common reasons for a diabetic to become hypoglycemic in the wilderness:

- ☐ They took too much insulin or too much of an oral agent.
- ☐ The patient ate too little in comparison to the diet they are on at home.
- ☐ The patient's exertion level is much higher than usual, resulting in higher glucose metabolism than expected.

Symptoms

Symptoms may look exactly like a stroke, so hypoglycemia should be considered as a diagnosis.

Rapid onset of confusion, irritability and even combativeness or agitation

Loss of coordination or inability to ambulate

Headache

Slurred speech

Weakness or numbness

Tremors

Diaphoresis

Seizures occasionally

Treatment

Treatment is glucose

- □ Give it immediately as hypoglycemia is a true emergency where minutes count.
- □ There are several methods to give glucose. The most common is oral glucose paste, however carrying a small tube of cake frosting will work as well.
- □ If the patient is unable to eat you may rub the glucose solution on the gums of the patient.

Glucagon can be given IM if you are unable to get the patient glucose.

Once you have gotten them out of the initial stage and the patient's mentation has cleared, feed them. Give them a meal that has complex carbohydrates and protein that will last for a longer period of time. These patients must be monitored closely for the next 6 hours to ensure that their hypoglycemia does not recur.

Evacuation Guidelines

All patients with hypoglycemia do not require immediate evacuation.

Evacuate those with hypoglycemia that returns despite treatment with glucose and a meal.

Evacuate those with hypoglycemia that may be due to an oral hypoglycemic (diabetic) agent. This is important as these patients can have persistent or recurrent hypoglycemic episodes for 24 - 48 hours that requires hospital management.

Evacuate those who do not have a rapid clearing of their neurological deficits.

HYPERGLYCEMIA

Hyperglycemia is less common in the backcountry.

Hyperglycemia requires treatment, but it is not as urgent as the brain has enough glucose.

Etiologies of hyperglycemia include

- □ Medication ineffectiveness, which most commonly occurs with insulin that is degraded due to the environment
- □ Increased stress, which leads to increased stress hormones
- □ Too much food or too little insulin
- □ Dehydration, which can worsen with the hyperglycemia and increase the release of stress hormones
- □ Infection

Symptoms

Fatigue

Hunger and thirst

Frequent urination, including nocturia (at night)

163

Blurred vision

Nausea and vomiting

Diabetics usually recognize these symptoms early

Treatment

The primary treatment in the wilderness is increased fluid intake. Most of these patients are dehydrated, and repletion of their volume will contribute greatly in decreasing their serum glucose to an appropriate level.

Be careful about giving extra insulin to these patients.

☐ Most patients have a sliding scale that they utilize to keep their sugar under control.

☐ If this does not appear to work, you may increase the amount of insulin they give themselves. However, you do not want to overshoot and make them hypoglycemic.

Search closely for the cause of their hyperglycemia. Infection is a common cause of patient's glucose imbalance.

Evacuation Guidelines

Evacuate those patients who have significant or worsening hyperglycemia.

High Altitude and Diabetes

High altitude is associated with severe diabetic ketoacidosis, though the reason is unclear.

Above 2500 meters freezing temperatures, hypoxia-induced lack of appetite, medication side effects and the higher incidence of mountain sickness can make diabetes difficult to control.

Diabetics CAN safely travel to high altitude but should be warned of this particular issue.

ALLERGIC REACTIONS AND ANAPHYLAXIS

There are three types of allergic reactions that exist on a spectrum: local, generalized and anaphylaxis. Any of these reactions can occur within seconds of exposure to an allergen.

Local

These are common in the wilderness setting

They are characterized by swollen and red areas of the skin that are usually pruritic.

Topical corticosteroids provide relief and should be carried in your first aid kit.

Diphenhydramine may be useful for the pruritus.

Cold packs may alleviate some of the pain or discomfort.

Generalized

A generalized reaction can come from any source.

Symptoms include pruritus, urticaria (hives), angioedema, and possibly bronchospasm.

Any of these may begin immediately or hours after the exposure occurs.

Treatment is to remove the patient from the allergen and to treat them with antihistamines and possibly steroids as discussed below.

Anaphylaxis

This is a true life-threatening emergency.

It begins like a generalized reaction but rapidly results in respiratory and/or circulatory collapse.

Anaphylaxis Symptoms

These are not subtle and include pruritus, hives, flushing, swelling of the tongue and lips.

The patient will have shortness of breath, wheezing, and tightness in the chest.

Nausea, vomiting, diarrhea, and abdominal cramping sometimes occur.

A drop in blood pressure may occur.

Anaphylaxis Treatment

Treatment must be immediate, as shock and respiratory arrest can occur in a matter of minutes. A delay of even several minutes can be life-threatening.

Epinephrine is the primary treatment
- ☐ An auto-injector that contains epinephrine is the most practical form of treatment.
- ☐ The dose is 1:1000 epinephrine 0.3 mg for adults and 0.15 mg for children.
  - There are many types of epinephrine auto-injectors available and all are reasonable to use as long as they have the appropriate dosing.
  - A common form is the EpiPen®
  - EpiPen®: This auto-injector also comes in both 0.3 mg and 0.15 mg (EpiPen JR®) dose forms.
- ☐ Give the IM injection directly into the thigh muscle, through pants if necessary. There is much better absorption when it is given IM in the thigh in comparison to the deltoid muscle.
- ☐ Be careful to hold the pen the correct way around, without your thumb on the tip, to avoid injecting yourself accidentally. Familiarize yourself with the pen prior to your trip to avoid confusion in an emergency.
- ☐ A 2nd dose of epinephrine may be required within 5 - 20 minutes after the first, depending on the severity of symptoms and the initial response to the epinephrine.

Antihistamines IV, IM or orally. There is no best antihistamine, although the non-specific antihistamines such as diphenhydramine (Benadryl) or chlorpheniramine are most commonly used.

An H$_2$ blocker such as cimetidine (Tagamet), ranitidine (Zantac) or famotidine (Pepcid) should be administered in addition to the other antihistamines.

Steroids should also be given. They can be given IV, IM or orally. An approximated dose is prednisone 1 mg/kg.

Inhaled beta agonists such as albuterol or levalbuterol can be used for wheezing.

Evacuation Guidelines

All patients with anaphylaxis require immediate evacuation from the wilderness.

Although the patients may rapidly improve with epinephrine and all of the other medications, they are at risk of a rebound anaphylaxis that may be worse than the initial illness.

Those with local and generalized reactions do not usually require evacuation unless their symptoms do not resolve with treatment or they have worsening symptoms.

ABDOMINAL EMERGENCIES

Appendicitis

Appendicitis may be a difficult diagnosis to make in the hospital setting when diagnostic testing is available, so you can imagine the difficulty with making the diagnosis in the wilderness setting.

Symptoms

Often starts as epigastric discomfort that may be associated with anorexia, nausea and possibly vomiting.

The abdominal pain progressively worsens over the next 6 to 24 hours as it localizes to the right lower quadrant.

The patient will develop initial tenderness in the right lower quadrant, which then progresses to peritoneal signs.

Patients may develop a fever much later in the disease process.

Treatment

Ensure that the patient has not already had their appendix removed.

Appendicitis is a surgical disease. All patients who you suspect of having appendicitis require evacuation.

Consider administering antibiotics such as fluoroquinolones and/or metronidazole if the patient is not going to be evacuated within four hours.

☐ This *may* help delay perforation or treat the patient if their appendix has already perforated.

☐ The argument against giving antibiotics is that it may interfere with making the proper diagnosis once the patient gets to the hospital. However, imaging studies, such as CT scan, can help differentiate the cause of the abdominal pain once the patient is in the hospital.

Evacuation Guidelines

Evacuate all cases of suspected appendicitis.

Severe Constipation / Fecal Impaction

This is much more common in the wilderness than people realize.

Why this happens:

- ☐ People become dehydrated easily, which leads to hard stools.
- ☐ Some people are shy and feel awkward defecating outdoors, the delay of which can lead to impaction.

Symptoms

No stooling for several days.

Gradually increasing pain, mostly in the left lower quadrant, is the usual presentation.

Masses are sometimes felt in the LLQ.

Treatment

High levels of hydration plus fiber.

Bowel stimulants are indicated.

Caffeinated drinks can stimulate bowel motility.

MiraLax is a tasteless powder that can be added to drinks. Consider bringing this on trips that involve children, as they are more likely to hold their stool than adults.

Evacuation Guidelines

Fecal impaction is not an indication for immediate evacuation, but it can lead to serious problems if not resolved.

Gallstones

Symptoms

Abdominal pain that is located in the RUQ and/or epigastrium.

The pain may radiate to the back or into the right shoulder.

Nausea and vomiting are common and may be the initial symptoms before the pain.

Treatment

Ensure that the patient has not had his gallbladder removed.

Pain relief with NSAIDs and possibly opiate analgesics depending on the amount of pain.

Consider an oral antibiotic if the patient has continuing pain and is awaiting evacuation. If the pain completely resolves there is no indication for antibiotics.

Evacuation Guidelines

- A "gallbladder attack" (biliary colic) alone is not an indication for evacuation unless the symptoms do not resolve over 6 to 12 hours.
- Evacuate those patients who have continuous or worsening pain, or intractable nausea and vomiting.

Gastritis / Gastroenteritis

Symptoms

- Nausea, vomiting and epigastric discomfort with gastritis.
- Nausea, vomiting, diarrhea and abdominal discomfort with gastroenteritis.
- Diarrhea may be watery and contain a mucus and blood.
- Patients may have significant malaise and fever.
- Dehydration may occur from an inability to take liquids and significant fluid loss from the diarrhea.

Treatment

- Large amounts of fluids that contain sugar and electrolytes. This should be given frequently in smaller than usual amounts due to the nausea/vomiting.
- Anti-emetics such as ondansetron, prochlorperazine, or metoclopramide may help with the nausea and vomiting. There are orally dissolving ondansetron tablets (Zofran ODT), which are very effective for the treatment of nausea and vomiting.
- GI anti-motility agents, such as loperamide (Imodium), may be used in those with frequent stooling. However, this is an area of controversy due to the concern of worsening illness in those with symptoms due to a bacterial infection. If you are going to use an anti-motility agent, it is best to prescribe antibiotics.
- Consider antibiotics such as the fluoroquinolones in those with bloody stools and fever.

Evacuation Guidelines

- Most patients with gastroenteritis will resolve their symptoms in 24 to 48 hours with symptomatic treatment.
- Those with intractable nausea, vomiting, and diarrhea who have significant dehydration, abdominal pain or fever should be evacuated.

Kidney Stones

Symptoms

- Sudden onset flank, back, or unilateral abdominal pain that is severe.
- The pain is colicky in nature and may radiate to the groin.
- The patient has difficulty finding a comfortable position and will be writhing in pain.

- On examination the patient will be uncomfortable, but their abdomen is generally non-tender without guarding.
- Gross hematuria may be present, but it is uncommon.
- The patient who has a history of kidney stones should be able to tell you if this is similar to previous episodes.

Treatment

- Pain relief with NSAIDs and possibly opiate analgesics depending on the degree of pain.
- Hydration is important, though more useful in the prevention of stones than their treatment.

Evacuation Guidelines

- The primary reason to evacuate someone is due to the amount of pain they are having.
- Most patients will require evacuation, but those achieving good pain control with NSAIDs may be able to stay out in the wilderness.
- Anyone with continued pain for several days however should be evacuated in order to obtain a formal evaluation.
- If the patient develops fever, they should be evacuated as soon as possible as they may have an infected kidney stone.

Ectopic Pregnancy

Symptoms

- Lower abdominal pain or abnormal vaginal bleeding in a sexually active fertile female.
- The pain may be in the midline or unilateral in location depending on where the ectopic pregnancy is located.
- Initially the pain may be mild in nature.
- Not all patients will have vaginal bleeding or specific vaginal symptoms
- An over-the-counter urine pregnancy test is very reliable and accurate in determining pregnancy. The best urine sample is the first morning void as it is the most concentrated.
- Always consider bringing several pregnancy tests along if you are the responsible health care provider on a wilderness adventure.
- An important differential diagnosis is a ruptured ovarian cyst, which presents similarly with unilateral pain but with a negative pregnancy test. A cyst that ruptures adjacent to a vessel may continue to hemorrhage and requires emergent surgical intervention.

Treatment

- Immediate evacuation is indicated in those patients you are concerned of having an ectopic pregnancy.

■ Consider Tylenol (or opiate pain medication if the patient has a normal blood pressure) for ectopic pregnancy. Avoid NSAIDs in patients with a positive pregnancy test as this is contraindicated in pregnancy and may worsen bleeding.

■ Consider NSAIDs for the pain of suspected ruptured ovarian cyst with a negative pregnancy test.

Evacuation Guidelines

■ This is a true medical emergency and immediate evacuation is required.

General Evacuation Guidelines for Abdominal Pain

■ Evacuate if abdominal pain has any of the following:
   □ The pain is associated with any signs or symptoms of shock.
   □ The pain persists for longer than 24 hours or gets progressively worse over a shorter period of time.
   □ The pain localizes and there are signs of guarding, rigidity and tenderness.
   □ Blood appears in the vomit, feces or urine.
   □ The pain is associated with a fever greater than 102 degrees F.
   □ The patient has a positive pregnancy test.
   □ The patient is unable to drink or eat.

QUESTIONS

1. You come upon a 56 year-old man who is having chest pain while hiking the Appalachian Trail. He has hypertension and takes a diuretic but has no other medical problems. He has no allergies. He has never had similar pain. He describes it as a moderate pressure on his chest that has been ongoing for over an hour. He is diaphoretic and appears short of breath but has no rash. He has a strong radial pulse with a heart rate of 52. Which one of the following is most appropriate in the management of this patient?

   a. Epinephrine 0.3 mg IM from an auto-injector
   b. Give his diuretic and wait to see how he responds
   c. Inhaled albuterol
   d. Nitroglycerin 0.4 mg sublingual
   e. Oral beta blocker (atenolol)

2. Which one of the following is a potential risk / side effect of giving nitroglycerin in the wilderness setting?

   a. Hypertension that is difficult to bring down
   b. Hyperglycemia in a diabetic by directly antagonizing insulin
   c. Hypoglycemia, requiring glucagon
   d. Hypotension with even one 0.4 mg tablet
   e. Wheezing and difficulty breathing in an asthmatic patient

3. A 30-year-old female with a known history of asthma complains of increased wheezing and difficulty breathing for the past two days. She states that this is a moderate episode for her and that it was brought on by the smoke from a campfire. She has improvement with her albuterol inhaler, but she has had to use it more often. Which one of the following should you add to her treatment regimen?

   a. Antibiotics
   b. Aspirin
   c. Clopidogrel
   d. Nitroglycerin sublingually
   e. Steroids orally

4. A 42-year-old male comes to you with the complaint of experiencing one day of right-sided chest pain and a cough productive of green mucus. He has chills and feels warm to the touch. He is a non-smoker who has no allergies or medical problems. He gets more easily winded when walking. His lungs are clear to auscultation with the exception of rales at the right base posteriorly. You are 3

days from getting him out of the wilderness. Which one of the following is the best course of action at this time?

    a. Epinephrine 0.3 mg IM

    b. Treatment with a fluoroquinolone antibiotic

    c. Treatment with an albuterol inhaler

    d. Treatment with an albuterol inhaler plus oral steroids

    e. Tylenol only

5. **A 27-year-old female is stung by a wasp while hiking with your group. She immediately becomes flushed and develops urticaria on her visible skin. Her eyes become very puffy and she is leaning forward having difficulty breathing. She has no known allergies or medical problems. Which one of the following is the first step in the management of this woman?**

    a. Albuterol inhaler 4 puffs every hour as needed for wheezing and shortness of breath

    b. Epinephrine IM 0.15 mg into the deltoid muscle

    c. Epinephrine IM 0.3 mg into the deltoid muscle

    d. Epinephrine IM 0.3 mg into the thigh muscle

    e. Steroids IM into the gluteal muscle

6. **You are biking with a friend who is an insulin-dependent diabetic. He becomes quiet and stops talking with you while you are on a break after a vigorous, complicated climb. When you approach him, he is unresponsive to your questions and is staring off into space. He is breathing and has a strong radial pulse. There is no method to measure his serum glucose. Which one of the following is the best way to manage your friend?**

    a. Administer glucagon subcutaneously

    b. Give him one-half his usual dose of insulin as a sliding scale.

    c. Put a cookie in his mouth and manually open and close his jaw to chew it for him

    d. Treat him with oral glucose paste and monitor him for improvement

    e. Treat him with water to treat his dehydration and to drive his sugar down

7. **Which one of the following is <u>not</u> used to treat the patient who has an anaphylactic reaction?**

    a. Aspirin

    b. Diphenhydramine (Benadryl)

    c. Epinephrine

    d. Ranitidine (Zantac)

    e. Steroids

8. **You are hiking in the mountains of Washington and in your group is a 16 year-old male in whom you suspect appendicitis. He has had pain for over 12 hours with nausea and vomiting. Your evacuation will last at least another 12 to 16 hours, if all goes well. Which one of the following should you consider treating the patient with?**
    a. Antibiotic such as a fluoroquinolone
    b. Anti-motility agent such as loperamide
    c. Bowel stimulants such as bisacodyl
    d. Steroids IM to calm the inflammation
    e. Steroids orally to calm down the inflammation

9. **There is a 21-year-old woman on a rafting trip with your group. She complains of left lower quadrant pain that has been ongoing for the past two days. She is sexually active but denies any vaginal bleeding. She has no urinary symptoms and denies any problems with stooling. She has mild tenderness to palpation in the left lower quadrant but an otherwise normal examination. Which one of the following is the best approach to the management of this patient?**
    a. Antibiotics such as a fluoroquinolone
    b. Evacuation as soon as possible
    c. Treatment with bowel stimulants such as bisacodyl
    d. Treatment with an anti-emetic agent such as ondansetron
    e. Treatment with MiraLax for constipation

Answers:
1. d
2. d
3. e
4. b
5. d
6. d
7. a
8. a
9. b

CHAPTER 11

Wilderness Dentistry

This chapter will train you to evaluate and treat oral and dental conditions that occur in the wilderness.

Objectives:

- To understand basic tooth anatomy
- To be able to describe etiologies and treatment of painful pulpitis
- To be able to recognize and treat failed dental restorations
- To be able to describe and treat various types of oral infections
- To be able to describe and treat a fractured tooth
- To be able to describe and treat an avulsed tooth

CASE 1

A 38-year-old male on a backcountry excursion injures a tooth while biting down on a piece of hard candy. He complains of sensitivity to cold and liquids on the left, lower pre-molar. On examination, you note that a filling is missing from the affected tooth. There is no bleeding or swelling.

1. What is the most likely complication that this climber will have if the tooth is not repaired?
2. What is the best way to repair the tooth?
3. Does this situation require antibiotics?

CASE 2

A 56-year-old woman is backpacking the Appalachian Trail when she develops a constant ache in her lower left first molar. The pain is made worse by cold and pressure. She denies trauma to the tooth. An examination reveals that the tooth has an intact large filling. The pain is made worse with percussion. There is no evidence of tooth fracture or gum swelling.

1. What is the most likely etiology for her symptoms?
2. What is the best way to manage this situation, other than pain management?
3. Does this situation require antibiotics? If you were going to use an antibiotic, which one would you select?

CASE 3

A 16-year-old climber is struck in the face by a falling rock, which dislodges his right, front, permanent, upper incisor. The rock knocked the tooth back into his mouth, and he possesses the avulsed tooth.

1. What is the first step in the management of this tooth avulsion?
2. Is this a tooth that should be replanted?
3. How would you clean this tooth if it fell into the dirt?
4. What is the best way to transport this tooth if you do not replant it?
5. Would your management be different if this was a primary tooth in a 4-year-old male?

BASIC DENTAL ANATOMY

- There are three primary regions of the tooth: enamel, dentin, and pulp.
- The supporting tissue consists of the gingiva (gum), periodontal ligaments (PDL), and bone.

Enamel

- Enamel is the outer layer of the tooth.
- It is the hardest substance in the human body and devoid of nerve endings.

Dentin

- Dentin is made up of tiny fluid-filled tubules. The tubules radiate through the dentin from the pulp, providing nutrients to the dental structures.
- If dentin is exposed, a person can experience pain when an applied stimulus makes the fluid in the dentinal tubules move.

Pulp

- The inner layer of the tooth is the pulp chamber, which consists of the neurovascular bundle, often referred to as the "pulp."
- When this area is exposed or traumatized, a person can experience pain.
- If a tooth is fractured down to the pulp, one may notice bleeding from the tooth.

ORAL INFECTIONS

Mouth infections can be viral, fungal, or bacterial. The first two are less frequent and generally not a major health threat in the wilderness. Bacterial infections can become a serious problem if not treated, in part because they have the potential to spread.

Herpes

- While there are several viruses that have oral manifestations, the herpes virus is the one most likely to be affect wilderness travelers.
- The virus is characterized by recurrent outbreaks of small, painful vesicles in localized clusters. These clusters may coalesce into larger lesions.

When the vesicles rupture, they leave a shallow, ragged, and extremely painful ulcer covered by a gray membrane and surrounded by an erythematous halo.

Outbreaks often occur during times of physical stress, which may include exercise and systemic illness.

One may reduce the incidence of an outbreak by using sun block.

Symptoms

Prodromal paresthesia or "tingle" in the dermatome of the impending herpes outbreak

Lymphadenopathy

Sore throat

Low-grade fever

Treatment

Analgesics (patients often require narcotics)

Acyclovir, valacyclovir, or famciclovir

Soothing mouth rinses, such as warm saline solution

Fungal

Fungal infections are most commonly found in individuals who are immunocompromised, debilitated or taking antibiotics.

The fungal infection most likely to be encountered is candidiasis, otherwise known as "thrush."

Symptoms

White patches on the mucosa that can be rubbed off, leaving a raw, red surface

Treatment

Nystatin or clotrimazole (Mycelex Troche)

Bacterial

A bacterial infection in the maxillofacial region can become a serious health threat. Such an infection should be treated aggressively. Oral infections generally spread slowly, but rapid spread to deep, fascial spaces may occur.

Regional lymphadenopathy is common. Osteomyelitis is uncommon even though bone is often involved.

Where definitive treatment is delayed, antibiotics should be started.

If the swelling is soft and fluctuant (ie an abscess is present), drainage will relieve pressure and prevent further spread.

Pulpitis

- Inflammation of pulp tissue (neurovascular bundle) is the primary cause of most toothaches, and is often the precursor for more serious dental and facial infections.
- Pain can range from mild to debilitating and can be steady or intermittent. Inflammation can arise for the following reasons:
  - ☐ Bacterial invasion (consequences of the tooth decay or "cavity" process)
  - ☐ Local irritation (e.g., a restoration being placed in close proximity to the pulp chamber)
  - ☐ Physical trauma (first causing inflammation of the pulp, and then reducing or eliminating blood supply to the tooth, which causes necrosis of pulp tissue)
- Pulpitis in early stages can be reversed. Early on, the tooth will be sensitive to a stimulus such as heat or cold or sweet or sugary food placed on the tooth. Once the noxious stimulus is removed, the tooth returns to its normal status. With irreversible pulpitis, the tooth will frequently remain achy or painful after the stimulus has been removed.
- Pulpitis can be classified into mild, moderate and severe. The amount of treatment needed varies with the severity of the toothache. Mild pulpitis is often reversible and can be treated simply by avoiding any stimulus. Severe pulpitis requires removal of pulp tissue or extraction of the tooth. This is usually not feasible in the wilderness and therefore warrants evacuation. Until that time, the patient must be managed to reduce pain and to prevent the situation from worsening.

Signs and Symptoms
- May range from mild, intermittent pain to severe, constant pain.
- Will usually have sensitivity or pain to stimulus (cold, hot, sweets, percussion).
- In early stages, it may be difficult to identify the offending tooth. In these cases, the tooth may look normal, or have a small cavitary lesion. In later stages, tooth decay may be quite obvious.
- Radiating pain may make it seem as if other teeth are involved
- Pain intensity may increase when the victim lies down

Treatment
- Remove any irritant or debris
- Temporarily fill any defect in the tooth
- Avoid stimulus that makes the tooth respond with pain
- Use NSAIDs and topical anesthetics as a first line for pain management and opiate analgesics for breakthrough pain
- A 2008 Cochrane review stated that antibiotics do not improve pain for patients with irreversible pulpitis (severe pulpitis requiring root canal). There do not appear to be any other indications for the use of antibiotics to treat pulpitis.
- All patients with pulpitis should see a dentist upon returning home. Patients with severe, unrelenting dental pain should be evacuated.

Complications

If necrotic pulp tissue escapes into surrounding tissue outside of the tooth, the infection can develop into an abscess. Abscesses in the backcountry need to be monitored very closely because the infection may spread into deeper anatomic areas.

Odontogenic Abscesses

Odontogenic infections can be caused by dental caries (cavity), deep restorations that approximate the pulp chamber, pulpitis, and periodontitis (gum disease).

An abscess from a tooth will follow the path of least resistance. Generally, it will stay localized and drain into the oral cavity. However, in some cases it may spread along fascial planes and into deep tissue spaces.

All abscesses should be monitored and treated. Any increased swelling or spread of infection is reason to evacuate the patient to obtain proper treatment.

Periapical Abscess

The abscess is confined to the apex of the tooth. Swelling may occur on the facial aspect of the jaw and the buccal vestibule adjacent to the offending tooth.

Signs and Symptoms

Pain

Swelling (localized)

Tooth sensitive to percussion

The affected tooth may be unresponsive to thermal changes because of pulpal necrosis

The patient may have a prior history of a toothache

Treatment

Pain management

Antibiotics are unnecessary unless cellulitis is present.

Drainage

- ☐ Periapical abscesses are typically managed by a dentist who will extract the tooth, perform a root canal, or conduct an incision and drainage.
- ☐ These measures are usually impractical, if not impossible, in the backcountry setting
- ☐ However, if a fluctuant area is appreciated, a stab incision to the area of maximal fluctuance may temporarily relieve the pain and serve as a temporizing measure.

Pericoronitis

This infection is found in the tissue around a partially erupted tooth. The most common site is the mandibular third molars ("wisdom teeth"). This infection seldom produces purulent drainage.

Signs and Symptoms
- Trismus (difficulty opening the mouth)
- Foul taste in mouth and halitosis
- Common in college-age patients as this is the age when wisdom teeth commonly erupt

Treatment
- Warm saline rinses (¼ tsp. salt in 8 oz. water) every two hours. May use chlorhexidine if available.
- Irrigate the area around the tooth and under the tissue flap
- Antibiotics
- Pain management

Periodontal Abscess

Proliferation of bacteria between the tooth and gingiva (gums)

Signs and Symptoms
- Swelling is near the gingiva where it meets the tooth, rather than in the vestibule
- The tooth may be sensitive to percussion and heat or cold

Treatment
- No incision is necessary. Drain through the gingival sulcus (between the tooth and gums) by dissecting the gingiva away from the tooth with a blunt instrument
- Follow up with warm to hot saline rinses

Facial Space Abscess

While most dental abscesses localize around a tooth, there is potential for the infection to spread into areas of the head and neck in such a manner that they may become life threatening. Due to proximity of the central nervous system and airway to the oropharynx, timely efforts are required to treat this condition. In the wilderness, immediate evacuation is indicated.

Sign and Symptoms

- Severe swelling
- Pain
- Trismus (difficulty opening mouth)
- Elevated temperature
- Rapid and weak pulse
- Difficulty swallowing
- Difficult or shallow breathing

Treatment

- Antibiotics
- Airway management
- Pain management
- Immediate evacuation

Antibiotic Use

- Odontogenic infections are typically polymicrobial. Anaerobes are prevalent, so penicillin has historically been the first choice for these infections.
- Increasing rates of resistance have led to the increasing use of clindamycin for oral infections.
- Indications for antibiotic use for oral infections:
  - ☐ Antibiotics are warranted in local infections for patients who are immunocompromised, have cellulitis surrounding the abscess, had an inadequate drainage of the abscess, or if a delay to definitive care is anticipated.
  - ☐ A patient who shows signs of disseminated infection, such as lymphadenopathy, fascial space involvement, or systemic symptoms, should be treated with antibiotics.
  - ☐ Compound maxillofacial fractures involving tooth-supporting bone warrant treatment with antibiotics.

FAILED DENTAL RESTORATIONS

When restorations (fillings or crowns) fall out or are removed, the surrounding tissue may have increased sensitivity to stimuli. Also, food may get packed between the teeth and irritate and inflame the gingiva (gums) leading to increased pain and infection.

Lost Filling

Signs and Symptoms

☐ Tooth sensitivity to stimulus (cold, hot, sweets). There is usually no pain in the absence of stimuli

☐ Sore tongue from rough or sharp tooth edge

☐ Food impaction between teeth, making tooth and gums sore

Treatment

☐ Remove any debris in or around the tooth

☐ Smooth rough or sharp edges with a file

☐ Temporarily fill any defect

   ☐ There are several commercially available temporary filling materials:
   - *Cavit* comes pre-mixed and will harden once placed in the mouth. Cavit can be thinned, if necessary, by mixing it with petrolatum jelly (Vaseline).
   - *IRM* comes in a powder/liquid form that requires mixing. The advantage of IRM is that it can be mixed to any consistency.

Complications

☐ Left untreated, bacterial invasion can begin the decay process that eventually leads to pulpitis and the need for endodontic therapy (root canal).

Lost Crown or Bridge

Signs and Symptoms

☐ Tooth sensitivity to stimulus (cold, hot, sweets)

☐ Food impaction around tooth

Treatment

☐ Clean out old cement from inside of crown

☐ Remove any debris around the tooth

☐ Check to make sure that the crown still fits

☐ Place a thin film of soft temporarily filling material in the crown and place the crown back on the tooth

☐ Have the patient bite down to squeeze out excess cement

☐ Note: You may need to thin the temporary filling material if it is too thick

☐ Have patient bite down to ensure that the replaced crown doesn't interfere with his or her bite

☐ Remove excess filling material

☐ Check the bite again

Complications

If decay is present under the crown, it may have gone unnoticed. If it is severe enough, the tooth may break off at the gum line and there won't be enough retention to cement the crown back into place. In this case, one could place a small amount of temporary filling material over the remaining part of the tooth to make it smooth, so that the tooth is less sensitive and the tongue won't become irritated.

DENTAL TRAUMA

Injuries to the tooth and supporting tissues are common during high-adventure activity mishaps, such as mountain biking, skiing, climbing, or rafting.

Trauma can be isolated to the tooth but it often involves the soft tissue and supporting tissue as well. Soft tissue consists of the lips, tongue, and cheeks, while supporting tissue is made up of bone, ligaments, and gingiva (gums).

History and Exam

Proper evaluation and history are helpful in a trauma situation. In addition to examination of the dental arches and surrounding tissue, the victim should be asked about loss of consciousness, nausea, vomiting, and dizziness to identify any possible head injury.

Clean the region well to unmask injuries hidden by blood or debris. Evaluate lacerations for any foreign material, including pieces of broken teeth.

Examine teeth for fractures and pulp exposures.

Evaluate the mandible and facial bones for any fractures.

Injuries to the Tooth

Tooth injuries consist of fractured or chipped teeth. A fracture can vary losing a chip of enamel to fracturing the tooth through the dentin and into the pulp.

Uncomplicated Crown Fracture

Signs and Symptoms

Visible chip on tooth

May see yellow tissue beneath the enamel, indicating involvement of the dentin

No visible pulp tissue or bleeding

Sensitive to stimulus (hot, cold, sweets)

Treatment
- Pain management
- Smooth sharp edges by placing temporary filling (IRM, Cavit, soft wax, or tape) over the tooth
- Avoid any stimulus that may aggravate the tooth

Uncomplicated Crown-Root Fracture

This fracture usually occurs with pre-molar and molar teeth, when part of the cusp has broken away but remains in the mouth because it is still attached to gingiva. There is no involvement of the pulp by definition.

Signs and Symptoms
- Loose piece of tooth
- Pain or irritation on biting

Treatment
- Remove loose fragment
- Cover the tooth with a temporary filling
- Pain management
- Avoid any stimulus that may aggravate the tooth

Complicated Crown Fracture

Signs and Symptoms
- Fracture involving exposure of pulp
- Sensitive to air, cold and other stimuli because of exposed nerve

Treatment
- Stop bleeding by biting on gauze
- Because the nerve has been exposed, the tooth is very sensitive, so the sooner the victim is taken to a dentist, the better
- Cover the tooth with a temporary filling
- Pain management

Complicated Crown-Root Fracture

Signs and Symptoms
- Fracture that exposes pulp
- Sensitive to air, cold, etc.
- Loose fragment of tooth attached to gingiva

Treatment
- Remove or stabilize fragment
- Proceed as for a complicated crown fracture

INJURIES TO PERIODONTAL TISSUES

Trauma to the oral cavity may not fracture a tooth. However, damage may occur to the supporting structures around the tooth, in which case the tooth will be displaced from its normal position. The following are possible scenarios that can affect teeth and the supporting tissues.

Subluxation

The tooth has increased mobility but has not been displaced from its original location. Symptoms may vary depending on the severity of injury to the supporting structures.
- Treatment consists of a soft diet, rest and NSAIDs for pain management, if necessary.
- When injured teeth are painful, temporary splinting may ease pain and enhance the ability to eat.

Intrusive Luxation

- The tooth has been pushed into the socket. The tooth is not mobile.
- Field treatment is palliative because the tooth is out of alignment.
- Endodontic and orthodontic treatment should be initiated within two weeks of the incident.

Extrusion Luxation

- The tooth is extruded partially from its socket and extremely mobile.
- Use gentle steady pressure to reposition the tooth, allowing time to displace any blood that has collected in the socket area. After reduction, the tooth should be non-rigidly splinted.

Lateral Luxation

The tooth is displaced laterally because of bone fracture and can get locked into a new position. If this happens, the tooth will not be mobile.

Reduce the tooth using the two-finger technique.

- ☐ With one finger over the apex, push toward the crown while the other finger places a small amount of pressure outwards to help position the tooth back into its socket. The tooth may snap back into position and be quite stable.

Splint if mobility is present after reduction.

Exarticulation (Avulsion)

Quick action is needed to increase survival of the tooth. The longer the tooth is out of the mouth, the less the chance for survival of the tooth.

Prognosis also depends on the health of the periodontal ligament (PDL) cells, some of which are on the root of the tooth (others are in the socket).

Do NOT scrub, curette, disinfect or let the root surface dry out; rinse the tooth with saline to remove debris.

Remove clotted blood from the socket, using gentle irrigation and suction. Avoid scraping the socket walls. Replace the tooth gently with steady pressure to displace any accumulated blood.

If immediate replantation is not possible, place tooth in the best transportation medium available.

Transport media (in order of effectiveness):

- ☐ Save-A-Tooth (Hank's balanced salt solution, which is a physiologically pH balanced saline)
- ☐ Milk
- ☐ Saliva. Do not place the tooth in the victim's mouth if there is a possibility he/she might aspirate it.
- ☐ Saline and water do not work well as transport solutions because they can damage the PDL cells. They should only be used to clean the tooth for immediate replantation and not for transportation.

Management of the Socket:

Gently aspirate without entering the socket; if a clot is present, use light irrigation to remove it.

Do not curette the socket.

Do not make a surgical flap unless bony fragments prevent replantation.

If the alveolar bone is collapsed and prevents replantation, carefully insert a blunt instrument into the socket to reposition the bone to its original position.

After replantation, manually compress facial and lingual bony plates (only if spread apart).

Splint or stabilize the tooth.

Splinting

- Once a tooth has been repositioned back into the socket, it will need to be splinted so that the ligaments can reattach.
- There are two types of splinting: rigid and non-rigid.
  - ☐ Rigid splinting is best for the bony segment fractures or jawbone fractures.
  - ☐ Non-rigid is the splinting of choice for tooth stabilization. In a backcountry environment, it may be necessary to improvise with material on hand. Fishing line or even floss could be bonded to splint teeth. Sutures can also be used to support the tooth by running the suture through the gingiva on the facial aspect of the tooth and then through to the lingual gingival, making a sling that will stabilize the tooth.

Injuries to Primary Teeth

- When dealing with first aid for primary teeth, the general rule is to remove the tooth if it is in the way.
- If a young child has sustained an injury that results in a tooth becoming dislodged or loose, the best treatment is simply to remove it.
- It is not necessary to replant avulsed primary teeth. If the displaced primary tooth does not interfere with occlusion, no treatment other than palliative is needed.

QUESTIONS

1. **27 year-old hiker notices a painful, tingling sensation on the right side of his upper lip. He has had this before, and it was followed by painful, blister-like lesions. What is the most appropriate treatment for his condition?**
   a. Acyclovir
   b. Cephalexin
   c. 1% Hydrocortisone Cream
   d. Prednisone

2. **An 18 year-old male gets hit in the mouth with a falling branch, knocking out his right, upper pre-molar. Which one of the following in the correct management of this injury?**
   a. Carefully rinse tooth in clean water, re-implant and splint in place
   b. Clean base of tooth with toothbrush and re-implant
   c. Do nothing. The tooth does not need to be re-implanted. It will not survive.
   d. Sterilize the tooth in boiling water and re-implant

3. **A 12 year-old girl falls off of a horse and loses her right, upper pre-molar. There are no other injuries. Which one of the following is the correct management of this tooth?**
   a. Carefully rinse the tooth with clean water, re-implant, and splint in place
   b. Do nothing
   c. Have the child hold the tooth inside her mouth until she can be seen by a dentist
   d. Place the tooth in Hank's solution and evacuate to a dentist and have the tooth re-implanted
   e. a, c, or d are all correct

4. **A 54 year-old climber is hit in the mouth by a falling rock. His left, upper, first molar is fractured. A small amount of blood is visible on the retained dental fragment. Which one of the following is the best management?**
   a. Attach the broken piece of tooth to the retained fragment with skin adhesive
   b. Cover the tooth with a temporary filling and evacuate to a dentist.
   c. Extract the retained dental fragment.
   d. Give prophylactic antibiotics

Answers:
1. a
2. a
3. e
4. b

CHAPTER 12

Wilderness Dermatology

This chapter describes dermatologic situations that may be encountered in the wilderness.

Objectives:

- Recognize poison oak, poison sumac, and poison ivy
- Describe prevention and treatment of poison ivy contact dermatitis
- Describe the recommendations for avoiding sunburn
- Understand the proper use of sunscreen lotion
- Understand the treatment of sunburns
- Describe dermatologic conditions in which evacuation to definitive medical care is necessary

CASE 1

A 45-year-old woman takes her hiking boots out of storage and joins some friends for a day hike. After returning home from a pleasant, uneventful trip, she develops an unrelenting itch and red rash on her right lower leg. The symptoms remind her of a rash she had last fall after hiking through dried brush. Strangely, the rash is in the same location on the same leg. Last fall she had been diagnosed with poison ivy allergic dermatitis, but this time she had hiked on an asphalt trail and had not brushed against any plants.

1. What caused the rash last fall?
2. Assuming she encountered no poison ivy on today's hike, what is causing the rash today?
3. How would you clean her boots to prevent future reactions?
4. How would you manage her current symptoms?

CASE 2

A middle-aged potato farmer is attempting to rid his field of the poison ivy that has caused numerous irritating skin outbreaks in the past. He builds a large fire and gathers trash, dead wood, and shrubs. He takes special care with the shrubs and handles them with thick vinyl gloves to prevent an outbreak. As he feeds the shrubs into the fire, he develops wheezing and progressive respiratory difficulty.

1. What is causing his respiratory distress?
2. How is he contacting the allergen?
3. What is the emergent treatment for his condition?

CASE 3

A 17-year-old boy is rock climbing in the desert with some friends. After lunch he is warm, so he removes his shirt and continues rock climbing through the afternoon. That night he has severe pain, warmth, and redness on his back. The pain is worsened with any contact to the affected skin.

1. What would have been the best prevention of his rash?
2. What treatments could relieve his symptoms?
3. What are the short-term and long-term outcomes of his sunburn?

POISON IVY

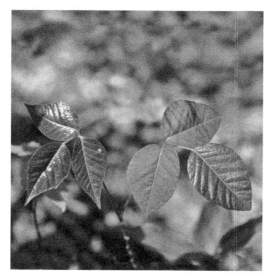

Poison Ivy: demonstrating the classical "leaves of three" appearance
(Photo courtesy of www.poison-ivy.org)

POISON OAK

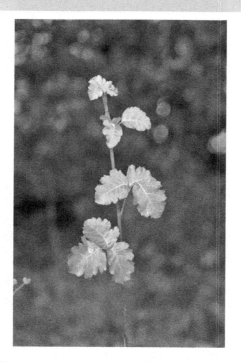

Poison Oak: with serrated edges easily confused with typical oak
(Photo courtesy of www.poison-ivy.org)

POISON SUMAC

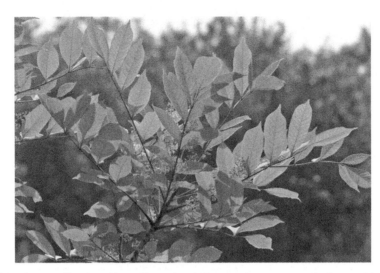

Poison Sumac: this deceptively attractive shrub is most commonly found in swampy regions
(Photo courtesy of www.poison-ivy.org)

POISON IVY RASH

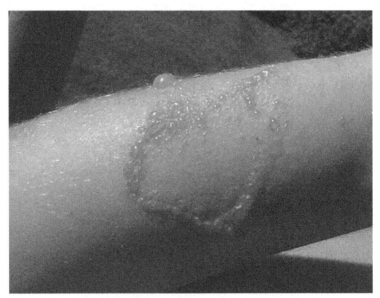

Poison Ivy Rash: scratching with resin under the fingernails
may cause the rash to appear in a linear pattern
(Photo courtesy of www.poison-ivy.org)

TOXICODENDRONS

Background

- Poison ivy, poison oak, and poison sumac belong to a genus of plants called toxicodendrons.
- Toxicodendrons grow in every state except Hawaii and Alaska.
- Poison oak, poison sumac, and poison ivy all contain a toxic resin called urushiol, which is responsible for the characteristic reaction.
- Urushiol is contained within the leaves, fruit, root and stem of the plant.
- Simply touching the plant does not cause a skin reaction. The plant must be traumatized in order to release the resin. Trauma as simple as drying or the leaves or raindrops can release the resin.
- Urushiol is remarkably adhesive and can cling to pets, garden tools, and clothing.
- Urushiol is quite heat stable and can attach to smoke particles when the plants are burned, making the potential for airway reactions a frightening possibility.
- The toxin is also very persistent, with reports of the resin attached to clothing causing allergic contact dermatitis years after it has left the original plant.
- 85% of the population will develop an allergic reaction if exposed to poison ivy, oak or sumac.
- Rash may appear after the first exposure, but on subsequent exposures the reaction is typically more pronounced and has a faster onset.

Poison Ivy

- *Toxicodendron radicans* is a climbing vine with three serrated-edged, pointed leaves that grows is found in every US state east of the Mississippi River. The three-leaf clusters have given rise to the popular adage "Leaves of three: let them be."

Poison Oak

- *Toxicodendron toxicarium/diversilobum* also has three leaves. It grows in the sandy soil of the southeast as a small shrub. In the western United States, poison oak is a very large plant that grows as a standing shrub or climbing vine.

Poison Sumac

- *Toxicodendron vernix* is a shrub or bush with two rows of 7 to 13 leaflets. It is most common in the peat bogs of the northern United States and in swampy southern regions of the country.

Disease Process

- Toxicodendron dermatitis is a type IV hypersensitivity reaction.
- Urushiol contacts the skin after direct encounter or contact through a secondary host (a pet, a piece of clothing, etc).

- Once urushiol contacts the skin it seeps through the protective epidermal level.
- The toxin is detected by antigen presenting cells that migrate to the lymph nodes and activate T cells. The cytotoxic T cells mount an attack that leads to the vasodilation and characteristic tissue response at the site of skin contact.
- Once an exposure has caused formation of clonal T lymphocytes, a subsequent exposure may cause a more rapid response.

Clinical Presentation

- The most common clinical presentation of toxicodendron exposure is a pruritic erythematous rash on an exposed part of the body.
- The rash often includes fluid-filled vesicles or bullae in a linear arrangement.
- The linear arrangement has led to the misconception that rupturing the fluid-filled vesicles while scratching causes spread of the reaction. In fact, the clusters are due to the area contacted by the toxicodendron.
- The vesicles do not contain urushiol and rupture of the vesicles does not spread the disease.
- In a first-time exposure, the appearance of skin lesions is commonly within 24 to 48 hours but may be delayed up to 21 days.
- In a sensitized patient, the rash appears between 4 to 96 hours after exposure.
- The time of onset of the rash can be difficult to describe because urushiol can cause a rash both due to contact irritation and allergic response.
- A small minority of the population are considered "exquisitely sensitive" to urushiol. These patient will develop the typical pruritis, erythema, vesicles and bullae within 6 hours of exposure. Systemic signs such as fever may also appear. These patients need immediate treatment.

Treatment

Prevention

- Avoidance of the toxicodendrons is the surest prevention of poison-ivy contact dermatitis. Full-length clothing helps prevent direct contact with the plants, but the urushiol resin can soak through protective clothing, even rubber or leather gloves. Vinyl gloves, however, are an effective barrier.
- Barrier creams such as bentoquatam, linoleic acid dimers, and barrier ointments have been marketed to prevent poison ivy contact dermatitis. These creams have varying efficacy and must be reapplied every few hours to maintain protection. Bentoquatam (Ivy Block) is safe and is probably the most well studied of these products. It prevents dermatitis in 68% of exposures, but like the other creams, it must be applied to the skin every four hours to maintain protection.

Early Treatment

Wash the area

A person with average allergic response can prevent immune reaction by washing off the resin within 20 minutes. The efficacy of rinsing the affected area seems to diminish as time passes.

Rinsing with copious amounts of cold water will help remove the resin without opening pores and enhancing absorption into the skin. Mild hand soaps and non-abrasive rubbing are also recommended.

Rubbing alcohol on a cotton applicator is effective at removing the urushiol resin both from skin and from tools and clothing. Take care to avoid reusing the cotton to prevent spread of the resin.

When cleansing, take special care to remove resin from the fingernails to prevent further inoculation when scratching.

Mild Disease

Mild dermatitis involves minimal exposure to urushiol causing small eruptions on the skin.

If available, the use of high-potency topical steroid creams before the formation of vesicles will offer relief and blunt the allergic response.

Avoid use of high-potency steroids on the face, genitals, and other areas of thin skin.

After vesicles have formed, topical steroids may not change the course of the allergic response but can relieve itching.

Symptomatic relief of the itching can be gained either by using oral diphenhydramine (25-50mg) or an equivalent dose of non-sedating antihistamines.

Several other products are marketed for topical relief of poison ivy dermatitis. The skin irritation can be soothed with calamine lotion or Aveeno oatmeal bath soaks.

Aluminum acetate (Burrow's solution) or Domeboro astringent solution may be applied to dry weeping areas for relief of pruritus.

- These topical products offer relief but do not alter the course of the dermatitis.
- Topical antibiotics and topical antihistamines should be avoided because these substances have a history of causing allergic dermatitis themselves and may complicate the irritation without offering any advantage.

Moderate Disease

Moderate contact dermatitis affects larger surface areas and causes significant distress.

Treatment should include topical steroids if given the opportunity to treat before vesicle formation.

After vesicle formation, relief may be obtained by oral Prednisone 60mg daily for 5 days then 40mg daily for 5 days, then 20 mg daily for 5 days.

Short-course prednisone therapy may cause a rebound of dermatitis once it is completed and should be avoided.

Symptomatic treatment as in mild disease is also appropriate.

Severe Disease

Any reaction that causes airway or genital swelling or involves a large amount of body surface should be considered severe disease and requires hospital care.

IV steroid therapy with methylprednisolone can prevent or significantly diminish the immune flare if patients present within two hours of exposure.

If patients present after this time, then the IV steroids must be followed by oral therapy as described above.

Disease Course

Most cases of poison ivy contact dermatitis are self-limiting and will resolve in 1 to 3 weeks without any treatment.

The vesicles will eventually rupture, crust over, and then heal.

The most common complication of toxicodendron exposure is secondary infection at the site of the lesion with Staphylococcus or Streptococcus skin flora.

Evacuation Guidelines

The majority of cases of toxicodendron allergic dermatitis can be adequately managed in the field.

The exception would be the exquisitely sensitive patient who develops severe allergic response or any exposure that involves the face, airway, or genital areas.

SUNBURN

Background

☐ Sunburn is inflammation of the skin that is caused by overexposure to the sun's ultraviolet (UV) rays.

☐ Sunburn is not only uncomfortable, but it predisposes patients to skin cancer.

☐ Approximately 32% of adults and 80% of young people report at least one case of sunburn in the previous year.

☐ Artificial "tanning" results in UV exposure and confers the same risk of skin cancer as sunbathing.

☐ Fair-skinned people are particularly susceptible to sunburn because their skin produces only small amounts the protective pigment, melanin. Even dark-skinned people, while they have a lower risk, can develop skin cancer.

Disease Process

☐ Two types of UV rays are clinically important in sun exposure: UVA and UVB

☐ UVA rays penetrate the skin deeply. They damage the DNA of the skin cells, contributing to the development of skin cancers. The tanning effect of the skin is also a response to UVA exposure. This is why tanning booths primarily emit UVA rays.

☐ UVB rays affect the more superficial layers of the skin, and are the chief cause of skin reddening and sunburns. They also play a role in the development of skin cancer, wrinkling, and tanning.

☐ There are no "safe" UV rays.

☐ UV rays strike the skin and cause multiple effects. Skin redness appears as the local blood vessels dilate and inflammatory substances (including histamine) are released.

☐ The tissue changes become apparent as redness develops over a period of 2 to 6 hours after exposure.

Clinical Presentation

☐ A sunburn is generally a clinically obvious diagnosis with redness in the sun-exposed areas.

☐ Symptoms can vary from mild redness and warmth of the skin to severe pain and blistering.

☐ The traditional classification of sunburn includes first-degree and second-degree sunburns.

☐ First-degree sunburns are those with redness and pain that may peel but heal within a few days.

☐ Second-degree sunburns also have redness and pain but may also have blisters and cause systemic symptoms such as fever, chills and headache.

Treatment

Prevention

Measures to limit sun exposure will prevent sunburn and its associated risks. Limit sun exposure to early in the day, trying to keep contact initially less than 15 minutes.

Avoid the sun between 10 a.m. and 4 p.m. UVB rays are more intense during this time of the day.

Use waterproof sunscreen on legs and feet since the sun can burn even through water. Wear an opaque shirt in the water because reflected rays are intensified.

Wear breathable full-length clothing, use wide-brimmed hats, and seek shade.

When the sun cannot be avoided, sunscreen should be worn.

Everyone six months of age and older should use sunscreen. Infants younger than 6 months of age should be kept out of the sun because their skin is thin and susceptible to burning. Sunscreens have not been approved for infants.

Traditionally, sunscreens have contained the chemical PABA, which screens UVB rays but not UVA rays. Newer broad spectrum sunscreens contain additives that also protect against UVA rays.

Sunscreens with ingredients such as benzophenone (oxybenzone), cinnamates (octylmethyl cinnamate and cinoxate), zinc oxide, avobenzone, sulisobenzone, salicylates and titanium dioxide provide the broad spectrum protection against UVA rays.

Sunscreen should be applied to dry skin 30 minutes before sun exposure.

Sunscreen must be reapplied after two hours or sooner if sweating or swimming. Even waterproof sunscreen loses effectiveness after about 80 minutes.

Sunscreens are rated according to their Sun Protection Factor (SPF). SPF measures how long it takes to sunburn while wearing protection compared to how long it takes to sunburn without protection. Wearing a sunscreen with an SPF of 2, a person who normally sunburns after 5 minutes without protection would take twice that long (10 minutes) to develop sunburn. That same person, if wearing SPF 10 lotion, would take 50 minutes to burn.

The American Academy of Dermatologists recommends the use a waterproof sunscreen with an SPF of at least 15.

First-Degree Sunburns

First-degree sunburns involve a limited surface area with symptoms of skin redness and pain.

The mainstays of therapy are pain control and skin care.

Pain control can be achieved with acetaminophen or with NSAIDs.

Diphenhydramine may also offer relief from itching and help the patient sleep.

Skin treatment can include any of the following measures that offer relief:

- ☐ Cool soaks in water or applying moisturizers such as aloe vera
- ☐ Topical pain relief with Aveeno lotion, Prax lotion, or Sarna lotion
- ☐ These medications may help alleviate symptoms, but they have not been shown to decrease recovery times.

- Topical steroids show little to no benefit.
- First-degree sunburns are uncomfortable and may cause superficial skin peeling, but they heal within a few days.

Second-Degree Sunburns

- Second-degree sunburns also have redness and pain but are more extensive, have blisters, and may cause larger systemic symptoms such as fever, chills, and headache.
- In addition to the therapies for first-degree sunburns, these patients may require stronger pain medications.
- Use of systemic steroids in severe sunburns has anecdotal and traditional support but has not been well studied. If used, treatment should commence early. 40-60mg per day of prednisone for 3-5 days is a suggested usage.
- Moderately burned skin should heal within a week, but even one bad burn in childhood carries an increased risk of skin cancer.

Evacuation Guidelines

If a large body surface area is involved, if systemic symptoms such as fever, chills, and headache are present, or if pain cannot be controlled then the patient should evacuated to definitive care.

QUESTIONS

1. **Poison ivy contact dermatitis can be caused by exposure to which parts of the plant?**
    a. The dried leaves during the fall
    b. The green leaves during summer
    c. The stem
    d. The root
    e. All of the above

2. **Appropriate treatment of poison ivy contact dermatitis includes which of the following?**
    a. NSAIDs
    b. Topical steroid creams
    c. Topical antibiotic cream
    d. Topical antihistamines

3. **Indications for evacuating a person with poison ivy contact dermatitis include:**
    a. Airway involvement
    b. Involvement of the hands, feet, or legs
    c. Itching with vesicle formation
    d. Previous exposure to poison ivy

4. **Which of the following are true of Urushiol?**
    a. It can attach to smoke molecules when burned
    b. It degrades and becomes inactive after one week
    c. It has seasonal effect, causing symptoms in the fall but not in the spring
    d. It is the active resin in poison ivy, and poison sumac, but not in poison oak

5. **Which of the following are true of UV light exposure:**
    a. UVB rays cause sunburn, but UVA rays are harmless
    b. UV exposure causes cell damage that can lead to cancer
    c. UV rays from tanning beds are not harmful
    d. UV rays are not a concern on cloudy days

6. **If a fair-skinned woman normally sunburns after 10 minutes in the sun, how long will she take to develop the same level of sunburn when wearing sunscreen (SPF 15)?**
    a. 3.3 minutes
    b. 150 minutes
    c. 30 minutes
    d. 1500 minutes

Answers:

1. e   5. b
2. b   6. b
3. a
4. a

CHAPTER 13

Eye Injuries and Disorders

This chapter will train you to recognize and initiate treatment of eye injuries and disorders in the wilderness.

Objectives:

- Competently evaluate injuries to tissues surrounding the eye and recognize which injuries can be treated in the wilderness and which ones require evacuation
- Be able to evaluate ocular injuries and understand their basic management in the wilderness
- Describe evaluation and treatment of the patient with a red eye
- Understand the differential diagnosis for visual loss
- Describe evacuation criteria for the patient with an eye injury or vision complaint

CASE 1

A 29-year-old male is fishing with friends at a river three hours away from the nearest hospital. They are a 10 minute walk from the trailhead. After a cast, the man falls down, writhing in pain. His friends notice that the fishing line is attached to the hook, which has penetrated the victim's eye. He has difficulty holding still and cannot open the eye because of pain and anxiety.

1. What is the next step in management of this patient?
2. What do you do with the fishing hook?
3. Can this be dealt with in the wilderness?
4. If evacuation is necessary, what is the best way to proceed?

CASE 2

A 59-year-old male complains of sudden decrease in vision in his left eye. He was fine several minutes previously, but then saw flashing lights in the left eye, followed by "floaters." He is able to see, but his vision seems decreased. On examination, his eye appears to be completely normal and he is easily able to count fingers at six feet in front of him.

1. What is the next step in management of this patient?
2. Can you manage him in the wilderness or does he need to be evacuated?
3. If evacuation is necessary, should you place a shield over his eye?

CASE 3

A 32-year-old woman is struck in the right eye by a rock while climbing up a cliff. Other than a small contusion on her eyelid, there is no external trauma. Examination of her eye shows normal counting of fingers at six feet and a very small layer of blood overlying the iris along the lower border of the cornea. The remainder of the exam is normal.

1. What is the injury?
2. What are the potential complications from this injury?
3. Is it reasonable to give the victim ibuprofen for pain?
4. Can you manage the victim in the wilderness, or does she need to be evacuated?
5. If evacuation is necessary, should you place a shield over her eye?

CASE 4

A 40-year-old woman has developed a red painful eye over the course of a day. You put several drops of proparacaine in her eye without any significant relief of pain.

1. What is the differential diagnosis for the pain?
2. What is the treatment for this, if available?
3. Does this patient require evacuation?

GENERAL APPROACH TO WILDERNESS EYE INJURIES

- ■ The initial step to approaching a patient with an ocular malady is to classify the etiology as traumatic or non-traumatic
- ■ Further division of these categories, and the management of each, will be discussed below.
- ■ To aid in evaluation of eye issues in the wilderness, a few items are required:
  - ☐ Penlight or flashlight
  - ☐ Blue-light penlight
  - ☐ Topical anesthetic such as tetracaine or proparacaine
  - ☐ Fluorescein dye (strips are preferred)
  - ☐ These items along with physical exam will allow one to diagnose most eye issues in the wilderness
- ■ Ophthalmic medications used in the wilderness:
  - ☐ Artificial tears
  - ☐ Ophthalmic topical antibiotics: fluoroquinolones (moxifloxacin, levofloxacin or ciprofloxacin) are first choice, erythromycin ointment
  - ☐ Oral fluoroquinolones or amoxicillin-clavulanate may be of benefit in certain cases
  - ☐ Cycloplegics (pupil dilators) such as cyclopentolate and scopolamine
    - ● This can reduce the pain caused by ciliary muscle spasm as is seen with a corneal abrasion and iritis.
    - ● Cyclopentolate is short acting, and scopolamine is long acting
  - ☐ Ocular steroids (prednisolone drops): although controversial, these may be helpful in some conditions during evacuation as an anti-inflammatory agent
  - ☐ Topical NSAIDs such as ketorolac
  - ☐ Pilocarpine drops for that rare time you need to treat glaucoma in the wilderness

TRAUMATIC OCULAR COMPLAINTS

- History and exam will determine if the trauma is periocular, ocular or both
- The initial determination to make is whether an open globe is present

Open Globe

- Present when there is a full-thickness injury to the cornea or the sclera
- Can be the result of a blunt or penetrating injury
- Physical exam findings may be obvious, such as
  - ☐ Aqueous or vitreous humor leaking from the wound
  - ☐ The globe may appear sunken due to loss of fluid.
  - ☐ The globe may protrude from the orbit if associated with bleeding behind the eye.
  - ☐ The pupil may appear irregular (see photo below)
- Once recognized, a protective shield should be placed over the globe, not a pressure dressing.
- No further exam should be done
- Do not apply pressure to the eye
- The patient should be given oral antibiotics if available. A fluoroquinolone is the drug of choice.
- Do not administer topical anesthetics or antibiotics
- Consider antiemetics to prevent the Valsalva mechanism associated with vomiting as this increases intraocular pressure
- Open globe injuries require immediate evacuation

Penetrating Foreign Body

- If a foreign object has penetrated the eye, do not try to remove it.
- Stabilize the object by taping a sterile dressing in a donut shape around the eye and then taping a cup or pair of glasses over the eye to prevent any jarring of the embedded object.
- You may consider patching the other eye shut to prevent eye movement if the victim does not have to use his or her sight to navigate out of the wilderness

Occult Ruptured Globe

- The presence of an open globe is not always obvious. Whenever there is trauma to or around the orbit, the eye should be assessed for signs of an open globe.

- Signs include a large subconjunctival hemorrhage, hyphema, corneal abrasion, or a peaked or ectatic pupil
- A suspected occult rupture should be treated the same as an obvious globe injury.

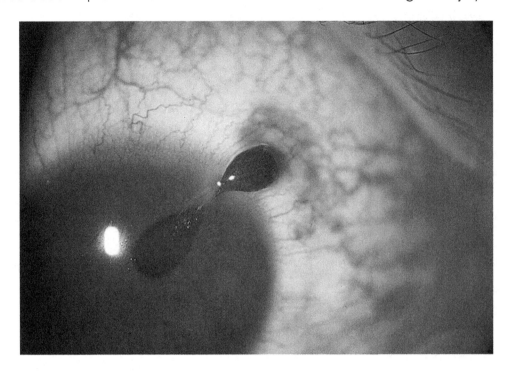

Open globe injury with an elliptical pupil and a portion of the iris herniating through the cornea

Superficial Lid Laceration

- A superficial lid laceration does not penetrate the full thickness of the eyelid and does not include the lid margins, the tarsal plate, eyelid musculature, or the eye itself
- Penetration of the eye by a foreign object must be ruled out.
- The eyelid does not contain fat, so presence of fat protruding from an eyelid laceration should make one suspicious for orbital trauma.
- Treatment of superficial lid lacerations is the same as that for other minor lacerations
    - ☐ Use clean gauze to apply pressure to the wound to stop the bleeding
    - ☐ It is important not to put pressure on the eye but rather on the surrounding bones of the orbit
    - ☐ After the bleeding stops, irrigate the wound with clean water or saline solution to remove dirt or foreign objects
    - ☐ The wound may be closed with suture or tape depending on availability of materials and provider experience
    - ☐ Do not use tissue adhesive (skin glue) to close lid lacerations due to the possibility of getting the material in the eye

☐ Cover the wound with a sterile non-adherent dressing or gauze

☐ Monitor daily for signs of infection

☐ Depending on the severity of the laceration, evacuation may be necessary for definitive repair

Complex Lid Laceration

A complex lid laceration penetrates the full thickness of the lid, includes the lid margins, or is within 5mm of the medial canthus (due to proximity to the lacrimal duct)

Penetration of the globe must be ruled out

Use sterile gauze to stop the bleeding. Irrigate the laceration with saline solution or clean water

Most health care providers are not comfortable closing complex lid lacerations. There is a considerable risk of poor cosmetic and functional outcome if the laceration is not closed appropriately. The wound should be treated with antibiotic ointment and then kept covered

Due to the need for repair, patients with complex lid lacerations should be evacuated

Blunt Orbital Trauma

Blunt force to the globe or surrounding bony orbit and soft tissues can fracture the thin bones that hold the eye in place

In most cases, significant periocular bruising and swelling will occur

There may also be restriction of eye movements, due entrapment of the muscle belly in the fracture. This most commonly affects the inferior rectus muscle as the floor of the orbit is much weaker.

Significant swelling, restricted eye movements, clear fluid leaking from of the nose, and decreased vision following blunt trauma to the orbit suggest considerable damage. The victim should be evacuated for evaluation and treatment.

Corneal Abrasion

Abrasions occur when the epithelial layer of the cornea is disrupted

A corneal abrasion may result in moderate to severe pain, tearing, and sensitivity to light

Patients often report having a foreign body sensation in their eye

Evaluation:

☐ Evaluate the eye to ensure there is not a globe perforation or foreign body on the cornea

☐ Apply a topical anesthetic. This will classically resolve all discomfort and also allows for further evaluation of the eye

☐ Apply fluorescein dye and examine the eye with a woods lamp if available. If present, a corneal abrasion will appear bright green when viewed with the UV light (see picture below).

■ Treatment:

☐ Common practice is to apply a topical ophthalmic antibiotic if available, particularly in contact lens wearers or abrasions from vegetative matter. If not available, the abrasion should still heal well.

☐ Cycloplegic drops (papillary dilators) may help ease the discomfort by halting ciliary spasm

☐ Topical NSAIDs may also be of benefit

☐ Artificial tears can provide substantial relief with minimal to no side effects

☐ Though seldom done in the hospital setting, consider patching the eye for comfort

  ● This is done by tightly taping a piece of gauze from the forehead to the cheekbone

  ● Eye patching is not a necessity and does not decrease time to recovery, but some victims report that this provides relief from their symptoms

☐ If the patient wears contact lenses, then he or she should not wear them until the abrasion is fully healed. They are at risk for developing a corneal ulcer.

■ The epithelial layer of the cornea heals rapidly, usually within 24 to 72 hours

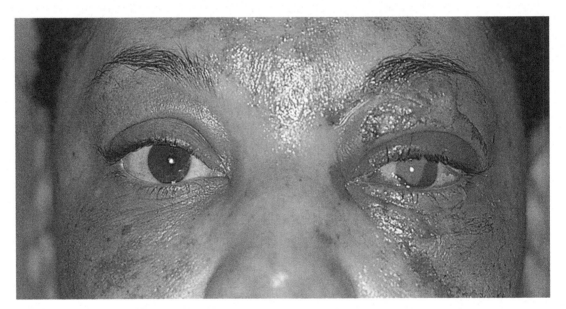

Large corneal abrasion of patient's left eye with fluorescein uptake

Hyphema

■ A hyphema is a collection of blood in the anterior chamber of the eye and can result from blunt or penetrating trauma

■ Hyphemas are best examined in the sitting or standing position, as the blood will settle, resulting in the formation of a meniscus in the anterior chamber. This allows the provider to determine how much blood is present. Small hyphemas can be difficult to appreciate when the patient is lying flat.

■ Hyphema is a serious condition that mandates evacuation due to its potential complications, which include acute glaucoma, vision loss, and rebleeding

Frequent reevaluation recommended given potential for rebleeding resulting in glaucoma and worsening status

Use an eye shield to protect the eye from any further trauma

The use of topical steroids, pupillary dilators, and pupillary constrictors remains somewhat controversial, though use could be considered to assist with pain management

Avoid aspirin, ibuprofen, or any other medications that may cause more bleeding

Control of nausea/vomiting is important as nausea/vomiting may result in increased intraocular pressure

Activity should also be restricted as much as possible during evacuation, though ambulation has not been shown to increase the risk of rebleeding

If able, elevation of head to 30 degrees promotes settling of the blood in the anterior chamber away from the visual axis while maintaining arterial blood flow compared to head fully upright

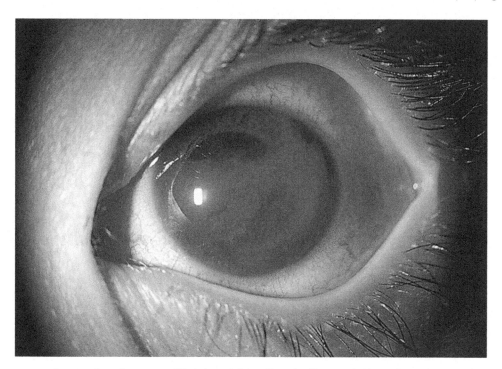

Large hyphema with blood fl oating in the anterior chamber

NON-TRAUMATIC EYE COMPLAINTS

Non-traumatic eye complaints are typically broken down into those with a normal-appearing eye, a "white eye" or a "red eye"

Acute Vision Loss in a Normal-Appearing Eye

Acute vision loss in a normal appearing eye is a serious condition.

The differential of acute vision loss in a normal-appearing eye includes:

- ☐ Retinal detachment
- ☐ Central retinal artery occlusion
- ☐ Central retinal vein occlusion
- ☐ Optic Neuritis
- ☐ Artery ischemic optic neuropathy (temporal arteritis)
- ☐ Vitreous hemorrhage

There is no definitive treatment available in the wilderness for any of these issues.

The immediate concern is evacuation of the patient.

Acute Red Eye

The acute red eye is often further subdivided into two groups:

- ☐ Those who have no pain or have their pain relieved by the application of topical anesthesia, thus indicating the issue involves the surface of the eye only
- ☐ Those who have pain that is not relieved by topical anesthesia, which indicates the problem lies deeper within the eye

Red Eye with No Pain or Pain Relieved by Topical Anesthesia

Differential:

Subconjunctival hemorrhage

Conjunctivitis

Corneal ulcer

Corneal erosion

HSV (herpes) keratitis

UV keratitis

Conjunctival foreign body

Dry eye

Episcleritis

Subconjunctival Hemorrhage

Subconjunctival hemorrhage is accumulation of blood in the space between the conjunctiva and sclera

This results in an extremely red-looking ("bloodshot") eye but is rarely a serious condition

This condition may occur spontaneously or as a result of increased intrathoracic pressure, which occurs with straining or coughing

It normally resolves over a period of a few days to two weeks without treatment

If this occurs from trauma, examine the eye for other more serious injuries, such as a foreign body or perforation

Conjunctivitis

The major causes of conjunctivitis are viral, bacterial, and allergic

Conjunctivitis is usually self-limiting and requires no treatment.

In the wilderness, the most practical treatment for the symptoms of these conditions is cold compresses using snow, ice or a cool wet cloth if available

Since the cause of conjunctivitis may be difficult to diagnose, providers will often prescribe topical antibiotic ointment or drops in case there is a bacterial cause

If topical antibiotics are unavailable in the wilderness, or if inflammation becomes worse after a few days of treatment, it may be appropriate to evacuate for evaluation and treatment

If a red eye is accompanied by decreased visual acuity or if the cornea becomes opaque or cloudy, evacuation is necessary because these symptoms may denote a more serious ocular disease

Corneal Ulcer

This represents an acute corneal defect caused by an infection

This is commonly seen in contact lens wearers

They also can occur as a result of a superinfected corneal abrasion

These are usually very painful

Topical anesthesia will relieve most of the pain of the ulcer, though a small amount may remain due to the pain caused by ciliary muscle spasm

Fluorescein uptake will be noted on exam

Contact lenses should not be worn if an ulcer is noted

Treatment is topical fluoroquinolones and evacuation

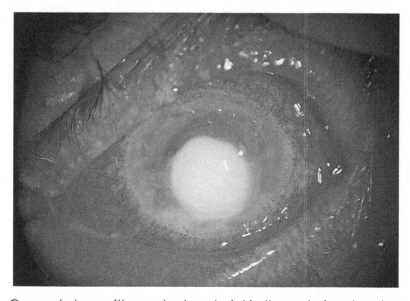

Corneal ulcer with purulent material in the anterior chamber

Corneal Erosion

- This is an atraumatic corneal defect
- On exam, this will appear similar to a corneal abrasion
- There is often a history of prior episodes or prior history of corneal surgery
- This occurs due to a defect in healing of the cornea
- Symptoms may be noted on awakening in the morning, as the opening of the lids may pull corneal membrane off the basement layer
- Treatment in the wilderness is the same as that for a corneal abrasion
- This case may be helped with lubrication from erythromycin ointment, particularly at night

HSV Keratitis

- Corneal infection that results from HSV inoculation
- Results in severe eye pain, similar to an ulcer or abrasion
- On fluorescein staining a dendritic lesion will classically be noted (see picture below)
- There may be a history of prior herpetic infection
- The patient should be evacuated for treatment. If you have oral or topical antivirals, you can start them while coordinating evacuation.

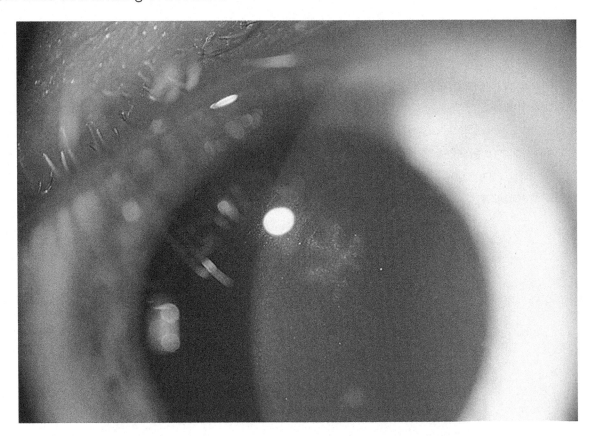

Herpes infection of the cornea with a dendritic lesion

UV Keratitis

- Caused by UV exposure and is essentially a sunburn of the cornea
- Symptoms begin about 6 to 10 hours after the sun exposure and victims typically are not aware that damage is occurring during the time of actual exposure
- Victims are usually very uncomfortable and their pain is worse with light exposure
- Sunglasses or eye patching may help with the discomfort
- Scopolamine or cyclopentolate may be helpful by reducing ciliary spasm
- Prevention is the key with this exposure. When travelling on snow or water, it is important to wear sunglasses or glacier goggles in order to prevent corneal damage.
- Altitude is a significant risk factor as UV damage is more significant at altitude.

Conjunctival or Corneal Foreign Body

- When patients have a foreign body sensation in their eyes, it is important to do a thorough examination to find it, this includes everting the upper and lower lids
- If a foreign body cannot be seen but you continue to suspect one may be present, irrigation with artificial tears or sweeping with a cotton swab may be successful
- After removal, the eye should be treated as for a corneal abrasion
- Do not attempt to remove foreign objects embedded in the cornea. If an object persists in the cornea or cannot be removed from the conjunctiva, apply a strip of bacitracin ointment to the lower lid.
- **Evacuation will be necessary because corneal foreign bodies can cause permanent scarring and conjunctival foreign bodies can become infected.**

Dry Eye

- This is a frequent wilderness problem due to wind exposure as well as the dry conditions associated with high altitude
- It is a diagnosis of exclusion, and other conditions such as foreign bodies, ulcers and abrasions must be ruled out before blaming dry eye for the patient's symptoms
- There may be a history of previous dry eye
- Treatment is with artificial tears
- Lubricating ointments can also be helpful
- Goggles and glasses that protect from the wind are also helpful

Episcleritis

- This is a benign inflammation of the eye lining between the sclera and the conjunctiva
- There is no discharge

There is no pain, photophobia, or change in vision

The presence of anything beyond very mild discomfort means another diagnosis

Episcleritis resolves without treatment and evacuation is not required

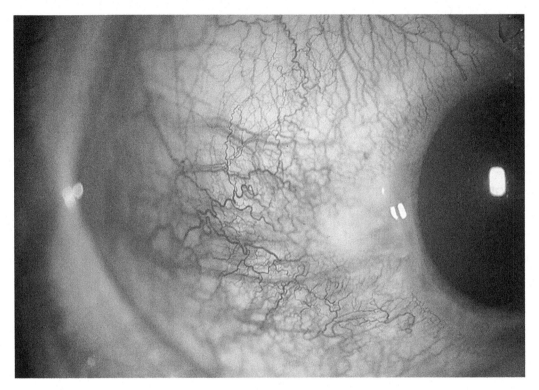

Episcleritis

Painful Red Eye (NOT Relieved with Topical Anesthesia)

Differential:

Iritis

Acute angle closure glaucoma

Scleritis

All etiologies require evacuation

Iritis (nontraumatic)

Iritis can occur after any corneal trauma as well as from non-traumatic causes

Non-traumatic iritis is associated with a number of systemic infectious and inflammatory diseases

The eye is red with marked ciliary flush

Photophobia is seen

Consensual photophobia is often present

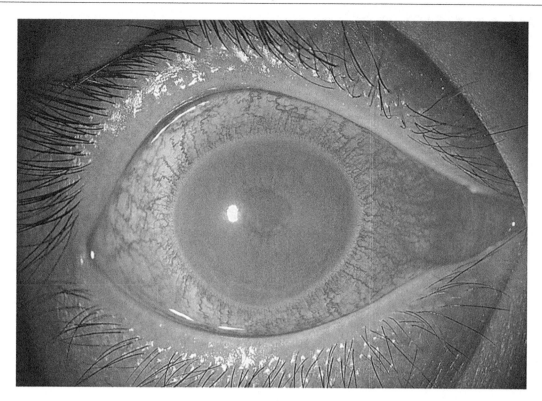

Iritis with ciliary flush and cloudiness of the cornea

Glaucoma

This is seen in individuals typically over age 50

Diagnosis is made in the clinical setting by measuring intraocular pressure, but in the wilderness you should be suspicious for angle closure glaucoma if the patient's pain is deep, not relived by topical anesthesia and is associated with a pupil that is fixed in mid-dilation and a steamy (cloudy) cornea.

Nausea and vomiting are often present

Treatment is with topical pilocarpine and/or timolol if available

Acetazolamide, if carried, can also be given

Evacuate emergently, as prolonged elevated ocular pressure does result in loss of vision

Scleritis

Appears similar to iritis

May require a slit lamp to differentiate

Wilderness treatment is the same as with iritis

MISCELLANEOUS CONDITIONS

Perioribital/orbital cellulitis

- Can be difficult to differentiate
- Periorbital is localized inflammation/infection to the anterior soft tissue surround the eye
  - ☐ Typically caused by spread of infection from blepharitis, conjunctivitis, sinusitis, or more commonly in the wilderness from a scratch or insect bite
  - ☐ If localized superficially, can be treated with oral antibiotic that covers for *Strep*, MRSA, and *Haemophilus influenza B* in the wilderness
- Orbital cellulitis is a deeper associated infection surrounding the eye, which is more serious
  - ☐ Associated with pain with ocular movements
  - ☐ May have fever and a change in vision
  - ☐ Evacuation as soon as possible is strongly recommended while initiating oral antibiotics

Altitude Associated Conditions

- People who have had corneal surgery may have decreased vision at altitude second to hypoxia causing corneal edema
  - ☐ More commonly associated with radial keratotomy
  - ☐ Generally resolves completely with descent
- Retinal hemorrhages
  - ☐ Often correlated with AMS
  - ☐ Difficult to diagnose at altitude
  - ☐ If occurs on the visual axis, recommend descent and evacuation

EVACUATION GUIDELINES

- Evacuate immediately if the globe has been perforated
- Evacuate immediately if there is sudden loss of vision, particularly in a normal-appearing eye
- Evacuate as soon as possible if there is a complex lid laceration or hyphema, or if the cornea becomes cloudy
- Evacuate as soon as possible any acute red eye condition where the pain is severe and not relieved with topical anesthesia
- Evacuate corneal ulcers as soon as possible
- Few red eye conditions that do not have pain or improve with topical anesthesia should be evacuated. Corneal ulcer, HSV keratitis, or retained conjunctival foreign body are of the few that should be evacuated.

QUESTIONS

1. **You are on a camping trip when a 60-year-old male member of your party awakens in the morning up with a red eye. He does not complain of vision loss and, in fact, does not notice any problem until you bring it to his attention. What is the next best step?**
   a. Apply ointment and patch the eye
   b. Evacuate immediately
   c. Irrigate the eye with saline or clean water
   d. Monitor for signs of vision loss or pain

2. **On a youth wilderness excursion, a young man is struck in the forehead with a tree branch during a robust game of tag. The victim falls on the ground and complains of severe eye pain. A small dry twig is lodged in the white part of the eye and does not fall out. Before evacuating, what should be done?**
   a. Apply ointment and patch the eye
   b. Do not remove the twig and tape a shield over the eye
   c. Give the patient aspirin or ibuprofen for the pain
   d. Remove the twig and patch the eye

3. **The morning after a long day of river rafting, a 58-year-old female complains of having seen light flashes during the night even with her eyes closed. Now, in the daytime with her eyes open, she sees dark dirt-like spots in one field of vision. What is the next best step?**
   a. Apply ointment and patch the eye
   b. Evacuate immediately
   c. Irrigate the eye with saline or clean water
   d. Monitor over time for signs of vision loss

4. **It is beginning to become dark on a trail and you accidentally walk into a low-lying branch that scrapes your eye. You feel intense pain that makes it difficult to open your eye. During the brief moments when you eye is open, you notice your vision to be unchanged. What is the next best step?**
   a. Apply direct pressure to the eye
   b. Apply ointment, patch the eye, and evacuate immediately
   c. Apply ointment and reassess in the morning
   d. Rinse the eye with river water, apply ointment, patch the eye, and reassess in the morning

Answers:
1. d
2. b
3. b
4. c

CHAPTER 14

Animal Bites and Stings

This chapter will train you on general issues, injury prevention and wilderness treatment of animal bites and stings when encountering the following land and marine creatures:

- Domesticated Animals
- Wild Animals
- Venomous Snakes
- Mosquitoes
- Spiders
- Ticks
- Hymenoptera
- Scorpions
- Jellyfish
- Stinging fish
- Sea snakes

CASE 1

You and a friend are camping in the Appalachians. You awaken to roars and thumps outside your tent. Looking out the tent flap, you see your friend on the ground in the fetal position as a black bear knocks him around. You see potato chips scattered all over the campground.

1. What is the best approach to stopping the bear from attacking your friend?
2. Would your approach be different if you were in Alaska and it was a grizzly (brown) bear?

CASE 2

You are camping with a friend when he comes running out of the woods being chased by several bees. After he runs approximately ¼ mile, the bees stop chasing him. Your friend comes to you with approximately 10 stings, several of which still contain a stinger with the sac attached. He does not have any breathing problems or airway swelling. He feels slightly dizzy, but does not appear to be sick. He has no problems breathing.

1. What is the best way to remove the stingers from the wounds?
2. If you have an EpiPen®, should you treat your friend with it?
3. Does he require evacuation from the site or should you just observe him?

CASE 3

A 24-year-old female has been swimming off the Gulf Coast when she notes the onset of an immediate stinging sensation on an arm and leg. Approximately 30 feet away you notice what appears to be a number of small "sails" floating on the water. On examining her, you notice a papular erythematous rash that has a "tentacle-like" appearance.

1. What should be the immediate treatment on the beach?
2. What is the cause?
3. What signs of severe envenomation is one able to notice?

DOMESTICATED ANIMALS

General

The majority (80% to 90%) of domesticated animal bites are from dogs.

Cat bites account for 5% to 15% of domestic animal bites.

Victims of bites are often pet owners or members of the pet owner's family.

Wilderness Care

Conduct a primary and secondary survey to ensure the victim is stable.

Direct pressure should be used to stop bleeding.

Wounds that do not break the skin can be treated with ice and anti-inflammatory medications.

The wound should be irrigated and debrided as soon as possible, especially if the victim is more than one hour from definitive medical care.

- ☐ Sterile water is not required, but the cleaner the water, the better.
- ☐ Irrigation should be done under "high" pressure (7 to 8 psi).
- ☐ Debride the wound with a soft clean cloth or sterile gauze.
- ☐ Dress the wound with an antibacterial ointment and a clean cloth or sterile gauze.

Wound Closure

Whether to close a bite wound, as well as the timing of closure, is an area of ongoing debate. This is covered more thoroughly in the wound management chapter.

Wound Infections

Infection is common with animal bites. Specific microbes and antimicrobials are discussed below.

Bites are tetanus-prone wounds, so ensure that tetanus immunization is up-to-date.

Rabies

Rabies is a concern when dealing with both domestic and wild animal attacks.

Management of a wound at risk for rabies should include the following:

- ☐ Good wound cleansing that should include the use of soap and water when possible. This is the one time when you would clean a wound with soap as the positive effect of being virucidal (killing the rabies virus) outweighs the risk of inhibiting wound healing.

- ☐ Additionally, the wound should be irrigated with Zephiran (1% benzalkonium chloride) or 1% povidone iodine. Both of these act as virucidal agents that may eliminate the rabies virus before it can enter muscle cells.
- ☐ Consider the need for rabies immune globulin and vaccination. While not a cause for immediate evacuation, the need for these treatments may necessitate shortening a trip.
- ☐ The Center for Disease Control (CDC) has a 24-hour helpline that can assist in determining the need to administer the vaccine. The CDC can be contacted by clinicians at 1-877-554-4625 or via the web at http://www.cdc.gov/rabies.

Dog Bites

Background

Dogs younger than one year are responsible for the highest incidence of bites.

The highest incident of dog bites occurs in children in summer months.

Prevention

Never leave a child alone with a dog.

Do not pet other dogs without permission.

Do not lean over and pet a dog on the head.

Do not physically separate fighting dogs; instead, use the spray from a water hose.

Never take a bone or toy away from an unfamiliar dog.

Do not approach a nursing dog.

Teach injury prevention regarding dogs to children from an early age.

Know the look of an angry dog and avoid animals that display barking, growling, bared teeth, flattened ears, erected tail, or hair standing on end.

Never pet or step over a sleeping dog.

Treatment

Treat the victim using victim management and wound care as outlined above.

Pasteurella multocida is a common pathogen found in wound infections from dog bites.

Simple wounds from dog bites have similar infection rates to other domesticated animals.

Prophylactic antibiotics are not necessary for most dog bites.

Antibiotic indications:

- ☐ Signs of infection
- ☐ Bite on face present for > 24 hours OR bite on extremity > 8 hours without adequate irrigation and cleansing
- ☐ Immunocompromised state for the victim
- ☐ Crush injury or significant contamination of wound
- ☐ Bite wounds of the hands or feet

Antibiotic treatment, if indicated, as above:

- ☐ Amoxicillin-clavulanate
- ☐ Clindamycin + fluoroquinolone if penicillin allergic
- ☐ Clindamycin + trimethoprim/sulfamethoxazole (TMP/SMX) if penicillin allergic in children

Cat Bites

General

- Cat bites have a higher infection rate in comparison to other domestic animals.
- Greater than 60% of cat bites are on the hand or finger; these wounds may be deep puncture wounds, which are difficult to clean.
- 70% of cat bite infections are due to *Pasteurella*.
- Cat scratches and bites on less risky areas may be watched closely.
- Indications for antibiotics are the same as with dog bites as outlined above.
- Antibiotic treatment
  - ☐ Amoxicillin/clavulanate
  - ☐ Clindamycin + fluoroquinolone if penicillin allergic
  - ☐ Clindamycin + trimethoprim/sulfamethoxazole (TMP/SMX) if penicillin allergic in children

WILD ANIMALS

General

- The incidence of wild animal bites is difficult to ascertain as many minor wilderness bites and attacks are not reported.
- In Asia and Africa, thousands of people are killed yearly by attacks from lions, tigers, elephants, hippos, crocodiles and snakes.
- In North America, large animals, like bears and cougars, kill very few people.
  - ☐ In Yellowstone National Park, for example, a visitor is more likely to be struck by lightning than to sustain serious injury from a large animal.

Prevention

- Animal behavior holds the key to prevention of most animal attacks.
- Aside from large carnivores, most animals do not attack humans unless provoked.
- The most common examples of human provocation of wild animals occur during time of animal capture or restraint.
- Even a very shy animal can inflict a life-threatening injury if it is cornered.

If contact with an animal is likely or necessary, a close observation of the animal's behaviors and cues should be undertaken to avoid mishap.

Treatment

Treatment of wild animal attacks is similar to treatment of a domestic animal attack.

In general, larger animals should raise more suspicion of blunt and penetrating trauma, including deep arterial damage, nerve damage and internal organ damage.

Antibiotic choice follows that of domestic attacks, with the exception of attacks that occur in natural bodies of fresh water (alligator or crocodile bite), where antibiotics should also be directed against *Aeromonas hydrophila*, or in salt (ocean) water, where antibiotics should also be directed against *Vibrio* species.

Bear Attacks

Background

North American bears include the brown (grizzly and Kodiak), American black and polar bears.

Bears are fast (running up to 40 mph), large (140 to 1,400 pounds) and have a keen sense of smell and hearing.

A bear's sight ability is equal or less in acuity to that of a human.

Bear attacks are more common in the summer months when wilderness visitors are more numerous and bears are not hibernating.

The most common scenario that ends in a brown bear attack occurs when there is a sudden and unexpected close encounter.

Victims are rarely killed.

The wounds are described as a mauling, but the bear often inflicts the injuries and leaves without inflicting wounds to its maximum capability.

Attacks that are more likely to be fatal include encroaching on a bear that is wounded, with a cub or near a carcass.

In contrast to the brown bear, black bears rarely attack because of close encounters. Black female bears with cubs are more apt to flee an area if the human shows aggression.

Prevention

Make noise, such as talking, and allow the bear(s) to move away from you.

Be cautious in environments where a bear may not be able to hear you, such as near loud streams and in uneven terrain.

Avoid common bear areas, such as streams with spawning fish, berry groves, and carcasses.

If spotted by a bear, allow it to see you as human by stepping forward to allow the bear a full view of you.

If able to avoid an attack, wait until the bear has left the area and then move in the opposite direction.

Pepper spray *may* be useful if discharged directly at a charging bear's head when it is within thirty feet. Pepper spray is NOT to be used as mosquito repellent. Pepper spray discharged in a camp may actually serve as a bear attractant.

If you encounter a **brown** bear, take the following actions:

- ☐ Do not look into the bear's eyes, as this is interpreted by the bear as a sign of aggression.
- ☐ Do not make any sudden movements.
- ☐ Do not run.
- ☐ Do not act aggressively toward the bear.
- ☐ Stand your ground, but be submissive.
- ☐ If attacked, quickly get into the fetal position with your neck protected, because attacking bears are "head oriented."
- ☐ If rolled onto your back, protect your face with your elbows.

If you encounter a **black** bear, take the following actions:

- ☐ Yell, throw things and act aggressively toward the bear. Black bears usually flee in response to aggression.
- ☐ If the black bear attacks, then you should continue to fight and kick against the bear as much as possible. The reason for this is that the bear is attacking you because he wants to eat you and has lost the fear of humans.

Treatment

The possibility of significant injury is high, so all bear attack victims should be considered blunt trauma victims and, therefore, candidates for immediate evacuation.

The CDC recommends rabies immunization for all victims of carnivore attacks. However, no cases of rabies have been reported as a result of bear attack. For specific recommendations, contact the CDC as instructed at the beginning of the chapter.

Cougar Attacks

The North American cougar (mountain lion, puma) are coming into contact with humans with increasing frequency.

Cougars are most commonly encountered in the western United States.

Cougars hunt by stealth, then pounce and break the victim's neck.

As with lions, cougars can be scared off by utilizing aggressive behavior toward the animal. This is less likely in the case of a cougar with a cub or with a wounded cougar.

When confronted by a cougar, face it, talk very loudly, and make yourself appear as a threat.

Do not turn and run away from a cougar.

If you have small children with you, pick them up, as the cougar preferentially attacks children.

If the cougar attacks, fight back using anything available, including rocks, sticks, and bare fists.

SNAKES

General

Background

North America has two native types of poisonous snakes:

- ☐ Pit vipers (subfamily Crotalinae)
- ☐ Coral snakes (family Elapidae)

The overwhelming majority of envenomations in the U.S. are from pit vipers.

Annually, there are approximately 9,000 snake bites reported to U.S. Poison Control Centers. This may underestimate the true number as many victims never present and there is no mandatory reporting.

Approximately 2,000 people are treated annually as envenomations.

From 1991 to 2001, there were 57 deaths attributed to snake envenomation in the U.S.

It is estimated that approximately 100,000 deaths from snakebites occur annually worldwide.

Pit vipers are found in 47 of the 48 contiguous states (all except Maine).

Pit Vipers

Background

In the U.S., pit vipers include multiple species of rattlesnake, the copperhead and the cottonmouth (water moccasin).

Pit vipers have specific recognizable anatomy:

- ☐ Triangle-shaped head
- ☐ Catlike, elliptical pupils
- ☐ Heat-sensing pits between eyes and nose

Venom is dispersed from ducts in the fangs.

Approximately 25% of pit viper bites are "dry" or without injection of venom.

Pit viper venom can be hemotoxic (attacking tissue and blood) and/or neurotoxic (damaging or destroying nerve tissue).

In the U.S., pit viper venom is hemotoxic. The one exception is the Mojave rattler, which has venom with primary neurotoxic properties.

Each snake has a varying potency of its venom based on multiple factors:

- ☐ Emotional state of snake
- ☐ Age of the snake
- ☐ Time of year that the bite occurs
- ☐ Location of bite
- ☐ Size, age, and health of victim
- ☐ Depth of the bite
- ☐ Amount of venom injected

Clinical Manifestations of Pit Viper Envenomation

- Severe burning at the bite site within minutes
- Soft tissue swelling outward from the bite
- Blood oozing from the bite
- Ecchymosis (local and distal)
- Nausea and vomiting
- Weakness
- Rubber, minty, or metallic taste in the mouth
- Numbness of mouth and tongue
- Fasciculations and paresthesias
- Increased heart and respiratory rates
- Respiratory distress in severe cases
- Hypotension and shock

Treatment

- Evacuate all victims of bites from venomous snakes while minimizing physical activity.
- Support of airway, breathing and circulation while transporting.
- Tight-fitting jewelry and clothing should be removed to avoid a tourniquet effect.
- The forward edge of swelling should be marked every 15 minutes for physicians to assess the severity of the envenomation.
- Treatment with antivenom should generally be reserved for the hospital due to potentially serious complications, including anaphylaxis.
- Snake bite treatment has been plagued over the years with poor suggestions and bad information. The following is **a list of things to avoid** because they are either harmful to the victim or do not work:
  - ☐ The Sawyer Extractor™ has been touted to remove up to 20% to 30% of injected venom if applied within two to three minutes of the bite. However, multiple recent studies show no evidence of decreased morbidity or mortality, and, in turn, there is a potential increase for tissue damage. Therefore, the Extractor is NOT recommended.
  - ☐ Do NOT use pressure immobilization. Simple immobilization is fine, but it has no proven benefit.
  - ☐ Electric shock therapy should NOT be used and can be harmful.
  - ☐ Local application of ice has not been adequately studied. Packing the affected limb in ice (cryotherapy) is contraindicated, as it may worsen necrosis.
  - ☐ Do NOT attempt to try to catch or kill the offending snake. Therapeutic recommendations for North American snake envenomations are the same for all species and attempts to capture a snake may result in additional envenomation and potentially another victim. Even a dead snake's jaw can clamp down and envenomate a human.
  - ☐ Do NOT use aspirin, as it may worsen bleeding.
  - ☐ Do NOT cut and suck on the wound, as this maneuver may infect the wound with oral bacteria and is ineffective at removing venom.

□ Do NOT use alcohol on the wound or as an oral analgesic.

□ Do NOT use a tight fitting tourniquet that restricts arterial or venous flow.

If available, two large-bore IVs should be established, and hypotension should be treated with normal saline or Ringer's lactate.

Analgesia will likely be necessary and should be administered, avoiding non-steroidal anti-inflammatory drugs and aspirin.

Although two types of antivenom are available, CroFab® has been shown to be more effective and safer than the polyvalent antivenom manufactured by Wyeth-Ayerst Laboratories.

CroFab® antivenom should be administered to all patients who have either or both of the following:

□ Signs of progressive local envenomation

□ Evidence of any systemic toxicity

Tetanus immunization should be updated if needed.

Evacuation

Victims of a pit viper bite should be emergently evacuated.

Coral Snake

Background

Coral snakes in the U.S. have a very distinct color banding pattern.

An easy way to remember the banding of the deadly coral snake is, "Red on black, venom lack; red on yellow, kill a fellow." In other words, a red band adjacent to a yellow (not black) band indicates a venomous species in North America. Color patterns of venomous coral snakes differ in other countries.

The bite of the coral snake typically involves a finger, toe, or fold of skin, because the coral snake is unable to widely open its jaws.

Clinical Manifestations of Coral Snake Envenomation

Mild, transient pain at the time of the bite

Minimal or no local swelling

Fang marks may be difficult to identify

Systemic symptoms will often progress rapidly once they appear

Nausea and vomiting

Headache

Abdominal pain

Diaphoresis and pallor

Paresthesias and numbness

Drowsiness

Euphoria

Treatment

Basic supportive treatment is the same as for pit viper envenomation.

Pressure immobilization has been studied on animal models and is used in Australia for elapid snake-bites but is not indicated for coral snake bites in the United States.

☐ Wrap the area snugly with fabric in a way that will impair lymphatic flow, but not venous or arterial flow.

☐ Any type of fabric, including an elastic bandage, works well.

☐ Monitor for subsequent swelling which might make the wrap too tight.

Antivenom administration should be planned for all victims of elapid bites, as symptoms initially may be minimal but progress rapidly.

Evacuation

All victims of a coral snake bite should be evacuated as soon as possible.

MOSQUITOES

Background

According to the World Health Organization in 2015

☐ About 3.2 billion people, nearly half of the world's population, are at risk of malaria.

☐ In 2015, there were roughly 214 million malaria cases and an estimated 438 000 malaria deaths

☐ Increased prevention and control measures have led to a 60% reduction in malaria mortality rates globally since 2000.

☐ Sub-Saharan Africa was home to 89% of malaria cases and 91% of malaria deaths.

Other mosquito-borne illnesses include encephalitis, yellow fever, dengue, chikungunya, zika, and lymphatic filariasis.

Mosquito-borne diseases found in the U.S. are eastern equine encephalitis, western equine encephalitis, St. Louis encephalitis, La Crosse encephalitis and West Nile virus.

If you are traveling to a location where you are unsure of the mosquito risk, consult the Centers for Disease Control and Prevention (CDC) website: http://www.cdc.gov/travel/index.htm. This website is very helpful for comprehensive, timely information on which immunizations (e.g., yellow fever) and prophylactic antibiotics (e.g., for malaria) are recommended.

Prevention

Mosquitoes are attracted by CO_2, lactic acid, warm skin, and moisture. They also gravitate toward the smell of soap, detergents, and perfumes.

Mosquitoes are most active at dusk, so staying indoors during that time will decrease contact.

Choose a campsite that is above and away from standing water.

Wear clothing with long sleeves and long socks with pants tucked into socks or boots.

Wear clothing that is tightly woven, such as nylon, and is loose fitting so that a mosquito cannot bite through the clothing.

Permethrin is a naturally occurring compound with insecticidal and some repellant properties that will remain on clothing for weeks when properly applied.

- ☐ Apply permethrin to clothing and bedding, especially mosquito netting.
- ☐ Do not apply directly to skin.

Insect repellent should be applied to uncovered skin.

DEET is the gold standard for insect repellents.

- ☐ It is sold in formulations of 5% to 35%.
- ☐ Use formulations of 10% or less in children and avoid use altogether in infants under 6 months of age.
- ☐ Use formulations of 30% to 35% in malaria areas on adults.
- ☐ Do not use sunscreens that contain DEET, as sunscreens need to be used liberally and often, whereas DEET should be used less often.
- ☐ When using both sunscreen and DEET, first apply the sunscreen then apply the DEET approximately 30 minutes later.
- ☐ Multiple non-DEET repellents have been studied. Though some have shown similar effectiveness, most do not provide protection for durations similar to those of DEET-based repellents.

Multiple other repellants have been studied extensively. Noteworthy ones include the following:

- ☐ Bite Blocker
  - A combination of multiple natural oils
  - It has not been as well studied as other products, but appears to have similar efficacy to 20% DEET.
- ☐ Citronella
  - Developed as a natural extract from Cymbopogon nardus grass
  - Effective for approximately 40 minutes but significantly less so than DEET
  - Sitting near Citronella candles may decrease bites by 42%. However, ordinary candles have been shown to decrease bites by 23%.
- ☐ Eucalyptus
  - Has an average protection times of 4 to 7.5 hours and is nearly as effective as DEET
- ☐ IR3535
  - Marketed in U.S. by Avon as "Skin-So-Soft Bug Guard Plus"
  - Studies demonstrate a half-life of 20 min to 6 hrs.
  - Overall, it's less effective than 12.5% DEET

- ☐ Picaridin
    - 20% concentration has been shown to have similar efficacy as 20% DEET for up to eight hours.
    - In the U.S., 7% Picaridin is marketed as "Cutter Advanced" and has similar efficacy to 10% DEET.
    - Picaridin has notably less malodor and less staining of materials than DEET.
- ☐ In a study in Alaska, individuals wearing permethrin-treated uniforms and DEET repellant had more than 99.9% protection over 8 hours, even under intense biting conditions
    - Unprotected persons received an average of 1,188 bites/hr.

In summary, from current studies, Permethrin-treated clothing plus DEET or Picaridin-based repellents confer best protection.

Treatment

Incubation period for mosquito-borne diseases is anywhere from 48 hours to one year or more.

Treatment recommendations for systemic symptoms after suspected mosquito bites vary depending on the area of travel and suspicion for resistant infection such as malaria. Consult the CDC website listed above or a travel medicine specialist before travel.

SPIDERS

Background

Many spiders are venomous, but only a few are dangerous to humans.
- ☐ Many spiders do not have enough venom to affect a human.
- ☐ Many spiders do not have fangs large enough to penetrate human skin.

Clinically, significant North American spiders include the following:
- ☐ Black widow
- ☐ Brown recluse
- ☐ Hobo

Black Widow

Background

The black widow is a female of the *Latrodectus* species.

It is characterized by black shiny skin and a red mark on the belly (often an hourglass shape).

It makes its home in irregular webs in sheltered corners of vineyards, fields, and gardens. It can also be found under stones, logs, vegetation, and trash heaps.

Clinical Signs of a Black Widow Bite

- A sharp pinprick is usually, although not always, felt.
- Faint red bite marks may appear later.
- Muscle stiffness and cramps of the bitten limb may ascend to include the abdomen and thorax.
- Additional symptoms include headache, chills, fever, heavy sweating, dizziness, nausea and vomiting, and severe abdominal pain.
- These symptoms occur within 30 to 60 minutes of the bite.
- Most victims of black widow bites have excellent long-term outcomes.
- Short-term problems include hypertension, autonomic instability, CNS dysfunction, and abdominal pain.
- One study showed that only 25% of bite victims progress to more serious symptoms.

Treatment

- Catch the spider, if possible, as even a smashed spider can sometimes be identified under the microscope of an experienced entomologist.
- Clean the bite with soap and water.
- Achieve pain relief with a cold compress and oral medications.
- *Latrodectus* antivenin may be used in the hospital for children and the elderly, but it is rarely used.

Evacuation

- The victim of a bite should be evacuated as soon as possible because envenomation can become very painful and the victim may warrant more medical attention than can be given in the wilderness.

Brown Recluse

Background

- *Loxosceles reclusa*, the brown recluse, is most commonly found in the southern states and up the Mississippi River Valley as far north as Wisconsin.
- The brown recluse may be difficult to identify, as it is generally nondescript, although some have a violin-shaped marking on the top front body portion.
- Its habitat includes small sticky webs under rocks and woodpiles. The brown recluse may also be found in warm human habitats including homes, warehouses, and sheds.

Clinical Signs of a Brown Recluse Bite

- The initial bite is usually painless. The victim is unaware that a bite occurred until it becomes painful, red, pruritic, and swollen two to eight hours after the bite.
- The majority of bites remain localized, healing within three weeks without serious complication or medical intervention.

Additional symptoms may include fever, weakness, vomiting, joint pain, and/or rash.

In more serious cases, the bite may become necrotic.

☐ It will have a white core surrounded by an erythematous patch of skin ending in a blue border.

☐ Within 24 to 48 hours, the central core will blister if the envenomation is more serious. This central core may become necrotic and continue to expand over a period of days to weeks.

☐ Spread is irregular and gravitational in configuration.

☐ In the case of necrosis, scarring is very common.

In rare, more serious envenomations, brown recluse venom has a direct hemolytic effect on human blood. It also effects platelet aggregation. If the reaction becomes systemic, the victim will have hemoglobinuria within 24 hours that lasts for up to a week.

Treatment

Catch the spider, if possible, to allow for identification.

Cleanse the bite with soap and water.

Elevate the extremity and loosely immobilize it.

Place a cold compress and give oral analgesics for pain control.

The victim is in no immediate danger unless systemic signs begin appearing. These include fever or blood in the urine.

Hospital management is only necessary if systemic symptoms occur.

Evacuation

There is no need to evacuate the victim in the absence of systemic symptoms.

Hobo and Funnel-Web Spiders

Background

Tegenaria agrestis, the hobo spider, was introduced to the U.S. in the early 1900s from Europe and/or west central Asia.

☐ In the U.S., it is now found throughout the Pacific Northwest.

☐ It is a 10 to15 mm brown spider with a yellow green tint on the dorsal abdomen.

☐ It builds funnel webs and is found near railroad tracks, under rocks, in woodpiles, and in debris.

Agelenopsis aperta, the funnel-web spider, is found in the southwestern United States.

☐ It builds large sheet-like webs and hides under rocks, logs, or in grass.

Clinical signs

Hobo spider bites may have local necrosis similar to that from a brown recluse spider at the bite site within 36 hours (50% of bites will have local necrosis).

Funnel-web spiders appear more likely to develop painful, non-necrotic lesions with systemic symptoms.

Bites from both spiders may lead to headache, visual disturbances, hallucinations, weakness, and lethargy.

Treatment

Treatment of bites attributed to either of these spiders is supportive.

Catch the spider, if possible, to allow for identification.

Cleanse the bite with soap and water.

■ Pain relief with a cold compress and oral medications.

Evacuation

There is no need to evacuate the victim in the absence of systemic symptoms.

TICKS

Background

Ticks transmit many diseases, including:

- ☐ Lyme Disease
- ☐ Rocky Mountain spotted fever (RMSF)
- ☐ Relapsing fever
- ☐ Colorado tick fever
- ☐ Ehrlichiosis
- ☐ Babesiosis
- ☐ Tularemia
- ☐ Southern Tick-Associated Rash Illness (STARI)

Tick paralysis, a non-infectious ascending paralysis similar to Guillain-Barré syndrome, may occur within five days after the tick attaches. Removal of the tick is curative.

Ticks are found in areas replete with weeds, shrubs, and trails.

They will often be found at forest boundaries where deer and other mammals reside.

Ticks will sit on low-hanging shrubs with legs outstretched until an animal passes.

Once host contact is made, they may take up to several hours to find a suitable spot to attach by their mouthparts.

Prevention

Check clothing and exposed skin for ticks twice daily.

Tuck shirts into pants and pants into socks.

Wear smooth, close woven, loose fitting clothing.

Soak or spray clothing with permethrin.

Wear DEET or similar quality insect repellent.

Treatment

Tick removal:
- ☐ Use thin-tipped tweezers or forceps to grasp the tick as close to the skin surface as possible.
- ☐ Pull the tick straight upward with steady even pressure.
- ☐ Wash the bite with soap and water, then wash hands after the tick has been removed.

Watch for local infection and symptoms of tick-borne illness (incubation period 3 to 30 days), especially headache, fever, and rash.

If Lyme Disease, RMSF, tularemia, or ehrlichiosis is suspected, a tetracycline such as doxycycline can be initiated while evacuation is being planned, if there are not contraindications. Treatment for other tick-borne illnesses is supportive, yet as these may be indistinguishable early in the course, initiating treatment while planning for evacuation is appropriate.

Treatment for tick paralysis is removal of the tick.

Colorado tick fever is caused by a virus; treatment is supportive.

The **DO NOTS** of tick removal:
- ☐ Do not use petroleum jelly
- ☐ Do not use fingernail polish
- ☐ Do not use rubbing alcohol
- ☐ Do not use a hot match
- ☐ Do not use gasoline
- ☐ Do not grab the rear end of the tick. This expels gastric contents and increases the chances of infection
- ☐ Do not twist or jerk the tick, as this will most likely cause incomplete removal of the tick

Evacuation

Most patients with tick bites do not require evacuation, especially if the tick is removed within 24 to 48 hours.

However, if the patient develops fever, headache, vomiting, petechial rash, or other signs of systemic illness, the patient should be urgently evacuated, as illnesses such as RMSF may be rapidly progressive.

For patients who present only with the classic rash of Lyme disease, erythema chronicum migrans (ECM), initiate treatment with doxycycline. As this is curative, in the absence of systemic symptoms, immediate evacuation is not necessary.

HYMENOPTERA

Background

- Hymenoptera is the order of insects that includes ants, bees, and wasps.
- More people die in the U.S. from bee, hornet and wasp stings than from any other animal bites or stings.
- One sting to an allergic person can be fatal in minutes to hours.
- Non-allergic victims may experience fatal toxicity if they sustain multiple stings.
- It takes between 500 to 1,400 simultaneous stings to cause death by toxicity in the non-allergic victim.
- Multiple stings have become more of a concern in the U.S. since Africanized honey bees ("killer bees") first arrived in 1990.

Clinical signs of Hymenoptera Sting

- A local reaction is the most common reaction. It consists of a small red patch that burns and itches.
- The generalized reaction consists of diffuse red skin, hives, swelling of lips and tongue, wheezing, abdominal cramps and diarrhea.
- Stings to the mouth and throat are more serious, as they may cause airway swelling.
- Victims of multiple stings often experience vomiting, diarrhea, dyspnea, hypotension, tachycardia, and syncope. In advanced stages of toxicity, the victim experiences increased muscle activity with hyperkalemia, acute tubular necrosis, renal failure, pancreatitis, coagulopathy, heart attack and stroke.

Prevention

- Do not wear sweet-smelling fragrances, such as certain after-shaves and perfumes. These may attract bees and other insects.
- Bee and wasps are attracted by rotten fruit and fruit syrups.
- Frequent cleaning of garbage areas and proper disposal of old fruit will decrease hymenoptera attraction.
- If an adult has had a full-fledged anaphylactic reaction, he or she should see an allergist for desensitization.
- A hymenoptera-allergic victim should wear medical tags and carry an EpiPen® or other epinephrine auto-injector.

Treatment

- Scrape away the stinger in a horizontal fashion.
  - ☐ Try not to grasp the stinger sac.
  - ☐ However, if one is unable to remove the stinger in a horizontal fashion, it is most important to remove it as soon as possible by any available means.
- Wash the site with soap and water.
- Place a cold compress or ice on the site.
- Give oral analgesics as needed for pain relief.
- Topical steroid cream can be helpful for swelling, as are oral antihistamines.
- If hives occur with wheezing and respiratory difficulty, then epinephrine should be given immediately.
  - ☐ Intramuscular epinephrine (1:1,000) at 0.3 ml for adults and 0.01 ml/kg up to 0.3 ml for children under 12.
  - ☐ The epinephrine injection can be repeated 5 to 10 minutes after the initial injection.
  - ☐ Beta agonist inhalers (e.g., albuterol) may help relieve the wheezing.
  - ☐ Oral steroids and antihistamines should also be added, especially in situations when epinephrine is used.

SCORPIONS

Background

- Scorpions are found in desert and semiarid climates between 50 degrees north and south latitude.
- Most scorpion stings result in only local pain and inflammation.
- In the U.S., the most medically important scorpion is the bark scorpion (genus *Centruroides*); found in the southwestern U.S., primarily Arizona and New Mexico.
- In North America, more serious scorpion stings occur in Mexico.
- The bark scorpion can be lethal to infants and elders.
- The bark scorpion can be found under wood piles, stumps, firewood piles, trees and in a moist indoor environment under blankets, clothing and in shoes.

Clinical Signs of Scorpion Sting

- Scorpions may sting multiple times.
- Except for the bark scorpion, most sting symptoms are similar to hymenoptera stings.

For the bark scorpion:

- ☐ The sting causes local pain followed by numbness and tingling.
- ☐ A neurotoxin released at the time of the sting is the cause of ensuing neuromuscular activity and autonomic dysfunction.
- ☐ Symptoms include paralysis, muscle spasms, breathing problems, vision problems, swallowing difficulty, and slurred speech.
- ☐ Death may result from loss of airway control, loss of respiratory muscle control, metabolic acidosis, hyperthermia and rhabdomyolysis secondary to muscle hyperactivity.

Prevention

Check for scorpions in clothing and shake out shoes when in areas common to scorpions.

Do not place your hands or feet into areas into which you cannot look directly.

Treatment

Clean the sting site with soap and water. Ice is indicated if available.

Place a cool compress for pain and swelling.

Systemic analgesia may be required, if available.

- ☐ If the scorpion is identified as NOT being a bark scorpion:
- ☐ Local treatment and monitoring similar to that for a hymenoptera sting is all that is required.
- ☐ Evacuation is not mandated unless the victim develops systemic symptoms.

If the scorpion is identified as a bark scorpion:

- ☐ Evacuate as soon as possible, because the victim may decompensate rapidly.
- ☐ The need for evacuation is more significant in children and elders.
- ☐ Antivenom is available for severe reactions.

Steroids are not useful unless there is an allergic reaction to the sting.

MARINE ENVENOMATION

Background

Marine creatures cause illness through a number of mechanisms, with the most common being the injection of venom (envenomation).

Marine creatures of most common medical concern can be broken down into several groups:

- ☐ Jellyfish and Portuguese man-of-war
- ☐ Stinging fish
- ☐ Sea snakes

Jellyfish and Portuguese Man-of-War

Background

These ubiquitous marine creatures cause envenomation through their nematocysts (stinging cells). When these cells contact skin, they fire venom-laden tubules into the victim's skin.

The greater the number of nematocyst that contact the victim, the greater the envenomation.

Envenomation can range from mild, which is the most common, to severe and life threatening.

Portuguese man-of-war (*Physalia* species) and the Indo-Pacific box jellyfish (*Chironex fleckeri*) have toxic venoms, with *Chironex* being the more dangerous.

Clinical Signs of Jellyfish and Man-of-War Envenomation

Mild envenomation

- ☐ Seen with most common jellyfish types
- ☐ Skin irritation is the major symptom
- ☐ The man-of-war and the box jellyfish can cause envenomation from mild to severe, depending on the degree of exposure to the tentacles.

Moderate envenomation

- ☐ Skin symptoms occur in addition to multiple organ systems.
- ☐ Neurologic: headache, vertigo, ataxia, nerve palsies, paresthesias, paralysis, coma, and seizures
- ☐ Cardiovascular: hypotension, arterial spasm, arrhythmias, and CHF
- ☐ Respiratory: rhinitis, bronchospasm, oropharyngeal and laryngeal edema, and respiratory failure
- ☐ Musculoskeletal: myalgias, arthralgias, and muscle spasms
- ☐ Gastrointestinal: nausea, emesis, and diarrhea
- ☐ Other: ocular symptoms and renal failure have also occurred

Severe envenomation

- ☐ Occurs most commonly due to highly toxic species

- ☐ Less commonly seen with the Portuguese man-of-war but can occur with significant exposure
- ☐ Presents as more severe manifestations of moderate envenomation
- Dermatologic signs and symptoms are the most common finding in jellyfish envenomations.
  - ☐ Paresthesias, pruritus, and "burning" or "stinging" pain
  - ☐ Red-brown tentacle marks are noted
  - ☐ Vesicles, urticaria, and petechiae can occur
  - ☐ In severe cases, ulceration and necrosis can occur
  - ☐ Systemic symptoms seen in more severe envenomations are as described above

Treatment

- Follow the MARCH primary survey.
- Rinse the wound with seawater.
- Remove tentacles with a gloved or otherwise protected hand.
- Acetic acid 5% (vinegar) should be poured on the sting and tentacles as described below:
  - ☐ It inactivates the nematocysts and toxin for jellyfish. Apply continuously until the pain resolves.
  - ☐ It may not decrease the pain of a Chironex (box jellyfish) sting but will halt the envenomation process.
  - ☐ It has been theorized to worsen the release of venom in Portuguese man-of-war stings, so it should be used with extreme caution on these stings or tentacles.
- Isopropyl alcohol can be utilized if acetic acid is not available. However, this should not be used for *Chironex*.
- Once inactivated, the nematocysts should be removed.
  - ☐ This is best done by applying shaving cream or baking soda and shaving off the nematocysts.
  - ☐ If nothing else is available, make a paste of sand and scrape it off with a straight edge.
- In man-of-war stings, hot water (45°C) may be utilized to effectively reduce pain AFTER removal of nematocysts and irrigation of the sting area.
- Cold packs may also decrease pain.
- Because of the severe toxicity of *Chironex*, antivenom is often used in the prehospital environment in geographic areas where the creature is ubiquitous.
- The **DO NOTs** of jellyfish and man-of-war stings:
  - ☐ Do not use freshwater to rinse the stings. Freshwater will cause more nematocysts to envenom.
  - ☐ Do not rub the area, as this will discharge more nematocysts.
  - ☐ Do not use isopropyl alcohol for box jellyfish stings.

Evacuation Guidelines

- Anyone with more than a minor envenomation and anyone with *Chironex* envenomation should be evacuated.

Stinging Fish

Background

- "Stinging fish" include many different fish with spines that possess a venom apparatus.
- Stinging fish include stonefish, lionfish, scorpion fish, stingrays, and catfish.
- The spines stick into the victim, break off and inject venom.
- These creatures are found worldwide in saltwater, with catfish also found in inland freshwater.
- Sea urchins, although not "stinging fish," cause similar envenomations.
- All have venom that is injected when one comes in contact with their spines, or in the case of a stingray, its barbed tail.
- All of these fish sting humans as a defensive measure, typically when accidentally grabbed or stepped on.
- The toxins of stonefish, scorpion fish, and lionfish can cause muscle and nerve paralysis.
- Stonefish venom has hemotoxic, neurotoxic, and cardiotoxic properties and is of such great toxicity that it has been compared to cobra venom.
- Antivenom is available for treatment of stonefish envenomation.
- The extent of envenomation depends on the number of spines encountered and the type of fish.
- Some parts of the venom of this group are heat labile.
- Typically, the venom-filled spines break off into the wound, causing a dirty wound and retained foreign body, which lead to wound infection.
- Sea urchin spines are brittle and break off easily, resulting in both envenomation and foreign bodies.

Clinical Signs of Stinging Fish Envenomation

- Immediate and severe pain is the common hallmark of a sting.
- Pain radiates centrally from the point of envenomation.
- Pain peaks in 30 to 90 minutes depending on the species and can last for hours to days if untreated.
- Wound areas may become ischemic, dusky, and cyanotic with surrounding areas of edema and inflammation.
- Stingray wounds also include a laceration component, as the tail has a serrated spine(s) that is thrust into the victim with significant force.

Treatment

- Follow the MARCH primary survey.
- Warm/hot water SHOULD be used for stinging fish treatment.
  - ☐ As soon as possible, the wound should be soaked in hot water at a temperature as high as can be tolerated; maximum temperature is 45° C.
  - ☐ The high temperature decreases pain.
  - ☐ The soaks should be done for at least 30 minutes.
- Soaks may be repeated if pain returns.

Control pain with narcotics as required.

Local anesthesia can be utilized for pain control.

The wound should be irrigated with warmed saline or potable water for initial wound care.

Antivenom is available in Australia for treatment of stonefish envenomation.

Evacuation Guidelines

Victims of a sting should be evacuated as soon as possible.

Sea Snakes

Background

Sea snakes (family Elapidae) are found in tropical warm waters worldwide. The Persian Gulf and Southeast Asian coasts are the areas of most frequent attacks.

Sea snakes are docile unless trapped or handled.

Almost all bites are due to stepping on, trapping, or handling the snakes.

Sea snakes have a variety of potent neurotoxins.

The venom of all varieties of sea snakes is similar to other Elapidae snakes.

Sea snake fangs are small and easily break off. Because of this, most sea snake bites cannot penetrate a wet suit.

Symptoms may not develop for a few hours after a bite. However, if no symptoms occur in eight hours then the bite has not resulted in significant envenomation.

Clinical Signs of Sea Snake Envenomation

A sea snake bite is typically painless or at most a "pricking" sensation.

Symptoms typically begin within two to three hours of a bite.

Symptoms are similar to terrestrial elapid envenomation.

Malaise or anxiety is initially noted.

Muscle aches and stiffness are noted, which then progresses to progressive flaccid or spastic paralysis.

Speech and swallowing difficulties develop.

The more severe the envenomation, the more rapid the onset of symptoms.

A lack of symptoms within eight hours of a "bite" means that significant envenomation has likely not occurred.

Treatment

The involved limb should be immobilized.

☐ The immobilization wrap technique utilized for terrestrial elapid bites can be utilized.

☐ Alternatively, a pressure dressing should be made of gauze placed directly over the fang marks and then covered with a circumferential pressure wrap, such as an Ace bandage.

☐ This bandage should be 15 to 18 cm wide and applied with enough pressure to inhibit venous, but not arterial, blood flow

■ Ice should NOT be applied to bite.

■ Incision and suction of the bite site should NOT be performed.

Evacuation Guidelines

■ All victims of sea snake bite should be evacuated immediately and considered for antivenom therapy if they display any signs of envenomation.

QUESTIONS

1. You come upon an 8-year-old Boy Scout who has sustained a large gaping laceration on his right forearm and hand as the result of a dog attack. What is the best way to minimize wound infection?
   a. Closure with 4-0 absorbable suture in a simple interrupted pattern
   b. Irrigate with sterile water, débride and pack
   c. Prophylactic treatment with amoxicillin/clavulanate
   d. Prophylactic treatment with a fluoroquinolone

2. True or False: When you accidentally encounter a black bear, you should immediately get into the fetal position and protect your neck.

3. True or False: When confronted by a cougar you should face it and appear very noisy as if you are a threat.

4. True or False: Once a snake has been killed, there is little risk in picking up the snake—in fact it is encouraged for identification.

5. Which one of the following is an appropriate tick removal technique?
   a. Light a match and burn the rear-end of the tick
   b. Lather the tick and surrounding skin with Vaseline to require the tick to come up for air
   c. Pour alcohol over the tick as an irritant
   d. Remove gently with tweezers grasping as close to the skin as possible

6. Which one of the following is an appropriate field first aid measure for snake bite wound care?
   a. Cut down the track of the bite with a clean knife and suck on the cut
   b. Give aspirin for the pain
   c. Evacuate the patient
   d. Place ice over the wound to decrease pain and swelling

7. A diver plays with a sea snake. He is not wearing gloves and notes a mild "pricking sensation" upon his hand. Which one of the following is most appropriate for management of this victim?
   a. A venous obstructing tourniquet should be applied at the level of the wrist
   b. He can be observed at the site for 8 hours and then evacuated if he starts to display symptoms
   c. The involved hand should have a pressure immobilization dressing applied
   d. Ice should be applied to the site to decrease any pain

8. **Which one of the following is correct regarding sea snakes?**
    a. Sea snakes have a large fang apparatus that can easily penetrate a wet suit
    b. Sea snakes do NOT have a toxic venom
    c. Sea snake bites always result in envenomation
    d. If symptoms do NOT develop eight hours after sea snake exposure, then the bite has not resulted in a clinically significant envenomation.

9. **Which one of the following should be performed as first aid for stinging fish envenomation?**
    a. Acetic acid poured vigorously on the injury site
    b. Cold water immersion of the affected part
    c. Hot/warm water immersion of the affected part
    d. Sodium hypochlorite (bleach) in a 1% solution

10. **A child inadvertently walks into several jellyfish in shallow water. He develops "burning" pain over both lower legs where he touched the jellyfish. Which one of the following is most appropriate to treat this child?**
    a. Rinsing with acetic acid (vinegar)
    b. Rinsing with hypochlorite (bleach) in a 1% solution
    c. Rubbing the area of the sting vigorously
    d. Wound rinsing with freshwater

11. **True or False: The stinger from a honeybee should be removed to prevent further toxin seepage, but the venom sac and stinger should not be touched at all because to do so will encourage the toxin to seep into the site.**

12. **A bite from which spider would be cause for immediate evacuation?**
    a. Black widow
    b. Brown recluse
    c. Hobo spider
    d. Tarantula

13. True or False: A DEET soaked wristband will repel mosquitoes for hours at a time.

14. True or False: Most scorpion stings in the U.S. are poisonous and require immediate evacuation.

Answers:

1. **b**
2. **False**
3. **True**
4. **False**
5. **d**
6. **c**
7. **c**
8. **d**
9. **c**
10. **a**
11. **True**
12. **a**
13. **False**
14. **False**

CHAPTER 15

Infectious Disease

This chapter will familiarize you with various infectious diseases that you may encounter in the wilderness setting.

Objectives:

- Understand the incidence and epidemiology of infectious diseases as they pertain to wilderness travel
- Describe common gastrointestinal infections that occur in the wilderness and be able to describe their clinical presentation, treatment and prevention
- Describe the clinical presentation, treatment and prevention of malaria
- Describe two ways to ascertain the risk of malaria on a proposed trip and the best way to find the correct preventive medication
- Explain the appropriate treatment and management of a person who sustains a bite from an animal that is worrisome for rabies
- Describe various tick borne diseases in terms of their clinical presentation and treatment

INFECTIOUS DISEASES AFFECTING THE GASTROINTESTINAL SYSTEM

- Surveys of climbers and commercial expedition companies suggest that gastroenteritis is the most common medical problem in the wilderness.
- Thirty percent or more of adventure travelers will experience diarrhea during their expedition.
- The vast majority of these cases are passed through fecal-oral transmission. This includes the intake of contaminated food or drinking water as well as the inadvertent ingestion of contaminated water during recreational play.
- Among the most common organisms causing symptomatic disease are: *Staphylococcus aureus*, *Salmonella* species, *E. coli*, *Campylobacter jejuni*, *Giardia lamblia* and viruses.
- Most diarrheal illnesses are divided into two categories: dysenteric and non-dysenteric.
  - ☐ Organisms causing non-dysenteric gastroenteritis usually colonize the inner-lining of the small bowel. This results in a non-bloody, high-volume, watery diarrhea.
  - ☐ Organisms causing dysentery usually invade the ileum and colon causing a lower volume of, but frequently bloody and leukocyte-containing, diarrhea.

Non-Dysenteric Gastroenteritis

Pathophysiology

- Non-dysenteric gastroenteritis is caused by a variety of organisms including: *Enterotoxigenic E. coli* (ETEC), *Vibrio cholera*, and viruses.
- In general, infection with one of these agents results in the secretion of water and electrolytes into the intestinal lumen.
- These enteric pathogens are typically spread by fecal-oral contamination, with contaminated food and water as the most common vehicles for transmission.
- *Enterotoxigenic E. coli* is by far the most common cause in developing areas, accounting for 30 - 70% of "Traveler's Diarrhea," while viruses are more common in the industrialized world.
- *Vibrio cholera* has been virtually eliminated in the industrialized world but disease outbreaks continue to occur in India and sub-Saharan Africa.
  - ☐ Approximately 1 in 20 of those infected will develop life-threatening disease characterized by explosive "rice water stools" produced at a rate of up to one liter per hour.
  - ☐ The rest have a mild, self-limiting diarrheal illness.
  - ☐ A vaccine is available, but the CDC does not recommend it for most travelers.

Clinical Presentation

- Symptoms include profuse watery diarrhea, abdominal cramping, and malaise.
- Nausea and vomiting are usually associated with viral etiologies.
- Adults are usually afebrile, but low-grade fever may be present.
- Incubation times from ingestion to clinical presentation usually range from 12 - 72 hours.

Treatment

- Non-dysenteric diarrhea typically runs a self-limited course with symptoms resolving within three to four days.
- The mainstay of treatment is rehydration with replacement of fluid and electrolyte losses.
- Oral intake should at least approximate fluid losses in stool.
- Most adults will do well by simply increasing their intake of clean water and supplementing this with saltine crackers.
- Moderately dehydrated adults and most children may require a specially prepared isotonic solution to replenish their fluid and electrolyte losses.
- A variety of oral rehydration solutions may be used:
  - ☐ U.S. Public Health Service Formula:
    - Glass 1
      - → 8 oz fruit juice
      - → ½ teaspoon baking soda
      - → ½ teaspoon honey or corn syrup
    - Glass 2
      - → 8 oz water
      - → 1 pinch table salt
    - Drink equal amounts from each glass alternating between the two.
  - ☐ WHO Oral Rehydration Solution (ORS) may be purchased as small packets in most developing countries.
    - Add one packet to a liter of disinfected or clean water.
  - ☐ For a WHO ORS equivalent, add the following to one liter of disinfected or clean water:
    - ¾ teaspoon of salt (two finger pinch)
    - ½ teaspoon baking soda (one finger pinch)
    - 2 to 3 tablespoons of sugar (three finger scoops)
    - ¼ teaspoon potassium chloride salt substitute (small pinch), if available
  - ☐ Sports drinks such as Gatorade or PowerAde may be used if diluted to half-strength with disinfected or clean water.
- Only disinfected water or juices should be used to prepare these solutions.
- Urine volume and color should be monitored as gross indicators of hydration status.

Antimotility agents:

- Antimotility agents provide symptomatic relief and serve as useful adjuncts to antibiotic therapy.
- Synthetic opiates, such as loperamide and diphenoxylate, can reduce frequency of bowel movements and enable travelers to ride on an airplane or bus while awaiting the effects of antibiotics.
- Loperamide (Imodium) may be used with non-invasive (non-bloody) gastroenteritis to reduce cramping and fluid losses.

Bismuth subsalicylate (Pepto-Bismol) is an effective treatment for travel-related diarrhea and has comparable treatment results to antibiotic therapy in mild to moderate cases. An appropriate adult dose of bismuth subsalicylate is 2 tablespoons or 2 tablets by mouth every hour up to eight doses in 24 hours. Loperamide appears to have antisecretory properties as well. Antimotility agents are not generally recommended for patients with bloody diarrhea or those who have diarrhea and fever.

Antiemetic medications:

Metoclopramide (Reglan), promethazine (Phenergan), or ondansetron (Zofran) can all be used to help relieve the nausea and vomiting associated with acute gastroenteritis.

Ondansetron has an oral dissolvable tablet (ODT) that is easy to use and very effective.

Antibiotics:

More severe cases of travel-related gastroenteritis may warrant empiric antibiotic therapy.

■ The CDC recommends antibiotics if patients experience three or more episodes of diarrhea in an eight-hour period.

   □ The treatment of choice is a fluoroquinolone (ciprofloxacin or levofloxacin) for a single-dose or 1-day therapy

   □ Azithromycin 500 mg by mouth daily for 3 days or trimethoprim/sulfamethoxazole 160mg/800mg DS tablets by mouth twice a day for 3 days may be used for cases when the use of fluoroquinolones is not an acceptable option (e.g. pregnancy or children).

   □ PLEASE NOTE: in May 2016, the US FDA is advising against the use of fluoroquinolones for patients with sinusitis, bronchitis, and uncomplicated urinary tract infections who have other treatment options.

   □ This advisory does _not_ include dysentery or GI disease but should be a consideration with prescribing.

   □ The safety review has demonstrated that fluoroquinolones are associated with disabling and potentially permanent serious side effects that can occur together. These side effects can involve the tendons, muscles, joints, nerves, and central nervous system.

Dysenteric Gastroenteritis

Pathophysiology

The organisms causing dysentery are invasive resulting in more severe symptoms, including bloody diarrhea and fever.

Up to 15% of travel related diarrhea is due to dysentery.

Causative organisms include _Salmonella_, _Shigella_, _Campylobacter_, enterohemorrhagic _E. coli_, _Yersinia enterocolitica_, and _Aeromonas hydrophilia_.

Most organisms causing dysentery are spread by a fecal-oral route, usually through contaminated food and water.

- ☐ *Salmonella* species are widespread and are commonly found in raw eggs, poultry, and meat.
- ☐ *Shigella* is highly contagious and is easily spread from person-to-person as ingestion of only a few organisms can cause infection.
- ☐ *Campylobacter* is a common contaminant of natural water supplies and is also common in unprocessed milk and raw poultry products.
- ☐ Enterohemorrhagic *E. coli* is transmitted in contaminated food and water, particularly under-cooked meats, such as hamburger.
- ☐ *Aeromonas hydrophilia* is spread through contaminated water and is more commonly observed in children.

Clinical Presentation

Acute onset of severe, intermittent abdominal cramps followed by diarrhea that may be copious.

The presence of fever, often as high as 104°F, along with the appearance of blood or mucous in the stool is used to distinguish invasive (dysentery) from non-invasive diarrhea.

Headache and myalgias are often present.

The patient may experience severe abdominal pain, especially in the lower abdomen.

Rebound tenderness and guarding may be present on physical exam.

Symptoms of bacteremia and sepsis may develop, especially in association with *Salmonella* and *Shigella* infections.

Incubation periods vary from 8 hours to 8 days, and symptoms may persist for 1-10 days.

Treatment

Fluid replacement with oral rehydration is the most important aspect of treatment.

Empiric antibiotic therapy should be initiated in suspected cases of bacterial dysentery.

The treatment of choice is a fluoroquinolone (ciprofloxacin or levofloxacin) for a single-dose or 1-day therapy. Please note the FDA advisory as noted previously

Azithromycin 500 mg by mouth daily for 3 days or trimethoprim/sulfamethoxazole 160mg/800mg DS tablets by mouth twice a day for 3 days may be used for cases when the use of fluoroquinolones is not an acceptable option (e.g. pregnancy or children).

Antidiarrheal medications such as loperamide (Imodium) or diphenoxylate with atropine (Lomotil) are classically contraindicated in the treatment of dysentery.

- ☐ The teaching has been that these medications should generally be avoided as they may allow for retention of toxic bacteria and may increase the carrier state for *Salmonella*.
- ☐ However, voluminous or frequent diarrhea is generally incompatible with most wilderness activities, so the antimotility agents are often used in this setting.
- ☐ If one elects to use antimotility agents, they should always be prescribed with antibiotics in order to lower the potential risks. There is little published data on this subject.
- ☐ According to the CDC: The safety of loperamide when used along with an antibiotic has been well established, even in cases of invasive pathogens

Bismuth subsalicylate (Pepto-Bismol) may also be used safely in cases of dysentery, but it slows the absorption of oral antibiotics.

Staphylococcal Enteritis

Pathophysiology

One form of gastroenteritis results from ingesting a heat-stable toxin produced by *Staphylococcus aureus*.

Staphylococcus colonizes human skin. Unwitting chefs contaminate their food with this bacteria if they do not wash their hands or wear gloves during food preparation and service.

The bacteria can grow in any food, but it flourishes in those that are high in protein such as mayonnaise, dairy and meat products.

The bacteria proliferate if left at room temperature (between 40 - 140°F). As they are allowed to multiply, the disease causing enterotoxin is produced.

The toxin is heat-resistant and cannot be neutralized by reheating or freezing contaminated food.

The ingestion of less than 1 microgram of toxin can result in disease symptoms.

Clinical Presentation

Staphylococcal gastroenteritis is characterized by the acute onset of nausea, severe vomiting, mild diarrhea and abdominal cramps. Severe cases may include headaches, myalgias and a drop in blood pressure.

Symptoms usually occur within one to six hours after the ingestion of contaminated food. This time-course separates it from most other causes of gastroenteritis, which typically take more than eight hours to produce symptoms.

Food poisoning by an enterotoxin is the likely culprit when multiple victims present with vomiting and diarrhea after consuming the same food.

Staphylococcal food poisoning is self-limiting and symptoms typically resolve within 24 hours.

Treatment

Treatment is supportive and based upon symptoms, with fluid and electrolyte replacement as the primary goal.

Anti-emetic medications may be used.

Antibiotic therapy is ineffective and unnecessary because the toxin is pre-formed and cannot be neutralized.

Prevention

The key to avoiding Staphylococcal enteritis is to ensure proper hygiene and sanitation when preparing food.

Hand sanitation with alcohol gels or hand washing with soap and water is essential for food handlers.

Food prepared in the wilderness must be consumed immediately after preparation and leftovers should be disposed of properly.

PROTOZOAL CAUSES OF DIARRHEA

Common protozoal causes of gastroenteritis include *Giardia lamblia*, *Entamoeba histolytica*, *Cryptosporidium*, and *Cyclospora*.

All are transmitted by the fecal-oral route via contaminated water and food.

Symptoms of protozoal infections vary widely from an asymptomatic carrier state, to acute dysentery and to chronic diarrhea.

Giardia is by far the most common cause of protozoal illness. It contaminates water sources in both the developing and industrialized world.

It is probably the most common cause of diarrhea in people backpacking in the United States.

Giardiasis

Pathophysiology

Giardia lamblia is a single-celled parasite that exists in a cyst form and a trophozoite form.

Infected individuals and animals pass the cyst form in stools. These cysts can survive in the environment for three months or longer.

Beaver, deer, dogs, cattle, sheep, and rodents are common carriers of *Giardia*, and many natural water sources may have *Giardia* cysts present despite being in remote or "pristine" locations.

Drinking contaminated water is the primary source of infection, with an infectious dose being as low as 10 to 25 cysts.

Once the cysts are ingested, they are partially digested by gastrointestinal enzymes. Each cyst divides to form two trophozoites, which cause symptomatic disease.

Clinical Presentation

About 50 percent of infected people will be asymptomatic. Some of these will go on to become chronic carriers.

Incubation time is one to three weeks after ingestion. Many travelers may develop symptoms well after returning home.

Diarrhea is the most common feature of giardiasis and is present in up to 90 percent of symptomatic cases.

The severity of diarrhea varies. Some may have mild to moderate amounts of foul-smelling soft stools, while others may experience copious and explosive bouts of diarrhea.

A characteristic "rotten egg" odor is associated with the intestinal gas and feces.

- Other symptoms may include malaise, bloating, abdominal cramping, nausea, vomiting, and low grade fever.
- Chronic diarrhea, lasting weeks to months, may develop and can have a cyclical pattern of worsening symptoms every few weeks.

Treatment

- All suspected cases of *Giardia* should be treated with antimicrobials.
- Metronidazole 250 mg by mouth three times a day for 5-7 days is standard therapy.
- Tinidazole 2 g by mouth x 1 dose is the first line medication in many countries. It is approved for use in the U.S. and reportedly has fewer GI side effects than metronidazole.
- Furazolidone 100 mg by mouth four times a day for 7 days may be used for children.
- No single treatment is effective in all cases, and multi-drug therapy may be needed in resistant cases.
- Symptoms may recur after an apparently successful course of treatment and should be treated in the same manner as the original infection.

Amebiasis

Pathophysiology

- *Entamoeba histolytica*, the cause of amebiasis, is a parasite found in water supplies around the world.
- It is particularly prevalent in tropical countries.
- Unlike *Giardia*, humans are the only reservoir for *Entamoeba*. Approximately 10 percent of the world's population is infected.
- The organism exists in cyst and trophozoite forms.
- Cysts are transmitted through fecal-oral contamination of food or water or through direct contact with an infected person.
- Ingested cysts become trophozoites that invade the colon wall and cause a variety of intestinal symptoms.
- Ingestion of as little as <u>one</u> cyst can initiate infection.

Clinical Presentation

- Most individuals are asymptomatic, and many become chronic carriers.
- Symptomatic individuals may develop alternating constipation and diarrhea, abdominal cramping, weight loss, anorexia, and nausea.
- More severe infections may develop weeks to months after infection, resulting in the classical symptoms of dysentery.
- Trophozoites may migrate to other locations in the body causing extra-intestinal metastases in the liver, skin, pericardium and brain.
- The liver is the most common site for invasion. These "sterile" abscesses result in fever, right upper quadrant pain, and weight loss.

Treatment

Consider treating for amebiasis in a patient with dysentery symptoms who does not respond to a course of antibiotics.

Diagnosis may be made by stool ova and parasite examination if the patient seeks medical treatment either during or after travel.

Antibiotic therapy for symptomatic disease includes metronidazole 750 mg by mouth three times a day for 10 days or tinidazole 2g by mouth daily for 3 days. This treatment should be followed by a course of iodoquinol, paromomycin, or diloxanide to eradicate the cysts and prevent the carrier state.

Cryptosporidium

Pathophysiology

Cryptosporidium is a protozoan organism that is present throughout the environment, including up to 97 percent of large streams, lakes and reservoirs in the U.S.

Transmission occurs through the ingestion of contaminated water and food.

The organism is resistant to iodine and chlorine disinfectants, but it can be killed by boiling water. Some filters are also effective.

Clinical Presentation

Symptoms include watery diarrhea, crampy abdominal pain, anorexia, malaise, and flatulence.

Immunocompetent patients usually have a self-limiting course lasting a few days. Children are generally more severely affected than adults.

Immunocompromised patients develop a more severe infection that can last from months to years. These patients can lose more than three liters of fluid per day.

Treatment

No effective treatment has been found, and the eradication of the infection is the result of the patient's own immune function.

Supportive therapy consists of fluid and electrolyte replacement.

Cyclospora

Pathophysiology

Cyclospora cayetanensis is a protozoan parasite that is most commonly transmitted in fecally contaminated food or water in developing countries, particularly Central and South America.

Clinical Presentation

The incubation period is approximately one week, so patients may develop symptoms after returning home from their vacation.

Infection typically causes watery diarrhea that may last for weeks.

Other symptoms include: anorexia, weight loss, bloating, abdominal cramping, flatulence, nausea, vomiting, myalgias, low grade fever, and fatigue.

Treatment

Antibiotic treatment with TMP/SMX 160 mg/800 mg DS tablets by mouth twice a day for 7 days is effective.

Water may not be reliably decontaminated by filtration or halide treatment and should be boiled.

OTHER GASTROINTESTINAL INFECTIONS

Hepatitis A

Pathophysiology

Hepatitis A virus causes acute inflammation of the liver and is the most common type of viral hepatitis.

The virus is transmitted by the fecal-oral route.

It is present worldwide but is more common in developing nations.

Clinical Presentation

The incubation period is 15 to 50 days from the time of ingestion.

Symptoms vary from mild gastroenteritis to fulminant liver failure.

Typical presentation includes: acute onset of fever, lethargy, anorexia, and nausea followed by darkening of urine (usually after 3 to 10 days), and jaundice.

Abdominal pain and vomiting, as well as itching and joint pain, may be present.

Physical exam may reveal hepatosplenomegaly.

Children usually have a more benign course than adults.

Symptoms usually resolve without treatment in several days to 2 weeks, with jaundice resolving after 3 to 4 weeks.

Chronic infection does not occur.

Fulminant liver failure is a rare complication, occurring in 0.5% to 1% of cases.

Treatment

Provide supportive care, and evacuate for advanced medical care if symptoms become severe.

No specific medical therapy is available.

Prevention

Hepatitis A vaccine is recommended for all travelers to developing nations. A single dose vaccine followed by a booster at 6-12 months provides protection for 10 years.

The vaccine is now part of the standard immunizations recommended for children. The first vaccine should be given between 1 and 2 years of age.

Unimmunized contacts of hepatitis A patients should receive an injection of gamma globulin.

Appropriate measures for hygiene and water disinfection should be followed vigilantly.

Typhoid Fever

Pathophysiology

Typhoid fever is a systemic illness classically caused by the organism *Salmonella typhi*.

S. paratyphi produces a similar illness, but it is usually of shorter duration.

Typhoid fever occurs worldwide but is most commonly contracted in developing nations.

Humans are the only hosts for *S. typhi,* and transmission occurs most commonly through ingestion of contaminated food and water.

Contact with chronic carriers of *S. typhi* may also lead to infection.

Once ingested, the bacteria penetrate the intestinal mucosa. From there, the bacteria invade the lymphatics, allowing it to spread systemically.

Clinical Presentation

The incubation period of *S. typhi* is 7 to 14 days.

Initial symptoms include fever, headache, dry cough, abdominal pain, and malaise.

"Pea-soup" diarrhea often occurs later in the course of the disease.

Although less common, constipation may also occur. It is caused by swollen lymphoid tissue surrounding the ileocecal valve.

The temperature rises slowly during the first week of the disease. During weeks two and three, a continuous high fever up to 104° F (40° C) persists. The fever is characterized by the relative bradycardia that accompanies it.

A characteristic rash of "rose spots," 2 to 4 mm macular blanching lesions, may appear on the trunk.

Physical exam may reveal splenomegaly and diffuse tenderness.

After three weeks, the fever typically begins to abate and symptoms begin to resolve spontaneously in uncomplicated cases.

Complications of typhoid fever include intestinal perforation, gastrointestinal hemorrhage, sepsis with multisystem failure, and pneumonia.

Treatment

Immunization is available in an oral or injectable form and is recommended when traveling to endemic areas.

Treatment of typhoid fever involves supportive care and management of fluids and electrolytes.

Antibiotic treatment reduces the duration of disease and decreases the complication rate.

☐ Antibiotic treatment of choice is ciprofloxacin 500 mg by mouth for 10 days. Resistance to this agent is increasing, particularly in Southeast Asia.

☐ IV antibiotic regimens include ceftriaxone 2 g IV q 24 hours for 14 days or ciprofloxacin 400 mg IV q12 hours for 10 days.

☐ Azithromycin 1 g by mouth once daily for 5 days is a reasonable alternative therapy.

☐ Chloramphenicol treatment has been used successfully in the past at a dose of 50mg/kg/day divided four times a day for 2 weeks. Increasing bacterial resistance and the rare incidence of aplastic anemia associated with its use have led to its designation as a second line therapy.

Dexamethasone may be beneficial in severe cases and should be given before the antibiotics.

Prevention of Gastrointestinal Disease

Proper hygiene and sanitation practices are essential in preventing infectious diseases of the GI tract.

The wilderness traveler must be vigilant to insure that food and water do not become contaminated.

Wash hands thoroughly with soap or hand disinfectant before preparing and eating meals.

Cooking and eating utensils should be cleaned with boiling water or bleach solution prior to each use.

Diet

☐ Avoid raw or undercooked meat, fish and seafood.

☐ When traveling internationally, avoid street vendors, raw vegetables, and fresh salads.

☐ Avoid unpasteurized milk, cheese, and other dairy products.

☐ Peeled fruits and vegetables are generally safe.

☐ Do not rinse food in water that has not been disinfected.

☐ Dispose of unused food properly.

Water

☐ Use appropriate methods of water disinfection

☐ When traveling internationally, avoid tap water and ice cubes made from untreated water.

☐ Purchase name brand bottled water.

☐ It is important that you always check the seal on any water bottle prior to drinking; if dining out, request that you break the seal and open the bottle yourself.

☐ Sometimes the vendors will recycle the bottles and fill them with tap water. Of course, they will bring the open water bottle to your table so that you will not recognize this trick.

Prophylaxis

☐ Bismuth subsalicylate has been shown to be safe and effective in prophylaxis of diarrheal illness, reducing incidence of disease by up to 65%.

☐ The recommended regimen is 2 tablets or 2 tablespoons four times daily.

☐ Side effects include darkened stools and tongue, and possibly constipation and nausea.

☐ Avoid concurrent aspirin use.

☐ In general, antibiotic prophylaxis is not recommended.

☐ In short term trips to high risk areas where circumstances may demand more aggressive strategies of prevention, the following broad spectrum antibiotics may be used:

- TMP/SM 160 mg/80 mg DS tablet by mouth daily
- Doxycycline 100 mg by mouth daily

Evacuation Guidelines

Any victim with moderate to severe abdominal pain that does not improve over 12 to 24 hours should be evacuated.

Victims unable to take sufficient oral rehydration fluids for more than 24 hours should be evacuated.

Anyone experiencing mental status changes, signs of significant dehydration, hematemesis, or copious bloody stools should be evacuated immediately.

Victims with signs and symptoms of dysentery who do not respond to appropriate antibiotic therapy in 24 to 48 hours should be evacuated.

MALARIA

Pathophysiology

Malaria is a parasitic infection caused by protozoa of the genus *Plasmodium*.

According to the World Health Organization in 2015:

☐ About 3.2 billion people, nearly half of the world's population, are at risk of malaria.

☐ In 2015, there were roughly 214 million malaria cases and an estimated 438 000 malaria deaths

☐ Increased prevention and control measures have led to a 60% reduction in malaria mortality rates globally since 2000.

☐ Sub-Saharan Africa was home to 89% of malaria cases and 91% of malaria deaths.

The infection is transmitted by the female *Anopheles* mosquito.

Once inoculated into the human bloodstream, the parasites travel to the liver, where they multiply.

The hepatocytes eventually rupture, releasing thousands of parasites which then invade individual red blood cells.

Five Species of Plasmodium That Cause Malaria

Organism	Distribution
Plasmodium falciparum	Worldwide, esp. sub-Saharan Africa, Amazon, Haiti, SE Asia
Plasmodium vivax	Worldwide, esp. Mexico, Central America, N. Africa, Middle East, India
Plasmodium ovale	West Africa
Plasmodium malariae	Worldwide

P. falciparum is the most virulent of the four species. It is also the most likely to have drug-resistant strains.

P. vivax and P. *ovale* has a hypnozoite stage, which remains dormant in the liver. These parasites can reactivate and cause symptomatic disease if not treated properly.

P. knowlesi, also called 'Monkey Malaria,' rarely infects humans.

Clinical Presentation

Symptoms typically present 1 to 2 weeks after exposure to an infected mosquito.

Initial symptoms include muscle soreness and low grade fever, which progress to paroxysms of shaking chills, high fever, and drenching sweats.

Cycles of chills and fever last several hours and may occur every 2 to 3 days, depending on the specific organism.

Headaches, myalgias, and backaches are also common and may be severe.

Other symptoms include nausea, vomiting, diarrhea, severe anemia, and darkened urine (a.k.a. Blackwater Fever.)

Severe *P. falciparum* infection may present with constant fever and high levels of parasitemia that can lead to cerebral malaria.

- ☐ Symptoms of cerebral malaria include high fever, confusion, coma, and seizures.
- ☐ Other complications of severe infection include pulmonary edema, acute renal failure, profound hypoglycemia, and lactic acidosis.
- ☐ Mortality rates of cerebral malaria are greater than 20 percent.

Physical exam may reveal splenomegaly and a tender abdomen in advanced infections.

Prevention

A combination of personal protective measures and chemoprophylaxis is essential to avoid malaria infection in endemic areas.

The *Anopheles* mosquito is most likely to bite between dusk and dawn.

- ☐ Limit exposure by using mosquito nets and wearing protective clothing impregnated with an insecticide such as permethrin.
- ☐ Light colored clothes with long sleeves and long pants are recommended.

- ☐ Insect repellent containing DEET (no higher than 35% concentration is necessary) should be applied to exposed skin.
- Consult with a travel clinic or the CDC recommendations to determine the appropriate chemoprophylaxis for the region of travel (http://www.cdc.gov/travel)
- Drug choice is based on the risk of chloroquine-resistant *P. falciparum* and patient contraindications (e.g. pregnant women, G6PDH deficiency). Chloroquine resistance is particularly common throughout sub-Saharan Africa and Southeast Asia.
- Options for chemoprophylaxis include:
  - ☐ Chloroquine
  - ☐ Doxycycline
  - ☐ Atovaquone/proguanil (Malarone)
  - ☐ Pyrimethamine / sulfoxime (Fansidar)
  - ☐ Primaquine
- Weekly drug regimens (chloroquine, mefloquine) should be initiated 1 to 2 weeks before traveling to an endemic area, while daily dosing regimens may be started 1 to 2 days before travel.
- It is important to continue medications after returning home, if prescribed, to prevent illness from reactivated *P. vivax* or *P. ovale*.

Treatment

- Malaria infection can occur despite careful behavior modification and chemoprophylaxis. For wilderness travel in endemic areas, appropriate medications should be taken for self-treatment.
- Recommended treatment regimens should be determined through consultation with a travel clinic or the CDC.
- Treatment should be initiated when signs and symptoms suggest malarial infection and medical care is not immediately available.
- Anyone suspected of having malaria should be evacuated, especially in areas where *P. falciparum* is common.

RABIES

Pathophysiology

- Rabies is caused by an RNA virus in the Rhabdoviridae family.
- The virus is transmitted in the saliva of infected animals.
- Only 1 – 3 deaths are reported annually in the US, but an estimated 55,000 people die each year from rabies worldwide, mostly in Africa and Asia. This is a rate of one person every ten minutes

In the US, over 90% of rabies occurs in wild animals, with less than 5% occurring in dogs.

In most developing nations, however, dogs account for up to 90% of reported rabies cases.

Any mammal can become infected with rabies. Bats are the most common vector for human infection in the U.S. Other major vectors include dogs, foxes, raccoons, skunks, coyotes and mongooses. Small rodents are unlikely to carry the disease as they will die before they can pass it on.

Following inoculation, the rabies virus travels through the peripheral nervous system to the central nervous system (CNS). Once in the CNS, the virus multiplies rapidly causing symptomatic disease.

Clinical Presentation

The incubation period varies from 9 days to more than a year, with most cases presenting within 20-90 days.

Incubation time is directly related to the location of the inoculation site and the distance the virus must travel before reaching the CNS. Rabies resulting from a bite involving the head or face has an average incubation period of 30 days, while a bite to the foot has an average incubation period of 60 days.

Prodromal symptoms are nonspecific and may include malaise, headache, fatigue, fever, irritability, insomnia, depression, nausea, vomiting, sore throat, abdominal pain, and anorexia.

Approximately half of patients experience pain, pruritus, or paresthesias at the inoculation site.

The prodromal period lasts from 2 to 10 days.

Following the prodrome, patients will develop signs of CNS disease.

Rabies exists in two forms, furious rabies and paralytic rabies. Humans more commonly develop the furious form.

- ☐ Furious Rabies
  - Hyperactivity
  - Disorientation
  - Agitation
  - Hallucinations
  - Aggressive or bizarre behavior
  - Hyperthermia
  - Tachycardia
  - Hypertension
  - Excessive salivation
- ☐ Paralytic Rabies
  - Progressive lethargy
  - Loss of coordination
  - Confusion
  - Stupor
  - Ascending paralysis

Both furious and paralytic forms of rabies are fatal, usually within a week of onset of CNS symptoms.

Treatment

- There is no proven therapy for treatment of rabies.
- Anyone suspected of exposure should undergo appropriate post-exposure prophylaxis (see below.)
- A single case report in 2005 described survival in a rabies patient who did not receive post-exposure prophylaxis.
  - ☐ Treatment included coma induction and antiviral treatment.
  - ☐ The patient sustained moderate neurologic sequelae but returned to independent functioning.

Prevention

- Wilderness travelers most at risk for rabies infection include spelunkers, professional hunters, wildlife workers, and those traveling to endemic areas for extended periods or to remote areas without medical care. These people should consider pre-travel vaccination.
- Pre-exposure vaccination:
  - ☐ International travelers might be candidates for pre-exposure vaccination if they are likely to come in contact with animals in areas where dog or other animal rabies is enzootic and immediate access to appropriate medical care, including rabies vaccine and immune globulin, might be limited.
  - ☐ The pre-exposure vaccination program consists of three 1.0-mL injections of HDCV or PCECV administered IM (deltoid area), one injection per day on days 0, 7, and 21 or 28
- Post-exposure prophylaxis consists of three steps:
  - ☐ Wash the wound immediately with soap and water followed by irrigation with a virucidal agent if possible.
  - ☐ Administer human rabies immune globulin (HRIG) 20 IU/kg. Current CDC recommendations call for the full dose of HRIG to be infiltrated at the site of the wound, if possible. If the location of the wound precludes infiltrating the full dose, the remainder should be injected intramuscularly at a site distant from vaccine administration using a clean needle and syringe.
  - ☐ Immunize with the intramuscular rabies vaccine (HDCV or PCECV). A 1-ml dose is given at 0, 3, 7 and 14 days.
  - ☐ If the victim has been immunized against rabies, then no HRIG is given but they should still receive the vaccine at days 0 and 3.
- Anyone suspected of rabies exposure should be immediately evacuated for appropriate medical treatment.
- Post-exposure prophylaxis should be given as soon as possible after a suspected contact with the virus.

TICK-BORNE DISEASES

Lyme Disease

Pathophysiology

- Lyme disease is caused by the spirochete *Borrelia burgdorferi*.
- It is the most common vector-borne disease in the United States.
- It is also endemic in Eastern and central Europe, northern Asia
- The bacteria are transmitted by the *Ixodes* ticks.
- Only 10% of bites from an infected tick will result in disease.
- 12 U.S. states report 95% of cases: Massachusetts, Connecticut, Maine, New Hampshire, Rhode Island, New York, New Jersey, Pennsylvania, Delaware, Maryland, Michigan, and Wisconsin

Clinical Presentation

Lyme disease presents with three distinct stages.

Stage I: Early Localized Infection

- ☐ Usually develops 3 days to 1 month after a tick bite.
- ☐ 95% of patients develop the classic rash called erythema migrans (EM). This is a characteristic rash that may be uniformly red or have a more complex "bull's eye" appearance due to central clearing.
- ☐ Other symptoms

● Malaise, fatigue, lethargy	80%
● Headache	64%
● Fever and chills	59%
● Stiff neck	48%
● Multiple annular lesions	48%
● Regional lymphadenopathy	41%

Stage II: Early Disseminated Infection

- ☐ Begins as the bacteria spreads through the bloodstream.
- ☐ Includes neurologic symptoms, such as radiculoneuritis (shooting nerve pain), cranial nerve palsies (especially CN VII), meningitis, and encephalitis.
- ☐ Cardiac problems, such as carditis and heart block, may also be present.

Stage III: Late Disseminated Infection

- ☐ Occurs months after an untreated or partially treated infection.
- ☐ Can develop chronic neurologic complaints: pain, vertigo, weakness, and cognitive impairments.
- ☐ Arthritis, usually involving the knee, is also often experienced.

Treatment

The Infectious Disease Society of America (IDSA) does not generally recommend antimicrobial prophylaxis for prevention of Lyme disease after a recognized tick bite. However, in areas that are highly endemic for Lyme disease, a single dose of doxycycline may be offered to adult patients (200 mg) who are not pregnant and to children older than 8 years of age (4 mg/kg up to a maximum dose of 200 mg) when all of the following circumstances exist:

☐ Doxycycline is not contraindicated.
☐ The attached tick can be identified as an adult or nymphal I. scapularis tick.
☐ The estimated time of attachment is ≥36 h based on the degree of engorgement of the tick with blood or likely time of exposure to the tick.
☐ Prophylaxis can be started within 72 h of tick removal.
☐ Lyme disease is common in the county or state where the patient lives or has recently traveled.

Otherwise, prophylactic antibiotics for tick bites are generally not recommended.

The following treatment regimens are recommended for early stages of the illness:

☐ Doxycycline 100 mg by mouth twice a day or 1-2 mg/kg twice a day
☐ Amoxicillin 500 mg three times a day or 25-50 mg/kg/day every 8 hours

Rocky Mountain Spotted Fever

Pathophysiology

Rocky Mountain Spotted Fever (RMSF) is a serious disease caused by the spirochete *Rickettsia rickettsii*.

The spirochete is transmitted by *Dermacentor* ticks (dog ticks and wood ticks).

Despite its name, most cases occur in southern and eastern states of the U.S.

It also occurs in Central and South America.

Reported mortality rates range from 3 - 5%.

Clinical Presentation

Most cases present during the spring and early summer, but infections can occur throughout the year.

The incubation period is usually 5-10 days.

Early symptoms may be non-specific and include mild chills, anorexia, and malaise, which then progress to the classic triad of fever, severe headache, and rash. Other symptoms include myalgias, bone pain, abdominal pain, and confusion.

The rash characteristically begins on the ankles and wrists, and spreads centrally. The palms and soles are also classically affected.

The rash starts out maculopapular, and progresses to a petechial morphology.

Patients may appear quite toxic, and the majority requires hospitalization.

Treatment

In addition to supportive care, the following treatment regimens are recommended:

☐ Adults: Doxycycline 100 mg by mouth twice a day

☐ Children: Doxycycline 2.2 mg/kg per dose twice per day, orally or IV

Use doxycycline as the first-line treatment for suspected RMSF in patients of all ages.

The use of doxycycline to treat suspected RMSF in children is recommended by both the CDC and the American Academy of Pediatrics Committee on Infectious Diseases.

Use of antibiotics other than doxycycline increases the risk of patient death.

At the recommended dose and duration needed to treat RMSF, no evidence has been shown to cause staining of permanent teeth, even when five courses are given before the age of eight.

Treatment should be continued for at least three days after defervescence.

Any patient suspected of RMSF infection should be evacuated immediately.

Lyme disease: erythema migrans   **RMSF: petechial rash**

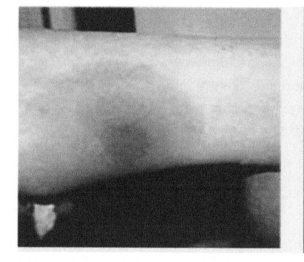
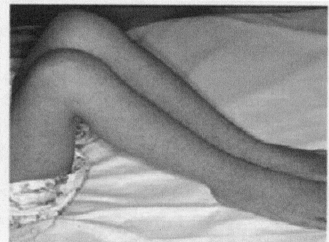

Ehrlichiosis

Pathophysiology

Ehrlichiosis is a rickettsial infection that presents similarly to Rocky Mountain Spotted Fever, but without the characteristic rash.

It is found primarily in the southeast and south-central U.S.

The disease is transmitted by the Lone Star Tick.

Clinical Presentation

Average incubation time is 5 - 10 days.

The characteristic symptoms are high fever and headache.

Myalgias, headache, and chills are common, while nausea, vomiting, arthralgias, and cough can also occur.

Rashes are rare.

Mortality rate ranges from 2 - 3%.

Treatment

In addition to supportive care, the following treatment regimens are recommended

☐ Adults: Doxycycline 100 mg by mouth twice a day

☐ Children: Doxycycline 2.2 mg/kg per dose twice per day, orally or IV

☐ All of the same issues regarding the use of doxycycline in the management of RMSF are the same for its use in ehrlichiosis.

Most patients are hospitalized for treatment.

Anyone suspected of this illness should be evacuated for appropriate medical care.

Tick Paralysis

Pathophysiology

Tick paralysis is an acute, ascending, flaccid motor paralysis caused by neurotoxic venom secreted from the salivary glands of ticks of both *Ixodidae* and *Argasidae* families.

In the U.S., most cases occur in the Pacific Northwest and the Rocky Mountain areas.

There is a similar tick paralysis in Australia that has greater morbidity

April through June are the highest months of risk in the U.S.

Clinical Presentation

Children are affected more severely as the neurotoxin is usually diluted in the larger blood volume of an adult.

Symptoms typically develop 5 – 7 days after tick attachment.

Early symptoms may include ataxia and paresthesias of the hands and feet.

This is followed in the next 24 – 48 hours by ascending paralysis and loss of deep tendon reflexes.

In cases where the tick is not identified early, Guillain-Barré syndrome is frequently blamed.

Treatment

Treatment involves removal of the tick and supportive care

To remove the tick, grasp as close to the patient's skin as possible with a forceps and pull firmly.

Symptoms usually resolve within 24 hours of removal.

In Australia, there is an antivenin to administer before removal of the tick. The antivenin is given because victims usually worsen after removal of the tick.

Colorado Tick Fever

Pathophysiology

Colorado tick fever is a viral illness transmitted by the wood tick, primarily during spring and early summer. Most cases occur in mountainous regions of the Western U.S. and Canada.

Clinical Presentation

The average incubation time is 3–6 days.

Symptoms include fever, chills, lethargy, headache, myalgia, ocular pain, photophobia, abdominal pain, nausea, vomiting, and a flat, papular rash.

The illness usually occurs in two stages, starting with a mild episode of symptoms lasting about 3 days. Symptoms then diminish briefly before a 1-3 day episode of more severe symptoms occurs.

5% – 10% of children develop meningitis or encephalitis.

Treatment

Treatment is supportive.

Persons with symptoms of Colorado tick fever should be evacuated for medical evaluation.

Tularemia

Pathophysiology

Tularemia or "rabbit fever" is caused by the bacterium *Francisella tularensis*.

It is contracted through exposure to ticks, deer flies, and mosquitoes; by contact with infected animals, such as rabbits, muskrats, foxes and squirrels; or by eating contaminated meat.

In the U.S., the most common vector of transmission is ticks although there have been recent outbreaks associated with deer flies.

The disease has been reported from all 49 continental states, but is most common in the south central states, mainly Arkansas, Missouri, and Oklahoma.

Clinical Presentation

Patients typically present with a history of fever, chills, and myalgias, followed by an irregular ulcer at the site of the inoculation, which may persist for months.

Regional lymphadenopathy develops, and these nodes may then become necrotic and suppurate.

Incubation time is 3 – 5 days.

Treatment

- The treatment of choice is streptomycin 10 mg/kg IM every 12 hours for 7 to 10 days. The daily dose should not exceed 2 g.
- The doses for alternative agents are:
  - ☐ Gentamicin 3 to 5 mg/kg IM or IV daily, given every eight hours for 7 to 10 days
  - ☐ Doxycycline 100 mg by mouth twice a day for 14 days
  - ☐ Chloramphenicol 25 to 60 mg/kg per day IV in four divided doses (not to exceed 6 g/day in adults) for 14 days

Borrelia – Relapsing Fever

Pathophysiology

- Relapsing fever is caused by spirochetes of the *Borrelia* genus.
- Both tick-borne and a louse-borne forms of the disease affect humans.
- The tick-borne form is transmitted by *Ixodidae* and *Argasidae* ticks.
- The disease occurs worldwide. Most U.S. cases occur west of the Mississippi River.

Clinical Presentation

- Incubation time averages around seven days.
- Symptoms include fever, chills, severe headache, lethargy, arthralgias, photophobia, petechiae, and splenomegaly.
- As the name implies, relapses of fever are characteristic:
  - ☐ The pattern is usually three days of symptoms with seven days between each relapse
  - ☐ There is an average of three relapses

Treatment

- Treatment is with doxycycline 100 mg by mouth twice a day

Babesiosis

Pathophysiology

- Babesiosis is caused by an intra-red blood cell protozoan parasite.
- It is spread by *Ixodes* ticks.
- In the U.S., most cases are reported from the northeastern coastal areas.

Clinical Presentation

☐ The incubation time is 1 – 3 weeks

☐ This disease causes a febrile illness that is worse in asplenic patients.

☐ Symptoms include malaise, fatigue, anorexia, shaking chills, fever, headache, and blood in the urine.

☐ Hemoglobinuria is a predominant sign.

☐ These symptoms are all similar to those of malaria, so inaccurate diagnoses may occur.

☐ The diagnosis is confirmed by a peripheral blood smear.

Treatment

☐ The treatment for mild cases is symptomatic.

☐ More severe cases may be treated with combination therapy of quinine/clindamycin or atovaquone/ azithromycin.

QUESTIONS

1. **Which one of the following is correct regarding gastroenteritis in the wilderness environment?**
    a. All victims should be started on antibiotics at the first episode of diarrhea
    b. Antimotility agents, such as diphyenoxylate, should be used on all cases of diarrhea
    c. Bloody diarrhea in conjunction with a fever of 104° F should be treated with oral antibiotics
    d. Enterotoxigenic *E. coli* accounts for 10% of "traveler's diarrhea"

2. **True or False: A person infected with malaria can be asymptomatic for days to weeks before developing symptoms.**

3. **Which of the following is the most appropriate treatment for Rocky Mountain Spotted Fever in a child?**
    a. Azithromycin 1 g by mouth daily
    b. Ciprofloxacin 500 mg by mouth twice a day
    c. Ceftriaxone 2 g IV every 24 hours
    d. Doxycycline 100 mg by mouth twice a day

4. **Which one of the following is responsible for most cases of rabies worldwide?**
    a. Bats
    b. Beavers
    c. Dogs
    d. Raccoons

5. **True or False: Rocky Mountain Spotted Fever is a self-limited disease and can be effectively managed in the wilderness.**

6. **Three hours after eating dinner, all members of your backpacking camp develop acute onset of vomiting and diarrhea. What is the most appropriate management?**
    a. Azithromycin 1g by mouth daily
    b. Immediate evacuation
    c. Metronidazole 500 mg by mouth three times a day
    d. Supportive care and oral rehydration solution

7. **A 16 year-old female is one week into a two-week camping trip in Colorado when she complains of weakness in her legs and difficulty walking up the hills. She was fine before the trip. On examination you find a symmetric weakness of the legs with absent Achilles and patellar reflexes. She has no rashes. Which one of the following is most appropriate in evaluating and treating this patient?**
   a. Amoxicillin 500 mg by mouth three times a day
   b. Doxycycline 100 mg by mouth twice a day
   c. Oral rehydration with a balanced salt and glucose solution
   d. Thorough evaluation for a tick with removal if one is found

Answers:
1. **c**
2. **True**
3. **d**
4. **c**
5. **False**
6. **d**
7. **d**

CHAPTER 16
Wilderness Medical Kits

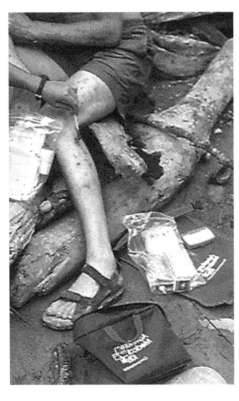
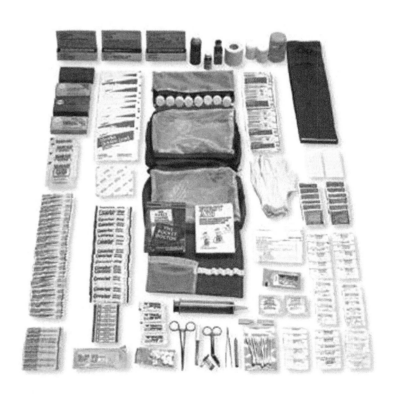

This chapter discusses general considerations, planning and preparation, and specific items that can be used for multiple purposes to treat ill and injured victims in the wilderness.

Objectives:

- Understand how to evaluate and anticipate injuries and illnesses inherent in a specific wilderness activity
- Plan for the types of individuals and special populations who will be going on a wilderness trip
- Construct a basic medical and survival kit
- Describe the PAWS method to help determine the appropriate supplies for a medical kit
- Understand the concept of using medications and equipment with multiple functions in order to minimize the amount of supplies in your kit
- Review the provided list of potential medications and equipment to assist you in developing a medical kit for a specific type of trip

GENERAL CONSIDERATIONS

- When constructing wilderness or travel medicine kits emphasis should be placed on items that will promote prevention of injuries and illnesses, enhance prospects for individual and team survival, optimize the ability of injured individuals to self-rescue, and failing self-rescue, to facilitate patient salvage. Bringing appropriate medical supplies into the wilderness is essential.

- A modular approach to kit construction may facilitate the identification of items that may make the difference between comfort, safety, effective treatment of illness and injuries, and timely rescue versus failure to achieve these goals.

- There is no all-purpose medical kit that provides adequately for every situation. Because there are so many variables to consider in packing a kit for a wilderness trek or expedition, it can become a daunting, time consuming and sometimes frustrating task.

- Our intent is to provide you with a framework and an approach to kit construction that will help guide you in developing medical kits for specific activities.

- Things to leave home or in your vehicle: Poorly constructed/stocked/"Rambo-ish" survival knives, axes, whetstones (nature provides sharpeners), heavy multi-tools with too many gadgets and items used for advanced medical procedures that are not applicable/sustainable in the wilderness environment head this list. Use your imagination.

TIP: Many outdoor enthusiasts engage in several different types of outdoor activities that span several environments and seasons. A modular <u>approach to medical kit</u>s is suggested. Such an approach allows the user to construct a core kit useful in most environments for most activities, adding items likely to have applications only in special environments, and removing those less likely to be used. Components may include:

- ☐ **An individual survival kit** (aimed at injury prevention and mitigation of survival situations to minimize potential injuries)
- ☐ **A core multipurpose medical kit carried by each individual in a party**
- ☐ **Environment specific medication and materials** (ex. aquatic, hiking, biking, altitude...)
- ☐ **Multifunction kit modules for groups that may separate into subgroups during trips**
- ☐ **Modules of extra consumable supplies to be cross-loaded** (distributed among party members) **for large groups, remote trips, and/or trips of long duration**

Understand your role on the team

- ■ By default, members of an expedition become a team. Teams may only be as strong as their weakest member. Remember that if you choose to serve as the medical care provider on an expedition it is your role to assist those in need. Accordingly, you may have to sit out parts of the trip (in which you would like to participate) to tend to ill or injured individuals.

- ■ Are you actually the designated medical advisor or a paid health care provider for the trip?
  - ☐ Consider insurance, licensing, and other legal ramifications of such a position
  - ☐ Add copies of required documents to your medical kit

- ■ Will there be there other medics / providers accompanying the trip, what is their experience level, and have they agreed to assist you/team members with routine care, only in the event of emergencies, or not at all?

- ■ Are you planning to be a non-medical member of a trip? Have you come to realize that some may come to you because of your medical knowledge even though you are not hired as a medical care provider?

Individual Preparedness

- ■ As an individual it is your responsibility to assure that you are prepared on number of levels. These include:
  - ☐ Personal preparedness, to include personal fitness, personal medications, and any 'special population' needs for those accompanying you (such as children, elders, those with special needs, etc.).
  - ☐ Review the contents of your personal survival, prevention and medical treatment kit for completeness and appropriateness in the context of the planned trip. Replace expired or consumed items.
    - Each person on the trip should carry a personal medical kit that contains the analgesics they prefer for aches, sprains and pain, basic bandages for blisters, wounds and scrapes.

274

Include any recommended activity specific supplies (altitude, water, desert, jungle) in addition to your personal medications.

- Ensure that those with chronic medical problems to bring extra medication. Ask about allergies or dermatologic conditions that only flare up during environmental changes such as hot/cold or dry/humid.

☐ Do not pack more than you can carry.

- Eliminate items that are of marginal utility or with which you are unfamiliar.
- Replace single use items with multi-purpose ones.

Medical provider preparedness: Medical providers charged with medical care for those on a trip should assure the following:

■ That each individual should be fit and prepared for the trip at hand well before departure.

■ Learn and anticipate all individual's medical problems and needs while planning for the trip.

☐ As a medical provider, you should know the age, past medical history, medications and allergies of each member of the group if you are going to be medically responsible for treating them. Have them fill out a brief health history and review it before the trip.

☐ It is highly recommended that you also carry an emergency dose of trip members' medications for any life-threatening condition.

☐ Make accommodations in advance for those who might not be able to participate in all activities, or refuse them participation on the trip. Pre-existing medical conditions, and those that develop or decompensate enroute, may hinder the overall objective of trip.

☐ Ensure that each member has appropriate personal survival and medical kits and an adequate supply of all personal medications (allowing extra medication for unplanned trip delays).

- By requiring this and making recommendations to the group prior to the trip, you will have to carry fewer group supplies. Others in the group be more personally responsible and self-sufficient.

- A potential downside to the use of personal medical supplies is that the medical leader may remain unaware of medical problems that arise until they escalate beyond the range of easy cures, proper mitigation, or even evacuation. To help avoid such situations, remind participants that you are there to keep them safe and ready to participate in all trip activities, not to disqualify them. Suggest that trip members report any and all use of items in their personal medical kits, and offer resupply of common items such as analgesics and blister bandages.

■ A creative approach to group monitoring will help medical leaders to minimize their workload and improve group safety and dynamics by aiding early and correct problem recognition (for example, analgesic use for headache due to dehydration or high-altitude cerebral edema – conditions that require more than analgesia).

On very long, remote or austere trips, and/or with large parties, robust and comprehensive medical kits are required. Just because you are the only medical provider, it does not mean that you have to carry all of the medical supplies. Group members should carry a component of the group survival and medical equipment ('cross-loading').

☐ Know with whom these items are loaded. Review the location and integrity of kit modules among the group before and after any "side trips" taken by a subset members of the group

☐ Distribution of kit components should account for members or teams in a group that may separate from the group so that essential items remain available to all members of the group. Be certain that 'Items that must be used together are NOT shipped separately.'

☐ This also helps to prevent the loss of all the medical supplies in the event of a single accident.

☐ Cross-loading of controlled medications (narcotics) is not recommended. Licensed medical care providers that sign for this material are solely (and seriously) responsible for its use and accountability.

Selection of medical kit items

Will depend on many aspects of the planned trip:

Your experience and training level: do not bring items you are unfamiliar with or have never used before. They are added weight if you are unwilling to use them, and they may be hazardous if you use them incorrectly

Type of activity (hiking, climbing, paddling, skiing, dog-sledding, SCUBA diving, etc.)

Will individuals carry the equipment, or will it be placed in a vehicle, watercraft, sled or airdropped?

Group size:

☐ Supplies loaded must be congruent with the group size.

☐ Will the group be broken down into smaller elements for movement?

Personnel on the trip: age, gender, ability and experience level for the activity.

Distance to be traveled: on foot, by paddling, by motor vehicle or other means like dogsled (be ready to do some running) or yak

Available means of evacuation: proximity, method, routes (on foot, all-terrain vehicle, aircraft with hoist capabilities, etc.), and reliability.

Be aware of communication methods to initiate rescue efforts and communicate during evacuation to an appropriate facility. Keep communications devices safely with critical equipment and provide backup means of communication whenever possible.

What weather/conditions will hinder or obviate evacuation?

Does the rescue service have additional supplies, access to equipment and personnel needed to diagnose and treat local or critical illness and injury? Examples include malaria, decompression injuries, snakebite anti-venom, and for trauma X-ray, CT, a trauma surgeon, a neurosurgeon...

Duration of the trip: locations and periods along the expedition that may permit resupply.

As examples:

■ A backpacking trip of seven days over remote, high, mountainous terrain requires a medical kit that is compact, lightweight and contains items that can treat emergencies related to high-altitude illness, cold exposure, avalanches, trauma, and geographically specific infectious diseases in the absence of available rescue or medical facilities.

■ In contrast, on a one-day river-rafting trip near a highway weight is less critical. A passing vehicle may aid evacuation to nearby advanced medical care. In the latter scenario, a kit with supplies to treat emergencies related to watersports-related injuries, cold exposure, and trauma would be appropriate.

■ **Medical kit items must be selected with multi-purpose use in mind** to conserve weight and packing space and to cover as many contingencies as possible.

   ☐ While having the right equipment is important, *it is impossible to carry all foreseeable items into the wilderness*. The ability to improvise is paramount in wilderness medicine.

   ☐ Examples of such versatile items include safety pins, gauze, duct tape, and SAM splints.

   ☐ Examples of multipurpose medications include diphenhydramine injection (anaphylaxis, allergy, antiemetic, sedative, local anesthetic), prochlorperazine injection (antiemetic, anti-motion sickness, sedative), or even common acetaminophen and opioid combination tablets (analgesic, antipyretic, antidiarrheal, sedative).

   ☐ Where practical, ultrasound is an extremely versatile tool in austere circumstances, and will be discussed later in the chapter.

■ **Consider immunizations and vaccines to be part of the team's preparations and kits.** Begin with enough time for multi-immunization vaccines to be completed (ex. Japanese encephalitis immunizations requires 2 injections 30 days apart). Vaccines to consider may include tetanus, diphtheria and pertussis, yellow fever, rabies and others. Consult the recommendations for travelers available on the CDC and U.S. Department of State websites.

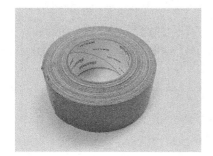 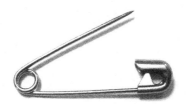 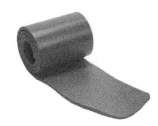

Prescriptions and Controlled Substances

■ It is recommended that all medications, especially prescription and controlled substances, be accompanied by the pharmacy prescription label with which they are issued.

   ☐ Check foreign laws before taking any medications abroad.

   ☐ For international travel it may be wise to keep a paper copy of the original prescription for medications carried as well.

■ On remote expeditions or when travelling to a foreign country it may be prudent to carry opioid analgesics or other controlled substances to facilitate performance of painful procedures, etc.

■ Special permission is usually required to bring narcotics into some countries!

☐ In some countries, unlicensed or unapproved importation of controlled substances without specific permission may be construed as drug trafficking and may even be punishable by death.

☐ Know the laws regarding exportation, importation and personal carrying of controlled substances before you travel!

☐ A list of controlled medication for U.S. providers can be found on the U.S. Department of Justice Drug Enforcement Administration (DEA), Office of Diversion Control website (http://www.deadiversion.usdoj.gov/drugreg/ Accessed 15 April, 2015). Becoming a registered provider requires filing a DEA form 224 for application and approval. Under some circumstances, additional paperwork and approval may be required in order to take controlled substances out of the U.S. Substances so registered may not be brought back into the U.S.

☐ United Kingdom (UK) providers can obtain a list of controlled substances through the UK Home Office Drugs Licensing Agency office. For example: a U.S. medical provider who wants to bring pseudoephedrine and ketamine for a diving trip in Australia is required to apply for a license and permit issued by the Office of Chemical Safety and Environmental Health (OCSEH); tmu@health.gov.au

TIP: The author has found it very helpful to consult a pharmacist familiar with controlled substance laws and DEA procedures for assistance in filing the correct paperwork when planning international trips. Keep at least two copies of the paperwork (one with and one separate from the medications in case of loss or theft while traveling). When carrying a large quantity of controlled substances for rescue/medical relief missions via commercial air carrier the author notifies the U.S. Department of Homeland Security (DHS) in advance of travel to facilitate screening through airport security checkpoints and has been well received by DHS being recognized by name and with expedited screening even when travel has been delayed.

■ When traveling with large supplies of medical equipment and medication it is important to carry an official letterhead document with your name and title and a list of medications. Copies of one's medical license and DEA registration may also be helpful. These simple precautionary measures will save you time and hassle during border crossings and in passing through customs agencies.

TIP: When definitive medical care is not usually more than a few hours away, consider carrying a lower ranking DEA scheduled or a non-scheduled analgesic with less abuse/diversion potential. Examples include agonist/antagonist opioid medications (such as nalbuphine, butorphanol and buprenorphine in escalating order of DEA schedule).

Physical Container for the Kit

■ There are numerous commercial options available in which to carry your medical supplies. In addition to these, there are several ways that you can make your own medical kit to fit your needs.

■ Important considerations for the physical container:

☐ Type of outside container: size, strength, and durability. Is it hard enough to protect fragile medical supplies from being dropped or smashed while traveling? Do you require a hard case, or are the materials you are carrying not breakage prone? Does the case need to be very flexible so you can fit it into your backpack or strap it to a horse?

● For most *backpacking*, a synthetic fabric organizer in a waterproof bag may be light and secure while allowing rapid access to emergency materials.

☐ Is the size appropriate enough to be able to carry all of the supplies you need? If you do not have to carry the kit on your person, then you may select a larger container and carry more supplies in it.

● Remember, however, that *controlled substances* must be under your direct control (and double locked) continuously if you are the responsible provider.

☐ Transporting medical equipment in larger containers may become a major issue if you have an unexpected vehicle breakdown. Using smaller commercial medical bags may be a better logistical option. Always consider a secondary option (backup plan) if lost in transit.

☐ Does it need to be protected from water? Cordura is an excellent material for most activities except water-related activities. It may be easier to pack and carry an Ortlieb waterproof rucksack for a *rafting* trip than carrying cumbersome waterproof containers.

☐ Will this kit protect the supplies from potential extremes of temperatures? This is an important consideration for *temperature sensitive medications* and in those trips in the desert, cold areas, and the mountains.

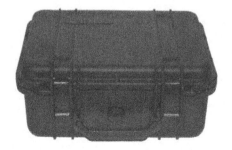 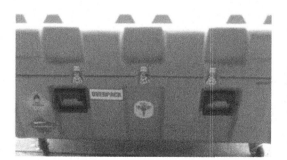 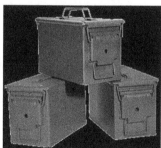

Specific Items

■ It is not practical to list each item that should be placed in every type of medical kit.

■ Some commonly used items are listed below.

■ Within the storage container, the author arranges his emergency medications in small zip-lock bags containing items likely to be used together in true emergencies so that they may be rapidly deployed. Sufficient amounts of medication should be carried based on the number of individuals along, the duration of the trip, the time to evacuation under adverse conditions, etc. Accordingly, no total quantity of each medication is suggested here.

☐ For example, items used to treat allergy/anaphylaxis will be grouped together:

Anaphylaxis	
Trained Provider/Initial treatment	**Untrained Provider/Follow-up doses**
Epinephrine 1:1000 and tuberculin syringe	Epinephrine Auto-injector
Diphenhydramine 50 mg/1 ml	Diphenhydramine (25 mg tabs)
Methylprednisolone 125 mg and syringe	Prednisone 60 mg dose (as 20 mg tabs)
Famotidine inj. 20 mg	Famotidine (20 mg tabs)

■ Other items are similarly protected, grouped and labeled according to use, including dose and frequency (one never knows when the medical care provider may become a victim and require care with the assistance of non-medical trip members). It is helpful to have stocking levels on the package to facilitate restocking if you make frequent trips of similar duration and group size. The labels may be organized in a computer database and printed on self-adhesive labels that can be affixed to small zip-closure plastic bags

For example:

Amoxicillin-clavulanate 875/125 mg
Skin and skin structure infections Urinary tract infection Lower respiratory tract infection Otitis media Sinusitis Diverticulitis
Adult dose: 1 tab orally every 12 hours
Contraindication: Penicillin allergy
Contains 20 doses

In planning for a modular medical kit approach, a **core individual medical kit for backpacking** and similar activities might contain some of the following items if the individual will be traveling alone or separating from the group often:

Container and zip –closure plastic bags to contain items	Bandaids #20, Assorted sizes	Steri Strips, ½ inch	Alcohol wipes#12	Benzoin, Applicators #4
Adhesive tape	Wound glue #2	Suture 4-0 nylon, 0-silk	Needles 25 ga x 1 ½ in 22 ga x 1 in, 18 ga x 1 ½ in	Syringes: 5 cc, Tuberculin
Small hemostat	Splinter forceps	Iris scissors	#10 & #11 scalpel blades	Safety pins
Triangular bandage	Ace/vet wrap	4 x 4 gauze pads	Iodine for water purification	Moleskin/ Second skin
Epinephrine 1:1000	Diphenhydramine Injection 50 mg	Cetirizine 10 mg tabs #20	Aspirin 81 mg, chewable 648 mg total	Ibuprofen 800 mg #20
Betamethasone Valerate 0.1% cream/ointment	Prednisone 20 mg #20	Hydrocodone/ APAP #12	Bupivicaine 0.5%	Loperamide 2 mg #20
Amoxicillin clavulanate 875/125 mg, #14	Ciprofloxacin 500 mg, #14	Metronidazole 500 mg, #20	Erythromycin ophthalmic ointment 1/8 oz	Tetracaine ophthalmic solution
Prochlorperazine 10 mg or Ondansetron ODT 8 mg	Bacitracin-poly-myxin ointment	Malaria prophylaxis	Meclizine 25 mg, #5 for motion sickness	Personal medications
Sunscreen SPF 30, waterproof	Insect repellent	Liquid crystal thermometer	Nitrile or sterile gloves	Vaccination card
Famotidine, calcium carbonate tablets, omeprazole	Ibuprofen	Topical antifungal (tolnaftate or similar)	Xeroform® gauze	Duct tape / safety pins

Controlled substances:

Analgesic(s) of choice for medically trained personnel: morphine, oxycodone, naloxone, ketorolac, opioid agonist/antagonist drug (see discussion above).

Parenteral and oral benzodiazepines such as diazepam may have a role in the treatment of seizures, sedation, anxiolysis for procedures, alcohol withdrawal and more.

If the individual will be in proximity to a large group for the duration of the trip, the contents may be cross-loaded; not every individual need carry all of the medications, though individual wound care supplies, comfort items, and supplies of analgesics and antidiarrheal medications are a wise investment. On long trips by large groups or in exceptional circumstances items not ordinarily practical or useful may add safety, capability or comfort for the group members. Some potential items are listed at the end of the next section.

PAWS

- The acronym PAWS is a general guideline and memory device for the selection and packing of a medical kit.
- **P**revention and procedures
- **A**nalgesics, antibiotics, antiseptics, anaphylaxis
- **W**ound care and weather considerations
- **S**urvival gear

Prevention/Procedures

Prevention

- Proper fitting boots, work gloves, and durable environmentally appropriate clothing and foul weather gear rank highly among the most important "preventive medicines" available. Be sure those on your trip are appropriately equipped!
- Having planned for a crisis situation prior to every having one is probably the most important thing you can do as a medical provider. A simple rehearsal of where medical equipment is, how to move a patient from point A to B, and communication with next higher care is crucial.
- A simple method to prepare for medical emergencies or survival situations is by using the "Rules of Three". In any extreme situation you cannot survive for more than
    - ☐ 3 seconds without situation awareness (scene safety) or common sense
    - ☐ 3 minutes without air (obstruction of airway) or blood (massive hemorrhage)
    - ☐ 3 hours without shelter (hypo/hyperthermia – extreme environments)
    - ☐ 3 days without water (dehydration – diarrhea)
    - ☐ 3 weeks without food (metabolic collapse)
    - ☐ 30 days without rest in a continuous heightened state (austere environment – combat)
    - ☐ 3 months without companionship/communication (losing the will to live).

■ Items listed here are considered for inclusion in your **prevention kit.**

    ☐ Water filter

    ☐ Water purification tablets

    ☐ Soap

    ☐ Gloves

    ☐ Sunscreen/lip balm

    ☐ Sunglasses

    ☐ Blister prevention and treatment

    ☐ Insect repellant and barriers (netting / treated clothes)

    ☐ Immunizations specific to your destination (before leaving)

    ☐ Oral rehydration packets

    ☐ Extra food and clothing

Procedures

■ There are certain tools of your trade that may be used in a variety of situations.

■ The level of comfort for each medical provider varies so the development of a specific list is more dependent upon those procedures a provider feels comfortable managing alone.

■ Items listed here are recommendations for consideration for inclusion in your kit.

Needles (2-3 sizes)	Oro/naso-pharyngeal airway	Safety pins	Tongue blades
Steri-Strips®	Zip-lock bags	Headlamp	Syringes for medications and wound irrigation
Zerowet® for wound irrigation	Scissors	Splinter removal forceps	Fluorescein, ocular anesthetic & cobalt blue filter light, ocular antibiotic
12G angiocath + stopcock	SAM® splint	Hemostat	Magill forceps
Scalpel and razor	Needle driver*	Sutures*	Foley catheter
Advanced airway	Bag-valve mask	Epistaxis kit	Ultrasound
Angiocatheter, large bore	Thoracostomy tube	Bone/dental wax	Dental repair kit (Cavit®, ZnO and eugenol, splint etc.)
Local anesthetic (bupivicaine for duration of action)	Optional: Near civilization, water sports, electrical injuries...	Pocket mask / CPR shield	IV start kit & fluids

Analgesics and antibiotics

Analgesics

Acetaminophen and NSAIDs should be a part of most kits.

Opioid analgesics may be required for some trips.

☐ The oral route should suffice in most situations but injectable (IV) medications may be required.

☐ Be aware of the laws pertaining to the distribution and transport of these controlled substances as they vary both nationally and internationally as discussed earlier.

☐ The best way to obtain opiates is by talking with your local pharmacist to ensure you are in compliance with the law.

Antibiotics

Select antibiotics that cover a wide spectrum of pathogens, thereby reducing the total number of items packed.

Common broad spectrum antibiotics to consider with some of their coverage:

☐ Doxycycline: lung, skin, and tick/mosquito borne infections

☐ Levofloxacin: HEENT, enteric, lung, skin, and urinary infections

☐ Amoxicillin /clavulanic acid: HEENT, lung, skin, enteric

☐ Azithromycin: HEENT, lung, skin, enteric organisms

If there are children on the trip, then you will need to consider medications that are safe for children as well as those formulations that children can take.

How and what medications to bring for a trek or expedition is individual based.

Depending on your travel plans ceftriaxone, ciprofloxacin, clindamycin, doxycycline, fluconazole, ivermectin, mebendazole and antimalarials such as chloroquine, mefloquine, atovaqoune/proguanil may have a role in your kit in addition to the items suggested above.

Although it's not strictly an antibiotic, topical permethrin 5% may be a major comfort in case of infestation with scabies or lice.

Anaphylaxis

Anaphylaxis is one of the true medical emergencies that one may see in the wilderness.

You should always be prepared to treat the anaphylactic patient.

At a minimum, you should have injectable epinephrine such as the EpiPen®, antihistamines, albuterol inhaler and oral steroids.

Acetaminophen	Ibuprofen	Opiate analgesic	Aspirin
Epinephrine injector or Epi 1:1000 and tuberculin syringe	Diphenhydramine (parenteral and oral)	Prednisone	Albuterol MDI
Ranitidine	Antiemetic (oral dissolving or suppository)	Oral rehydration salts	Loperamide
Simethicone	Doxycycline	Azithromycin	Levofloxacin
Amoxicillin with clavulanate	Ceftriaxone	Metronidazole	Dexamethasone
Glucose paste	Sedative - oral	Acetazolamide	Nifedipine
Anti-malarial / other anti-parasitic	Topical antifungal	Pseudoephedrine	Aloe vera
Cycloplegic	Ophthalmic antibiotic	Ophthalmic anesthetic	Saline eye wash
Topical antibiotic	Local anesthetic for wound closure	Glycerin suppositories	Topical steroid

Please refer to other chapters that specifically address the recommended medications for the different wilderness emergencies. This list gives additional items to consider.

Wound Care and Weather

Wound Care
- Regardless of the activity, abrasions and lacerations are among the most commonly experienced injuries. As a result, appropriate and adequate supplies for wound care are one of the most important parts of a medical kit.
- Having each person on the trip bring their own basic wound supplies will help to ensure that enough wound care supplies are available. Below are two different treatment options for basic wound care.

■ Curad Silver bandage (Band-Aid) is an over-the-counter (OTC) adhesive bandage with silver added for an antibacterial effect, which helps reduces bacterial growth (Staph. aureus, E. coli and P. aeruginosa) in the dressing for 24 hours. This is an effective and simple means to treat minor cuts, scrapes, abrasions, and lacerations in the wilderness setting.

■ Dermabond or New Skin liquid bandage create an antiseptic polymeric layer that binds to the skin possibly causing less trauma and complication than field suturing. 2nd Skin is a hydrogel bandage made from sterile water which also allowing visual wound healing without removing the bandage and risking exposure to bacteria.

■ * *Note: Closure of wounds in the wilderness is controversial. See the wound care chapter for more information.

Gloves	Wound closure strips	Tincture of benzoin	Alcohol swabs
Band-Aids	Moleskin or 2nd skin	Large trauma dressing	4X4 Gauze
Irrigation equipment	Povidone-iodine solution USP 10%	Antiseptic wipes	Antibiotic ointment
Sterile scrub brush	Knuckle bandage	Sterile dressing	Tape (cloth / duct)
Elastic bandage (Ace)	Q-tip	Eye pad	Triangular bandage
Gauze wrap	Tegaderm	Tissue adhesive (Dermabond)	1% lidocaine + topical lidocaine gel

Weather

In tropical climates the following survival items may be consider for inclusion in your kit:

Plastic sheet and surgical rubber tubing for solar still (and sling shot)

Extra water storage

Tinder and kindling (wet environments)

Fish hooks, weights, lures and braided line with fluocarbon leader

Topical antifungal agent

Solar blanket

Sun block/lip balm

Sun hat

Sunglasses

Rain gear

Hammock, lightweight

Tube tent

Insect head net / permethrin-treated clothing / DEET (insect repellent)

Oral rehydration electrolyte

In the desert water and shelter assume particular importance, as does your vehicle's equipment and repair kit.

In arctic climates high quality clothing and foul-weather gear is paramount. Do not skimp on these items or your shelter. Plan for adequate food and extra energy bars. Along with good judgement these are essential for survival. Don't forget a balaclava and sun protection items including glacier glasses and sunscreen.

In marine/fresh water environments assure that you have spare dry clothing, sun protection items, insect repellent, waterproofed food, dry tinder and kindling, fire starter, extra flotation devices and paddles. A raft repair kit may be relevant. Consider a fluorescent sea marker and exra flares.

Survival

- The potential for the group members to be separated and other worst-case scenarios need to be considered. Below is a table of items each group member should carry at all times.
- In any survival situation it is very important to STOP: Sit, Think, Observe, Plan.
- Take care of your boots and clothing. They are your shelter.
- Core survival items belong in your pockets (provided your clothing is in good repair). Examples include map, compass, knife, fire starter, etc.

ID/pencil/notepad	Knife (one hand operation) / multi-tool / wire saw	Compass/Map/GPS and (cold-weather stable) batteries	Nylon paracord (50 feet)
Personal medications	Waterproof strike-anywhere matches in waterproof matchbox	Metal match with magnesium, 3 in hacksaw blade, waterproofed tinder	Metal signal mirror and Fresnel magnifying lens
Plastic bag 38 in x 65 in, 4 mil, orange/ Tarp 6' x 8'/ Space blanket or Mylar sleeping bag	Iodine-based water purification method	Energy bars/Survival chocolate	Flashlight, LED or compact, hi and lo intensity, doubles as signal device
Whistle, high volume	Duct tape, several feet	Triangular bandage/ bandana	Chemlyte / Strobe/ Signal flares

Wire (for snares/ repairs)	Fishhooks and monofilament line	Nylon zip ties	Heavy foil or metal cup
Ace Wrap/Vet Wrap	Water bottle	Bug headnet/chemical hand warmer	For medical environments: N 95 mask, nitrile gloves

In-Vehicle Medical and Survival Kits

A medical kit to keep in the vehicle can serve as an extra kit while traveling to a trailhead and as a more comprehensive kit in the event of an evacuation or vehicle breakdown. Weather may change during the course of an expedition, and parked vehicles may become entrapped. In wet regions roads may turn muddy or wash out, and in woodlands trees may fall across roadways blocking egress. An in-vehicle kit may include and/or augment previously listed items in addition to the following:

Dry clothing / spare boots	Burn dressings / Splints / traction equipment	Spinal immobilization board	Work gloves
Ropes / rescue equipment	Blankets / dry sleeping bag	Extra food / water / cooking pot	Scissors
Flashlight	Battery cables / spare battery or booster / generator	Lighter / matches / tinder & kindling	Long burning candles (heat, light, fire starter)
Radio / CB / cell phone charger	Toilet paper / paper towels	Tarp to shade vehicle	Antifreeze/ motor oil / extra fuel / siphon
Foil / wind shelter	Tire chains / carpet strips (traction)	Fire extinguisher	Flares (6)
Fan belts	Cables / tow chain / winch	Wedge chocks / blocks	Stove / cookware / extra cooking fuel
Saw / chainsaw	Axe / pry bar / shovel	Mechanics tools / spare parts / repair manual	Jack / spare tire / Air pump

Additional Items to Consider: Large Goups and Long Trips

Other items for potential inclusion depending on the nature of your trip and group follow:
Equipment:

Pharmaceutical selection and dosing guide

Pocket medical reference

Finger and toenail clippers

Trauma shears

Sewing kit

Alcohol-based hand sanitizer

Chlorhexidine scrub or preps

Masks/splash protection

Morgan lens

Tourniquet

Chemical ice/hot packs

Digital thermometer (expanded range for hyper/hypothermia)

Glucometer, strips and calibration device

Urine dip sticks

Urine pregnancy test

Stethoscope

Watch with sweep second hand

Gamow Bag

Pulse oximeter

End-tidal CO_2 detector/monitor

CO detection device/monitor

Airway kit including laryngoscope and endotracheal tubes (timely evacuation available)

Cricothyrotomy kit

Chest trauma kit (large groups, long trips, evacuation available)

Medications:

Oxymetazoline

Silver nitrate cautery sticks

Docussate, glycerine suppositories, other laxative

Saline for irrigation

Hemorrhoid ointment

Albuterol

Epinephrine MDI (Primatene Mist®) or albuterol or albuterol/ipratropium

Nitroglycerin

Metoprolol

Diltiazem

Quinine

Antivenom (arthropods, snakes)

Rabies immune globulin (often difficult or impossible to locate in emergencies)

SPECIFIC ACTIVITIES AND KIT ADDITIONS

Specific activities or special patient populations may suggest additions to items stocked in basic or "core" individual and group kits.

If you plan to climb, and especially if you have accepted responsibility for team medical care, you should have training in rope rescue and mountaineering. Prospective cavers should have training in confined space rescue, and divers should be trained in dive rescue and dive medicine.

Climbing, Caving and Canyoneering
Rescue equipment for difficult evacuation, extra splints and wound care supplies, and extra water purification tools/supplies. Pelvic binder. Ankle splint.

Extreme Sports
These sports known as freesport, action sport, and adventure sport (i.e. BASE jumping), have a high level of inherent danger and require stabilization equipment such as spine board, C-collar, traction splint, and pelvic binder.

Mountaineering
Consider a Gamow® bag, extra sunglasses, avalanche safety and rescue equipment, AvaLung®, thermometer, and cold-exposure items (hand and foot warmers, space blanket, and aloe vera for frostbite).
For altitude-related illness consider acetazolamide, dexamethasone, sildenafil and nifedipine.
Cyclopentolate ophthalmic 1% drops may ameliorate ocular pain resulting from UV exposure.
Oxygen and administration devices.

Pediatric
Pack medications in chewable or suspension form (appropriate dosing according to weight), smaller sizes of equipment (ex. mask, airway, needles, Epi Pen Jr.®), Magill forceps, and tympanic membrane anesthetic.

Water Sports
Consider bringing water rescue equipment (extra flotation device, throw bag and line, rigging for a Z-drag, etc.), a bag-valve mask, extra sunscreen and insect repellent, water disinfection equipment, vinegar (for nematocyst inactivation on salt water trips), ciprofloxacin, and metronidazole.
Cervical spine collar

CHAPTER 17

Water Treatment

This chapter will discuss the treatment of water collected from a wilderness source to mitigate the risk of infection caused by its ingestion.

Objectives:

- Describe various waterborne pathogens that may cause illness from contaminated water
- Describe three pre-disinfection techniques to initiate the water purification process
- Describe techniques for point of use water disinfection and their limitations, to include filtration, chemical treatment, heat and ultraviolet irradiation
- Recognize the importance of basic hygiene as it relates to the prevention of gastrointestinal illness

CASE

A group of backpackers traverse a difficult ridge in the High Uinta Wilderness of northeast Utah. On reaching the other side, they are exhausted and thirsty. Having consumed all available water, they search for the nearest stream.

The icy cold waters are reasonably clear, so they fill their canteens and hydration bladders. As one of the most lightweight options, iodine and chlorine tablets were brought for water disinfection. Although very thirsty, they are careful to follow the directions on the tablet packaging before drinking the water. The remainder of the trip is uneventful.

About a week later, two of the hikers begin to experience abdominal cramping and watery diarrhea. One of them develops a low-grade fever of 100.6°F, yet her symptoms resolve over the next few days. The other hiker experiences more severe symptoms of nausea, vomiting, and weight loss. After several days, he is admitted to the hospital because of dehydration and requires IV fluid therapy.

During his evaluation, fecal specimens reveal microscopic oocysts but no white blood cells. There are no other specific signs or symptoms. An infectious disease physician conducts specialized testing, which confirms an infection with *Cryptosporidium*.

There is no effective treatment available for this illness; however, the hiker improves with supportive treatment and is discharged from the hospital.

BACKGROUND

Gastrointestinal illness from poorly treated water is a major cause of diarrhea and dehydration in the wilderness.

In a survey of wilderness hikers seven days into their trip, diarrheal illness was the second most common medical complaint (56%), closely following blisters (64%).

Basic definitions:

- ☐ Purify: remove taste, odor and smell
- ☐ Disinfect: remove or destroy pathogens
- ☐ Sterilize: destroy all life forms
- ☐ Filtration: mechanical process of forcing water through a membrane to remove pathogens

The goal of water disinfection is to kill or remove all enteric pathogens to an acceptably low number.

Unfortunately, judging water by its taste, appearance and collection location are unreliable methods for determining if it is safe for consumption.

MICROBIOLOGIC ETIOLOGY

Waterborne pathogens that may cause gastrointestinal illness fall into four major categories:

- ☐ Bacteria
- ☐ Viruses
- ☐ Protozoa
- ☐ Helminths (parasitic worms)

The likelihood of encountering any of these microorganisms depends on the location and exposure of the water source to contamination.

- ☐ Watershed areas with animal grazing and human contact have different risks than water that appears to come from an underground source. Some organisms may reside in particular soils or underground springs, while others may contaminate surface water by run-off from the rain.
- ☐ Generally, pristine watershed areas tend to be free of viral agents. However, with increasing human exposure, viral contamination becomes a greater concern.
- ☐ In the past, much attention has been given to the protozoan *Giardia lamblia* as a cause of wilderness gastrointestinal illness. However, most experts believe it is much more likely that bacteria cause the majority of wilderness gastrointestinal illness.
- ☐ In the wilderness, it can be very difficult to determine who or what has previously been in an area, potentially contaminating water sources. In order to be safe, one should adhere to the principle that all wilderness water sources are contaminated.

The table below categorizes some of the leading waterborne pathogens.

Bacteria	Viral Agents	Protozoa	Helminths
Escherichia coli *Shigella* *Campylobacter* species *Salmonellae* *Yersinia enterocolitica* *Aeromonas* species *Vibrio cholerae*	Hepatitis A Hepatitis E Norwalk agent Poliovirus Rotavirus	*Giardia lamblia* *Entamoeba histolytica* *Cryptosporidia* *Cyclospora* species *Blastocystis hominis* *Acanthamoeba* *Balantidium coli* *Isospora belli* *Naegleria fowleri*	*Ascaris lumbricoides* *Taenia* species *Trichuris trichiura* *Fasciola hepatica* *Strongyloides* species *Echinococcus* *Diphyllobothrium* species

PRE-DISINFECTION TECHNIQUES

Purification

- When water is initially collected, it is essential to minimize accumulated particulate matter.
- Organic and inorganic particles can interfere with the disinfection process, as well as make for an unpleasant drinking experience.
- All three of the following pre-disinfection techniques can be time consuming. Depending on the urgency of the situation, one will have to decide upon the most feasible technique(s).
- It is important to understand that these techniques help purify water but are not effective for disinfection by themselves.

Screening

- This technique is intended to remove the largest of the contaminants. It involves using a primary filter as a screen to hold back dirt, plant, and animal matter. Many commercially available filtration systems already have a "pre-filter" attached.
- Whether using a commercially available filtration system or improvising, when filling a container by dipping or pouring, one can screen out unwanted debris by pouring the water through a cloth, such as a bandana, handkerchief, or even a T-shirt.

Standing

- This technique requires the collected water to remain undisturbed for a period of time.
- During this time, particles that were small enough to pass through any screening material may fall or "settle out" to the bottom of the container.
- Within as little as one hour, even muddy or turbid water may show significant improvement.

After some settling has occurred, the clearer water can be carefully decanted from one container into another, leaving the sediment behind.

Flocculating

This technique can remove small particulate matter that normally stay suspended in water even after using the screening and standing techniques.

Adding specific chemicals promotes agglomeration of the particulates until a complex forms that is then large enough to precipitate.

One such chemical is "alum", which is often used in canning and pickling, and easily found in grocery stores. It is also a component of baking powder. The fine, white ashes from burned wood (rich in mineral salts) can also be used as a flocculating agent.

Add a "pinch" of flocculant for every gallon of water and then stir gently for about 5 minutes. After stirring, allow the water to stand and settle before decanting off the cleaner water.

DISINFECTION METHODS

Filtration

Filters screen out bacteria, protozoa, and helminths and their cysts and eggs. However, they are not reliable for eliminating viruses.

Viruses tend to adhere to other particles, or clump together, which may allow some of them to be removed by filtration. However, because they are so small (less than 0.1 micron), viruses cannot be eradicated by filters alone. Some filters are impregnated with an iodine element in order to destroy the viruses as they pass through the material. However, these additions are of questionable efficacy and lifespan.

Because filters work by trapping small particles in their pore matrix, they clog and become less effective over time. Operating a pump forcefully as it becomes clogged can push pathogens through the filter, thereby contaminating previously processed water.

Interpreting advertised filter specifications can be difficult.

☐ The best way to evaluate a given filter is to ascertain its functional removal rate of various organisms. For example, a filter labeled "effective against pathogens" does not truly describe its efficacy.

☐ Filters need to eliminate microbes down to the 0.2 micron range (absolute size, not nominal) to be effective for most pathogens, even though larger pore sizes of 0.3 to 0.4 microns may work for many applications.

For practical usage, filters should only be utilized as the sole disinfection method in areas where human contact with the risk of virus contamination is limited.

■ When uncertain, one should use a second method of disinfection (i.e. halogenation) as a final step.

Chemical Treatment

Halogenation

■ Iodine and chlorine can be very effective as disinfectants against viruses and bacteria.

■ However, their effectiveness against protozoa and helminths, as well as their eggs and cysts, varies greatly. For example, while *Giardia lamblia* is effectively killed, *Cryptosporidium* cysts are extremely resistant to halogen disinfection. The amount of halogen required is impractical for drinking.

■ Regardless of this limitation, the major problem with chemical disinfection is improper treatment by the user. Disinfection depends on both halogen concentration and contact time.

■ Factors that affect halogen concentration include water temperature, pH and the presence of contaminants.

☐ Chlorine is more sensitive to these factors and is thus less suitable for cold, contaminated water. In these conditions, halogens require increased contact time and/or concentration.

☐ Turbid water should be allowed to settle before halogenation because particulate matter can deactivate the available halogen, rendering disinfection incomplete.

☐ Household cleaners, such as bleach, vary widely in concentration and are not a recommended chlorine source for disinfection of drinking water as they have some efficacy against bacteria, but not viruses.

■ Another challenge with halogens is their unpleasant taste.

☐ This can be remedied in several ways, but must be done after disinfection.

☐ A "pinch" of ascorbic acid (vitamin C) has been shown to neutralize taste, closely matching that of distilled water.

☐ Flavored drink mixes, especially containing ascorbic acid, can also help mask the unpalatable iodine or bleach flavor.

☐ Activated charcoal is another option for reducing the chemical load after disinfection.

■ There has been concern that outdoor enthusiasts may be ingesting too much iodine over a prolonged period of use.

☐ Some studies have demonstrated changes in thyroid function after prolonged use, although the specific amount of time has not been clearly identified.

☐ A general guideline is to avoid using high levels of iodine (recommended tablet doses) for more than one to two months.

☐ Persons planning extended use may warrant thyroid function studies before leaving and again upon return.

☐ For safety, iodine should not be used by persons with thyroid disease or by pregnant women.

☐ Anecdotal research suggests that 10% povidine-iodine solution may have some potential use and efficacy as a water disinfectant

Chlorine Dioxide

Chlorine dioxide for consumer use has shown promising results. Many smaller municipalities have used this treatment method for years, but it has only recently been made available for consumer water disinfection. Liquid and tablet options are becoming increasingly available commercially.

Chlorine dioxide is chemically different from "chlorine." It has a wider range of effective pH and often does not require more than simple mixing.

Treatment also imparts a much less offensive taste compared to the halogens.

Finally, it is one of the only chemical disinfectants shown to be effective against *Cryptosporidium*.

Sodium Dicholoroisocyanurate

Sodium dicholoroisocyanurate is a chemical cleansing agent and disinfectant that can be found in some modern water purification tablets and filters.

Despite its past and current use for water treatment in some developing countries, the results from several anecdotal studies suggest that although its use does improve water quality and reduce bacteria levels.

Heat

Enteric pathogens, including cysts and eggs, are readily destroyed by heat. The thermal effectiveness for killing pathogens depends on a combination of temperature and exposure time. Because of this, lower temperatures can be effective if the contact time is longer. Pasteurization applies this science with carefully controlled temperature. However, without a thermometer, it is too difficult and risky to gauge temperature short of boiling.

The boiling point of water at sea level is 100°C (212°F). At this temperature, disinfection has generally occurred by the time the water boils. This is because most organisms are effectively killed at temperatures below *this* boiling point (see table). However, since it is difficult to determine the exact temperature of the water, boiling is the safest way to ensure that an appropriate temperature has been reached.

One important characteristic of boiling points is that they decrease in temperature with increased elevation. For instance, water boils at only 86°C (187°F) when at an elevation of 14,000 feet (4,300m). Some physicians believe this does not make an appreciable difference in water disinfection times.

The CDC recommends boiling water for at least 3 minutes if one is located above 6,562 feet (2000 m).

Using heat properly is a very reliable method for water disinfection. Remember to use a pot cover to preserve fuel when heating water. Also, bring the water to a rolling boil to wash back down any pathogens on the inside of the container and assure the surface of the water has reached the boiling point.

Effective Times for Disinfection Using Heat

Pathogen	Thermal Death
Giardia lamblia, *Entamoeba histolytica* cysts	After 2 to 3 minutes at 60° C (140° F)
Cryptosporidium oocysts	After 2 minutes at 65° C (149° F)
Enteric viruses	Within seconds at 80° to 100° C (176° F to 212° F)
Bacteria	Within seconds at 100° C (212° F)
Hepatitis A virus	After 1 minute at 92° C (198° F)

Irradiation

Ultraviolet Radiation (UVR)

UVR has recently gained popularity as a portable means of water disinfection.

It is proven to disinfect water against bacteria, viruses, protozoa and their cysts, including *Cryptosporidium*.

In situations where the water is clear, it could be used as the sole form of disinfection.

If the water is cloudy or turbid, the water should be filtered of debris in order to allow the UV radiation to contact all of the water as the debris could block the UV rays.

UVR may allow a liter of water to be disinfected in less than 2 minutes.

SteriPEN is a commonly used UVR water disinfection tool.

UVR has several potential drawbacks to consider.

- ☐ Extra batteries may be needed for the longer trips.
- ☐ Cold weather may affect the battery life and output.
- ☐ Due to their complexity, failure or damage to the device in the wilderness could occur so one should have an additional backup mechanism.

Bottled Water

The safest option for hydration, if possible and practical, is to bring potable water into the wilderness.

However, one must realize that buying "bottled water" in many countries of the world does *not* ensure safety.

- ☐ "Bottled water" in developing countries may be contaminated tap water
- ☐ If buying water in a country with potentially contaminated water, one should ask to break the seal on the bottle to help protect against the reused water. This is not fool proof as dishonest venders may still seal the cap with glue.
- ☐ Carbonated drinks, such as sodas or sparkling water, are safest since the bubbles indicate that the bottle was sealed at the factory.
- ☐ Drinking containers and ice cubes may also be sources of waterborne pathogens.

Summary of Treatment Method Efficacy

Infectious Agent	Heat	Filtration	Chemical
Bacteria	+	+	++
Viruses	+	-	+
Protozoa and cysts	++	++	+
Helminths and oocytes	++	++	-

PREVENTION

- Proper hand hygiene and using clean eating utensils will help prevent gastrointestinal illness.
- Several studies have shown that hikers are much less likely to develop diarrheal illnesses when they practice proper hygiene.
- Eating and cooking utensils should be cleaned thoroughly using warm, soapy water after each use.
- The same results can theoretically (and possibly more easily) be accomplished with an alcohol-based hand sanitizer. Recall that hand sanitizer is only effective when there is no visible contamination of the hands. Therefore, any visible foreign matter should be removed as much as possible prior to use.
- Consider using diluted bleach to disinfect serving areas and in the final rinse water for dishes and utensils. Use enough to give a distinct chlorine smell.
- Proper human waste management is also necessary to protect water sources from contamination. Waste should be buried 8-10 inches in depth, at least 100 feet from any water drainage, and downhill from any groundwater sources. Large groups should use a portable latrine.

QUESTIONS

1. **Which one of the following pathogens is considered to be the most likely cause of wilderness gastrointestinal illness?**
   a. Ascaris lumbricoides
   b. Bacteria
   c. Giardia lamblia
   d. Viruses

2. **For an extra margin of safety, the CDC recommends boiling water for more than 3 minutes above what elevation?**
   a. 3,500 feet
   b. 5,000 feet
   c. 6,500 feet
   d. 10,500 feet

3. **Which of the following is the LEAST likely to be found in pristine watershed areas?**
   a. Cryptosporidium
   b. E. coli
   c. Giardia lamblia
   d. Hepatitis A

4. **Which one of the following is usually NOT removed by filters?**
   a. Bacteria
   b. Entamoeba cysts
   c. Giardia
   d. Viruses

5. **When choosing a filter, it is important to:**
   a. Choose one that includes activated carbon
   b. Find specific information on the functional removal rate of organisms
   c. Have a nominal pore size of 0.2 microns
   d. Make sure it is "effective against Giardia"

6. **True/False: Filters impregnated with halogens are very effective at killing viruses.**

7. **Which one of the following CANNOT hinder halogen disinfection of water?**
   a. Adding ascorbic acid or flavored drink mix before adding the halogen
   b. Cold water temperature

    c. Using chemicals before the expiration date

    d. Visible particulate in clear water

8. **True/False: Use of iodine is safe for someone with a pre-existing thyroid condition if it is well controlled by medication.**

9. **Which of the following is the best method for water disinfection?**
   a. Chemical halogenation that properly follows directions
   b. Water filtration with a 0.2 micron absolute pore size
   c. Ultraviolet irradiation
   d. The best method depends on the particular location and group size

10. **True/False: One can effectively reduce the risk of diarrheal illness in the backcountry by properly cleaning hands after urinating or defecating.**

Answers:

1. b
2. c
3. d
4. d
5. b
6. False
7. c
8. False
9. d
10. True

CHAPTER 18

Diving Medicine

In this chapter you will learn about the potential complications of diving and the medical treatment for them

The agenda for this chapter is as follows:

- Review pathophysiology of diving injuries
- Review barotrauma
- Discuss care of overpressure syndromes
- Review decompression sickness (DCS) and other gas dysbarisms

GENERAL OVERVIEW

Diving medicine is an expanding field, with over 3.5 million recreational divers in the United States alone.

Accurate data is difficult to obtain, as there is no official regulation of the industry.

■ There are approximately 177,000 new dive certifications in the U.S. annually, among the 4 largest dive organizations.

The incidence of decompression sickness (DCS) is approximately 2.8 cases per 10,000 dives.

DCS afflicts an estimated 1,000 U.S. divers annually, as recorded by Divers Alert Network (DAN) http://www.diversalertnetwork.org/ .

Types of Diving

There are many types of diving, although open circuit SCUBA is the most common amongst recreational divers.

Breath-hold and/or Freediving

☐ This is the simplest and oldest form of diving, and uses no breathing apparatus or supplemental air.

☐ Freediving is considered an extreme sport and includes 8 different types of breath-hold diving sanctioned by the AIDA, the official international freediving federation.

☐ The submergence is limited to the time the diver can hold his or her breath.

☐ The greatest medical risk associated with breath-hold diving is hypoxia which can result in loss of consciousness and drowning.

☐ The world record for depth achieved on a breath-hold dive is 214 m / 702 ft in 2007, using a weighted sled to speed descent and a lift bag to assist ascent. The record for a completely unassisted (i.e. without weight, rope, or fins) freedive is 101 m / 331 ft in 2010.

SCUBA

☐ SCUBA is an acronym for Self Contained Underwater Breathing Apparatus.

☐ SCUBA diving uses an air filled tank with a pressure regulator that supplies compressed air on an open circuit to the diver at a pressure equal to the ambient water pressure.

Rebreather/closed circuit diving

☐ This form of diving uses a device that captures a diver's exhaled breath, removes carbon dioxide, and replenishes oxygen before giving the air back to the diver to breathe once again.

☐ Classically used by military combat divers but is starting to gain popularity in civilian diving.

Mixed-gas diving

☐ This refers to diving using a breathing mixture other than compressed air (21% oxygen, 79% nitrogen).

☐ It employs varying concentrations of oxygen and nitrogen or the substitution of an inert gas, such as helium, for nitrogen.

☐ Mixed gases are commonly used for commercial/technical deep diving because they reduce or eliminate the risk of nitrogen narcosis.

☐ Enriched Air Nitrox diving uses a higher concentration of oxygen and lower concentration of nitrogen, and is increasingly popular in recreational diving. Benefits include extended bottom times before decompression is required, and lower risks of decompression sickness and nitrogen narcosis for a given dive profile; however, there is an increased risk of oxygen toxicity.

☐ The world record for open circuit SCUBA diving was set with mixed gases in 2014, reaching a depth of 332.35 m / 1090 ft 4 $^{41}/_{64}$ in. The record using only atmospheric air with 21% oxygen is 155 m / 508 ft 6 $^{23}/_{64}$ in.

Surface-supplied (tethered) diving

☐ A diver's breathing gas is pumped via hoses from a surface source or from a submerged diving bell at a pressure equal to ambient water pressure.

☐ Most often used in commercial or military settings such as "hard hat diving."

Saturation diving

☐ After 18 to 24 hours at a given depth, the diver's tissues establish equilibrium with the breathing gases, resulting in no further decompression obligation no matter how long the diver stays submerged.

☐ Divers stay in living quarters at depth in order to complete their assigned underwater mission. Example: Aquarius Reef Base underwater laboratory.

☐ Decompression schedule to reach surface again may require several days.

One-atmosphere diving

☐ This form of diving limits the exposure pressure to 1 atmosphere absolute (equivalent to the ambient pressure at sea level), eliminating any decompression obligation or possible pathology associated with diving under pressure.

☐ Diving systems range from one-man pressure suits such as the Atmospheric Diving Suit to multiple-person submersibles.

Dysbarism

Dysbarism refers to medical conditions resulting from changes in ambient pressure.

Dysbarism may affect divers, caisson (compressed air) workers, aviators, and astronauts.

It can lead to a number of issues including barotrauma, overinflation injury, decompression syndrome and gas toxicities.

Diving Physiology and Laws

Pressure is defined as the amount of force acting per unit area.

Atmospheric pressure is the average pressure exerted by the entirety of the column of air above the earth's surface, measuring 1 kPa or 760 mmHg (14.7 PSI) at sea level. This is also referred to as 1 atmosphere (1 atm).

- The total pressure at any depth is pressure from column of water plus atmospheric pressure. This is known as Atmospheres Absolute or ATA.
- Pressure gauges read zero at sea level; they have been adjusted to remove the effect of atmospheric pressure. This is "gauge pressure."
- Water
  - Each foot of seawater adds 0.445 PSI of pressure to the atmospheric 14.7 PSI at sea level.
  - Every 10 meters / 33 feet of seawater therefore adds 14.7 PSI, or 1 ATA.
  - Calculated ATA = (Depth/33)+1
  - At 33 feet of depth, the body experiences 2 ATA absolute pressure.
  - At 66 feet of depth, the body experiences 3 ATA absolute pressure.
- The change in pressure is linear with depth, but the greatest relative change is near the surface. This is important in the expansion/compression of gases or gas-filled cavities.
- Four laws of physics govern the physiologic effects of pressure on the body.
  - Pascal's Law:
    - Pascal's law states that pressure applied to any part of a fluid is transmitted equally through the fluid. Although liquids and gases are both considered fluids by Pascal's Law, liquids are non-compressible, while gases are compressible under pressure (see Boyle's law, below).
    - Most of the human body is a liquid and thus is not generally directly affected by the increased pressure under water. The air filled cavities are affected because of the compressibility of air (Boyle's Law).
  - Boyle's Law:
    - Boyle's law states that the pressure and volume of a gas are inversely related.
    - As pressure increases with descent, the volume of a gas bubble decreases, and as pressure decreases with ascent, the volume of that gas bubble increases.
    - Air-containing spaces act according to Boyle's law. This predominantly means the lungs, middle ear, sinuses and gastrointestinal tract.
  - Dalton's Law
    - Dalton's law states that the total pressure of a mixture of gases is equal to the sum of the partial pressures of the gases. This law can be used in conjunction with Henry's law to make different mixtures of gases (Nitrox) to decrease or avoid gas toxicities during a dive.
  - Henry's Law:
    - Henry's law states that as the partial pressure of a gas increases, more of that gas will be dissolved in a given liquid.
    - As depth increases, the amount of nitrogen dissolved in the body will increase and can lead to nitrogen narcosis. If the rate of ascent of a diver is too fast, the gases dissolved in the tissue, mostly nitrogen, will come out of solution as bubbles, resulting in decompression sickness.

Pressure in air-filled spaces of the body is in equilibrium with the pressure of the environment and other air-filled spaces.

☐ These spaces remain in equilibrium with the changing environmental pressure unless the passageway that allows equilibrium with the rest of the environment becomes obstructed.

☐ If this occurs, disequilibrium develops and barotrauma can result.

BAROTRAUMA

Barotrauma is tissue damage resulting from pressure disequilibrium.

The most common medical problems in diving are related to barotrauma.

Many types of barotrauma: mask squeeze, sinus squeeze, ear canal squeeze, middle ear squeeze, inner ear barotrauma, tooth squeeze, suit squeeze, lung squeeze, and GI barotrauma.

Mask Squeeze

As a diver descends, ambient pressure increases and the volume of air in the facemask decreases, according to Boyle's law.

Mask-pressure equilibrium is maintained by nasal exhalation during decent, which adds air to the facemask.

Failure to exhale into the mask during descent results in a relative negative pressure within the mask, pulling the face into the mask, and rupturing capillaries.

This results in skin ecchymosis, subconjunctival hemorrhage, lid edema, and rarely hyphema.

This generally resolves over several days to a week without treatment; cold compresses and analgesics may be used if symptomatic. May dive when resolved.

Barotitis Media (Ear Squeeze)

This is by far the most common diving medical problem, affecting 10 to 30% of divers during any single dive and >90% of consistent active divers at some point in time.

Symptoms include progressive ear pain during descent, a sensation of fullness, and reduced hearing in the affected ear after the dive.

At a depth of 2.5 ft, a 60 mmHg pressure gradient is generated across the ear drum, resulting in slight pain from stretching and inward bulging of the tympanic membrane (TM).

A depth of 4 ft results in a 90 mmHg pressure gradient.

☐ This collapses the medial one-third of the eustachian tube, resulting in the inability to maintain equal pressure within the middle ear, as well as increased pain.

- □ At this pressure gradient, attempts to equalize middle ear to ambient pressures by Valsalva or other maneuvers may not succeed, forcing the diver to ascend in order to reduce the ambient pressure.
- Depths of 4.3 - 17 ft are associated with 100-400 mmHg gradients, which may rupture the TM.
    - □ TM rupture relieves the pain of ear squeeze, but cold water entering the middle ear will cause severe vertigo with nausea, vomiting, and disorientation underwater.
    - □ Vertigo resolves within minutes to hours.
    - □ Rupture of the TM with water entering the middle ear can lead to polymicrobial infections
- Barotitis media is preventable by early (starting immediately upon leaving the surface) and frequent equalization maneuvers.
- Any eustachian tube dysfunction from an upper respiratory infection, allergies or smoking predisposes to barotitis media by interfering with equalization.
    - □ Topical and oral decongestants may be used before diving to facilitate equalization.
    - □ Any diver unable to equalize should not dive until they are able to do so.
- Treatment for barotitis media includes decongestants and analgesics, as well as an antihistamine if an allergic component exists.
    - □ Combining an oral decongestant with a long acting topical nasal spray (e.g.: 0.5% oxymetazoline) for the first few days is most effective.
    - □ Repeated gentle autoinflation of the middle ear can help to displace any fluid collection through the eustachian tube.
    - □ Systemic and otic antibiotics are indicated for TM perforation, since water should be considered contaminated.
    - □ Diving should be avoided until full resolution, including healing of any TM perforation.
    - □ The majority of TM perforations heal spontaneously within 1-3 months. Surgical repair can be considered if healing has not occurred within 1 month; most commonly performed for >10-20% rupture.

Barosinusitis (Sinus Squeeze)

- This is caused by the same basic mechanism as barotitis media.
- If there is inability to equalize the air pressure in any paranasal sinus (frontal sinus most common, followed by maxillary) during descent, a relative vacuum develops in the sinus cavity.
- The relative negative pressure causes mucosal congestion, edema, and hemorrhage, along with severe pain.
- The process may be reversed on ascent, resulting in a "reverse squeeze," with expanding air volume in a sinus causing pain and tissue damage if not released. Will usually "self-correct" blowing the obstruction out and relieving the pressure.
- Blood and mucus in the mask is a telltale sign of reverse sinus squeeze.

- Treatment for barosinusitis is the same as for barotitis media; systemic antibiotics are indicated for signs of sinusitis, including fever and purulent nasal discharge.
- Upper respiratory infections, symptomatic allergic rhinitis, sinusitis, nasal polyps and significant nasal deformity may predispose to barosinusitis.

Labyrinthine Window Rupture

- A severe but rare form of inner ear barotrauma resulting from an overly forceful Valsalva maneuver or very rapid descent, which may lead to permanent deafness or vestibular dysfunction.
- May result in inner ear hemorrhage, Reissner's membrane rupture, oval or round window fistulas, and perilymph leaks.
- Classic triad of symptoms is roaring tinnitus, vertigo, and hearing loss.
- Other symptoms may include fullness of the ear, nausea, vomiting, nystagmus, pallor, diaphoresis, disorientation, and ataxia.
- Treatment includes bed rest with the head elevated to 30 degrees, avoidance of strenuous activity or straining, and symptomatic therapy.
- Any suspected inner ear barotrauma should be evaluated by ENT specialists.
- Deterioration of hearing, worsening vestibular symptoms, or persistence of significant vestibular symptoms after several days warrant urgent ENT evaluation, as well, and possible surgical exploration and fistula closure.
- Diagnostic dilemma may exist if a diver complains of tinnitus, vertigo, and hearing loss after diving, since this could indicate labyrinthine window rupture (recompression contraindicated) or inner ear decompression sickness (discussed later, urgent recompression indicated). Careful history is most important since inner ear DCS occurs only after ascent, while labyrinthine window rupture usually occurs during descent. **When in doubt, always recompress.**

PULMONARY BAROTRAUMA

- Gas within the lungs begins to expand with ascent, with the greatest volume changes occurring at the shallower depths.
- If the diver does not allow the expanding gas to escape, a pressure differential develops between the intrapulmonary space and ambient pressure.
- This results in over-distention and rupture of the alveoli, and allows air to escape into the local tissues or systemic circulation; causes various forms of pulmonary overpressure sequelae.
- Most commonly occurs in divers with a history of rapid and uncontrolled ascent, as might result from running out of air and/or panicking, sudden uncontrolled positive buoyancy (e.g.: dropping weight belt, inadvertent inflation of buoyancy control device), or breath holding during ascent in inexperienced divers.

May also result from a localized overinflation of the lung (e.g.: bleb, air trapping from bronchoconstriction, alveolar mucus plug).

Fatal pulmonary barotrauma has resulted from breath holding during ascent from a depth as shallow as 4 to 6 feet.

Mediastinal Emphysema

Also called pneumomediastinum

This is the most common form of radiographically evident pulmonary overpressure syndrome (POPS), and results from air dissecting along perivascular sheath and bronchi into the mediastinum.

Symptoms:
☐ May be asymptomatic
☐ Substernal chest pain (most common symptom when symptoms are present)
☐ Subcutaneous emphysema may be palpable in neck and anterior chest
☐ Dyspnea is typically not present except in severe cases
☐ Hoarseness and fullness present if air dissects from mediastinum into neck
☐ Hamman's sign, pericardial "crunch" sound synchronous with each heartbeat, is rare, but may be present when air is present around the heart (pneumopericardium)

Radiographs will confirm the diagnosis.

Treatment is conservative.
☐ Avoidance of further pressure exposure and observation
☐ Supplemental oxygen may be useful in severe cases
☐ No need to recompress if no other symptoms present

Pneumothorax (PTX)

Rupture through the visceral pleura, with accumulation of air in the pleural space, can occur, although it is uncommon since the visceral pleura is stronger than the pulmonary interstitium. Only 5 to 10% of divers with arterial gas embolism (AGE) have radiographically evident pneumothorax.

Signs and symptoms may include pleuritic chest pain, dyspnea, and decreased breath sounds on the affected side.

Treatment is the same as for pneumothorax of any other cause.
☐ Supplemental oxygen and observation.
☐ Chest tube is indicated for large or tension pneumothorax, air transport in unpressurized aircraft or if recompression is required for concomitant injuries.
☐ Non-decompressed pneumothorax can develop into tension pneumothorax during ascent from recompression treatment in hyperbaric chamber.

Arterial Gas Embolism (AGE)

This is the most feared complication of pulmonary barotrauma.

This is the most common cause of death and disability among sport divers.

Results from air bubbles entering the pulmonary venous system from ruptured alveoli.

☐ These bubbles then migrate via left atrium into the left ventricle, aorta and arterial system.

☐ The bubbles then shower distally and can obstruct blood flow in the distal vessels.

☐ Coronary involvement typically produces EKG changes and elevation of cardiac enzymes, but rarely myocardial cell death.

☐ Passage into carotid or vertebral arteries may result in an ischemic stroke. The neurologic symptoms that occur depend on where the air causes obstruction, thus they can be myriad, multi-focal and deadly.

AGE typically develops during ascent or immediately after surfacing. Symptoms of AGE may develop up to 10 minutes after surfacing, but are most often evident within 2 minutes.

AGE will not occur later, as alveolar and bronchial pressures and volume will equal atmospheric as soon as surface breathing starts.

Any symptoms, especially sudden loss of consciousness, occurring immediately upon a diver surfacing are due to AGE until proven otherwise.

Approximately 5% of AGE patients suffer immediate death that is not responsive to CPR or recompression; autopsy usually shows complete filling of the central vascular system with air. Death is theorized to be due to a catastrophic reflex cardiac arrhythmia not amenable to resuscitation.

Treatment:

☐ Urgent recompression is the priority. No adjunctive therapy should delay this.

☐ High-flow supplemental oxygen (100% O2 by non-rebreather facemask at 15 L/min).

☐ Intravenous crystalloid infusion to maintain urine output at 1-2 ml/kg/hr.

☐ Maintain the patient in a supine position.

● Trendelenburg and left lateral decubitus positions are NOT recommended. Historically, these positions were recommended, but this recommendation has proven ineffective.

☐ Lidocaine may be given as a 1mg/kg initial dose followed by a 2–4 mg/min IV infusion. Research data is limited, but the general consensus is that it may be helpful.

☐ Treatment with recompression may be effective for AGE even if the recompression cannot be performed until up to 24 hours later.

☐ Recompression reduces bubble diameter and volume, allowing return of hyper-saturated blood to the obstructed areas.

☐ Even if neurological symptoms have resolved, the patient should still be treated with recompression.

If a patient requires air evacuation to reach treatment, unpressurized aircraft should fly no higher than 500 ft. above ground level.

- Recompression therapy in a hyperbaric chamber follows a number of protocols developed specifically for treatment of AGE. Most US facilities follow US Navy Dive Tables.
- DAN can provide advice on treatment of dive injuries as well as the location of the nearest hyperbaric chamber if required.

INDIRECT EFFECTS OF PRESSURE

Nitrogen Narcosis

- Also known as rapture of the deep, the narcs or inert gas narcosis.
- Development of intoxication due to increased partial pressure of nitrogen in compressed air which dissolved into tissues at increased depth.
- As the partial pressure of nitrogen increases with depth, cellular membranes, specifically neuronal membranes, are affected by the absorption of the inert gas into their lipid component.
  - ☐ The greater the lipid solubility, the greater the narcotic potency of that gas.
  - ☐ $NO_2 \gg N_2 \ggggg He$
  - ☐ Helium, due to its low lipid solubility, is essentially non-narcotic and therefore is commonly used as a substitute for nitrogen in deep diving.
- It causes anesthetic-like euphoria, overconfidence and diminished judgment and cognition, which can lead to serious errors in diving techniques, accidents, and drowning.
- Typical nitrogen narcotic/anesthetic effects by depth:
  - ☐ 70 - 100 ft: lightheadedness, loss of fine sensory discrimination, giddiness, and euphoria
  - ☐ >150 ft: increasingly poor judgment, impaired reasoning, overconfidence, and slowed reflexes
  - ☐ 250 - 300 ft: auditory and visual hallucinations, and feelings of impending blackout
  - ☐ 400 ft: loss of consciousness
  - ☐ Significant individual and diurnal variability in depth of onset and severity of symptoms.
  - ☐ Experienced divers may experience some acclimatization.
  - ☐ Sport divers should dive to a maximum of 100 ft to avoid this complication.
- Treatment consists of ascent to shallower depth (<70 - 100 ft), where symptoms clear quickly.

Oxygen Toxicity

- High partial pressures of oxygen are toxic. May result from breathing oxygen-enriched mixtures during diving, receiving oxygen therapy in hyperbaric chambers, and using regular air at great depth.
- Oxygen primarily causes toxicity to the lungs and CNS through several different mechanisms.

Pulmonary Toxicity

- This is theorized to primarily result from tissue damage due to the formation of oxygen-free radicals, but the pathophysiology has not been proven.
- Oxygen toxicity is a function of time and partial pressure of oxygen:
  - ☐ 0.5 ATA of O_2 –oxygen toxicity will not occur
  - ☐ 1 ATA of O_2 – 20 hours (breathing compressed air at 130 ft = 0.21 x 5 atmospheres)
  - ☐ 2 ATA of O_2 – 6 hours
- Symptoms of pulmonary toxicity
  - ☐ Substernal chest discomfort on inhalation that progresses to burning pain
  - ☐ Persistent coughing
  - ☐ Prolonged toxicity can lead to a permanent loss of vital lung capacity

CNS Toxicity

- Theorized that it results primarily from oxidation of enzyme systems.
- CNS oxygen toxicity is also called the "Paul Bert Effect" after the first individual to describe it in the late 1800s.
- CNS toxicity requires much higher oxygen exposure than that causing pulmonary toxicity and occurs at 2 ATA or higher of partial pressure of oxygen. This requires significant depth (>280 feet at 21% oxygen), or oxygen-enriched breathing mixture at lesser depths. Closed Circuit rebreather units can have O2 toxicity at 30 to 50 feet depending on time at that depth.
- Most people can tolerate 100% oxygen for 30 minutes at 2.8 ATA at rest in a dry chamber.
- Symptoms of CNS toxicity:
  - ☐ The earliest symptoms are typically twitching of the facial muscles and small muscles of the hands, but unconsciousness and seizures may occur without warning.
  - ☐ Acronym **VENTID-C**. **V**isual disturbances (blurred or double vision), **E**ars (tinnitus or roaring sound), **N**ausea, **T**witching (primarily muscles of face), **I**rritability, **D**izziness, **C**onvulsions
  - ☐ Seizures – these are not inherently dangerous and typically resolve when the partial pressure of oxygen is reduced, but may lead to drowning when they occur underwater.
- Treatment:
  - ☐ Remove oxygen mask in hyperbaric chamber at first sign of toxicity.
  - ☐ Maintain constant chamber pressure during seizure to prevent possible pulmonary barotrauma, may ascend once seizure has ceased.
  - ☐ Anticonvulsants are not required for seizure control.
  - ☐ If occur underwater, move up to reduce partial pressure. If unconscious and rescued by buddy then keep mouthpiece in and slowly ascend. There are a few different protocols for buddy rescue which are covered in dive certification classes.

DECOMPRESSION SICKNESS (DCS)

In mid-19th century, tunnel and bridge laborers working in caissons pressurized with compressed air were noted to sometimes develop joint pains and paralysis after leaving the high-pressure environment. Now known to be DCS; referred to as "caisson disease" at the time.

■ DCS is caused by formation of inert gas bubbles within both the intravascular and extravascular spaces after a reduction in ambient pressure and inadequate decompression.

Rapid decompression, due to a rapid decrease in ambient pressure from fast ascent or omission of needed decompression stops, causes nitrogen (inert gas) to come out of solution and form bubbles in tissue and venous blood.

Bubble formation leads to cellular distention and rupture, mechanical stretching of tendons and ligaments, intravascular and intralymphatic occlusion, congestive ischemia/infarction, and lymphedema.

Intravascular bubbles also produce activation of intrinsic clotting, kinin, and complement systems, resulting in platelet activation, lipid embolization, microvascular sludging, increased vascular permeability, and interstitial edema.

The deeper and longer one dives, the more inert gas dissolves into body fluids/tissues (based on Henry's law), requiring more time for it to come out of solution safely during ascent (decompression).

DCS onset occurs after surfacing.

☐ Often occurs within one hour (rarely within minutes like AGE) and the majority of DCS cases (95%) are seen within 6 hours.

☐ In rare cases, it may not be noted for 24-48 hours.

The incidence of DCS is 1/7500 dives.

DCS was classically described as only Type I or II but is now further divided into subtypes under Type I and II to better help describe and treat:

☐ Type I - Musculoskeletal DCS, Cutaneous DCS, and Lymphatic DCS

☐ Type II - Neurological DCS, Pulmonary DCS, and Inner Ear/Vestibular DCS.

Musculoskeletal DCS

Most common form of DCS (70%); often referred to as "bends."

Can involve any joint, although shoulders and elbows are the most common.

Pain is often referred to as boring or deep, dull ache.

Movement worsens the pain, which makes it difficult to differentiate from other musculoskeletal causes based on history or exam.

Some studies suggest inflating a BP cuff to above 200 mmHg over the joint may partially relieve the pain of DCS but not musculoskeletal. However, a lack of pain relief does not rule out DCS.

Must differentiate local from radiating pain. If pain is radiating it is neurologic DCS.

Neurologic DCS

- The spinal cord is most commonly involved in divers where the brain is involved with aviation personnel. Effects the lower thoracic to lumbosacral segments more often.
- May start insidiously as back pain then progress to paresthesias/paralysis.
- Symptoms can be dynamic and not follow single nerve pathways, because the bubbles can come out of solution in multiple different areas.
- DCS of the brain produces a variety of symptoms, which may be indistinguishable from AGE, and include dizziness, vertigo, altered mentation, generalized weakness, visual defects, ataxia and loss of balance.

Pulmonary DCS

- Uncommon but very serious, form of DCS, also referred to as "chokes."
- Probably represent massive pulmonary gas emboli with mechanical obstruction of the pulmonary vascular bed by bubbles.
- Symptoms begin when 10% or more of the pulmonary vascular bed is obstructed.
- Symptoms include burning chest pain, especially on inspiration, dyspnea and nonproductive cough.
- May rapidly progress to cardiovascular collapse.

Cutaneous DCS

- Pruritus is the most common skin manifestation of DCS and does not require recompression.
- Cutis marmorata, a mottling or marbling of the skin, is a harbinger of more severe DCS and recompression treatment should occur as if it DCS Type II, which will follow a different recompression table than Type I.

Inner Ear or Vestibular DCS

- Symptoms include dizziness, vertigo, nystagmus, tinnitus, nausea, and vomiting.
- Referred to as the "staggers."
- High risk for residual inner ear damage despite appropriate treatment.
- Most often seen in saturation divers due to poor blood supply and slow off-gas from inner ear.
- **Isobaric DCS** is similar: while making a rapid ascent on Heliox, or when switching from slow to fast diffusing gases on ascent from very deep dives can get DCS.

DCS Treatment

- The primary treatment is recompression as soon as possible.
- High-flow supplemental oxygen should be provided.

- Oral or intravenous fluids should be provided to maintain urine output at 1-2 ml/kg/hr.
- Air transport should utilize low flying aircraft and/or fly at <1,000 feet above the starting elevation.
- Diazepam may be beneficial in treating vertigo associated with vestibular DCS.
- The following treatment adjuncts are <u>NOT</u> recommended:
  - ☐ Aspirin and other non-steroidal anti-inflammatories were routinely used for DCS in the past but are no longer recommended.
  - ☐ Steroids and lidocaine are also not recommended for use in DCS treatment. This is in contrast to AGE, where lidocaine use <u>may</u> be helpful.
  - ☐ Anticoagulants are not recommended.

DCS Prevention

- Dehydration is the greatest risk factor to predispose to DCS.
- Dive computers or dive tables should be correctly utilized, obeying depth limits and bottom times, allowing sufficient decompression stops, and waiting an appropriate surface interval times between dives.
- Flying after diving should be delayed for 12-24 hours or more after surfacing, depending on the depth and duration of the dives.

Risk Factors for DCS Include:

- Obesity
- Advanced age
- Cold
- Smoking
- Flying after diving
- Dehydration
- Hypercapnia
- Repetitive diving

Contraindications to diving

- Absolute
  - ☐ Seizure disorder: *seizure free for 5 years relative
  - ☐ Symptomatic CAD
  - ☐ Previous spontaneous pneumothorax
  - ☐ Bullous lung disease

- Relative
  - ☐ URI
  - ☐ Pregnancy
  - ☐ History of POPs
  - ☐ HTN – due mainly to medication side effect
  - ☐ Patent foramen ovale (PFO)

Divers Alert Network (DAN)

- The definitive go-to network for dive medicine information as well as consults on dive injuries.
- They can also provide information on the hyperbaric chamber nearest to your location.
- 1-919-684-9111 available 24/7/365. They will accept collect calls. If out of the USA check for the DAN number.

QUESTIONS

1. During initial open water SCUBA training, a student panics from seeing a shark nearby, and bolts for the surface. The dive boat crew finds him floating on his back with his buoyancy control device fully inflated. He is unconscious, but breathing. Which one of the following is the most likely diagnosis?
   a. Cerebral arterial gas embolism
   b. CNS decompression sickness
   c. Panic induced nonfatal drowning
   d. Shallow water blackout

2. An otherwise healthy SCUBA diver is making an initial descent to a reef, when he develops moderate pain in the right ear at a depth of 6 feet. He is unable to equalize/clear his ears by moving his jaw back and forward. What is the best course of action?
   a. Abort the dive until decongestants or topical nasal spray can be taken
   b. Ascend until able to equalize, then resume descent with frequent clearing
   c. Continue descent at a slower rate, since pain will resolve spontaneously at greater depth
   d. Maintain current depth and clear the ears using forceful Valsalva maneuver

3. When a freediver descends from the surface to 33 feet of seawater, the volume of his lungs at this depth is what fraction of his lung volume at the surface?
   a. 2/3
   b. 1/2
   c. 1/3
   d. 1/4

4. Which of the following medical conditions is an absolute contraindication for diving?
   a. Atrial fibrillation on anticoagulation
   b. History of myocardial infarction
   c. History of spontaneous pneumothorax
   d. Insulin dependent diabetes mellitus

5. As a diver descends from a depth of 100 ft to 200 ft, the increased partial pressure of which of the following gases is most likely to result in lightheadedness, euphoria, poor judgment, and impaired reasoning?
   a. Carbon dioxide
   b. Helium
   c. Nitrogen
   d. Oxygen

6. **Which one of the following statements about decompression sickness in SCUBA divers is correct?**
    a. DCS can be effectively ruled out if a diver follows his/her dive computer properly
    b. Most common form of DCS primarily affects the central nervous system
    c. Musculoskeletal DCS most commonly affects the knees and ankles
    d. Spinal cord DCS most commonly affects the lower thoracic and lumbosacral cord

Answers: 1A 2B 3B 4C 5C 6D

APPENDIX

Additional Educational Material

CHAPTER 19

Wilderness Medicine in Australasia

Objectives:

- Recognize specific problems related to Wilderness Medicine practice in Australasia
- To be aware of venomous animal and insect bites and stings and their wilderness management
- Recognize the differences in management when compared to bites and stings in other areas of the world
- Have an awareness of the frequency of cold water immersion and its management

CASE 1

You are trekking in central Australia when one of your group steps on a dark coloured snake that turns around and bites him on his lower leg. The snake then rapidly moves off into the nearby undergrowth. It is mid morning and you are on a dirt road track; three hours walk from the nearest town. You have a satellite phone with the group.

1. What are the first priorities for treating this wound?
2. How would you prevent spread of the venom?
3. How could you tell if the bite was from a venomous snake?
4. What would be the best way to evacuate the victim?

CASE 2

Whilst snorkeling in the sea off the north coast of Australia one of your party spots a jellyfish and swims up to it to get a closer look. He gets too close and one of the tentacles brushes against his right arm. He gets immediate severe pain in his arm and screams and thrashes about in the water. He is able to make it to a nearby beach but is in agony lying on the sand.

1. What might you use, if available to treat the pain?
2. Should you remove any cysts attached to his skin?
3. Does this victim need to be evacuated to a hospital?
4. Is pressure immobilization effective treatment?

CASE 3

It is spring and you are kayaking across Lake Wakatipu, Queenstown New Zealand. You are half way across the lake when you encounter strong winds and capsize. You are unable to get back into your kayak, which has sunk and you are a 5km swim from dry land. You are wearing a PFD and medium weight clothing. The water temperature is 10°C.

1. How long are you likely to survive in the water?
2. Can you plan to self-rescue by swimming to shore?
3. How long before hypothermia sets in?
4. If help arrives before you drown, are you safe once rescued?

BACKGROUND

Australasia is a region comprising of Australia, New Zealand and New Guinea together with some smaller islands within the Pacific Ocean. A large geographic region, it contains much unique fauna and flora. The climate varies from sub-Antarctic to Tropical, dry desert to tropical rainforest and alpine regions. All the countries of Australasia have extensive coastlines and access to the Pacific Ocean.

ANIMAL BITES

Australasian Snakebites

All significant Australasian snakes belong to the elapidae family; they are found throughout Australia and New Guinea (but not New Zealand) and include the Brown snake, Black snake, Tiger snake, Death Adder and Taipan. Wilderness treatment of bites is the same for all of these snakes and differs significantly from the treatment of viperidae found in North America and other parts of the world.

All snakebites should be treated as a potential envenomation. Although a significant proportion of bites may be "dry bites" without envenomation, it is impossible to be certain which bites will lead to clinical toxicity.

The core wilderness management of elapid snakebites is pressure immobilisation. The venom from elapidae is thought to be spread through the lymphatic system and this can be significantly impeded by the application of a pressure dressing to the affected limb (the majority of bites occur on a limb) combined with immobilisation.

A pressure dressing should be applied to the whole effected limb with an elastic bandage or similar with a pressure described as similar to that used for a sprained ankle. It probably makes little difference if the bandage application in begun above or below the bite, but should cover the whole limb. The bite site is not cleaned and a dry dressing only applied (this may help later when a swab is taken from the bite site to identify the appropriate anti-venom to use). The limb must then be completely immobilised with splinting if necessary and the victim should rest completely and await evacuation via appropriate transport. The pressure bandage should never be removed until the victim is in a hospital and monitored with immediate access to resuscitation facilities and anti-venom available.

INSECT BITES

Australasian Spider Bites

The most common venomous spiders in Australasia belong to the latrodectus species, (related to the North American Black Widow spider). Latrodectus Hasselti is the Australian Redback spider, easily identifiable by a red stripe on its black body. Latrodectus Katipo, the New Zealand Katipo is notable for being both rare and also New Zealand's only native venomous insect. The bites are very similar to Black Widow bites. Deaths are rare. Clinical features include significant local pain, which may respond poorly to conventional painkillers and systemic upset including nausea, vomiting and abdominal pain. There is no effective wilderness management and symptomatic bite victims should be evacuated to a healthcare facility where they can be treated with antivenom if required.

The Funnel Web spider (Atrax species) is unique to Australia, being found on the Eastern side of the country. It is a large ground dwelling spider, the males of the species being especially active and aggressive during the breeding season. Its bite is responsible for a number of deaths. The acidic venom causes immediate pain and deaths are often due to immediate cardiovascular collapse. There is no effective wilderness treatment for the bite, supportive care should be provided if available and the victim transported as rapidly as possible to the nearest healthcare facility able to treat the bites.

Other spider species in Australia can cause morbidity but not mortality. Again evacuation is required for any symptomatic bite.

MARINE ANIMALS

Australasia has some very unique and interesting marine organisms capable of causing significant morbidity and mortality. The warm climate in much of the region, extensive coastline and clean, clear water are attractive for many water sports.

Sharks and crocodiles are responsible for occasional deaths. Management should follow that for other wild animal bites bearing in mind that injuries may be severe and the safety of rescuers must be of concern. Trauma may be complicated by associated submersion injury.

Jellyfish are common in tropical regions and stings may cause severe morbidity and mortality. The two major species are the Box jellyfish and the Irukanji. Box jellyfish tentacles contacting skin can cause severe and immediate pain and on occasion cardiovascular collapse and death. The pain is caused by small nematocysts, which can be inactivated by the application of acetic acid (vinegar) for at least half a minute. Remaining cysts should be carefully removed from the skin by scraping. All envenomation require evacuation and pain control may be very difficult to achieve. Irukanji syndrome may have a delayed onset of symptoms and more systemic effects such as abdominal pain, nausea and vomiting.

Stingrays have barbed spines on their tails capable of causing both mechanical penetrating injury (such as cardiac penetration and death as in the case of Steve Irwin) and also toxin mediated and infectious injury. Wounds are extremely painful and the pain does not respond well to normal painkillers. The toxin is heat labile and immediate relief of pain can be obtained by placing the wound in water heated to 40-45 Celsius (104-113 Fahrenheit). This may be very difficult to achieve in the wilderness setting. The spines are also prone to breaking off in wounds and can cause foreign body reactions and serious infection. Evacuation is to a healthcare facility is recommended for all such wounds. Good wound care is important and prophylactic antibiotics should be considered if there is likely to be a delay in transfer to definitive care.

Stonefish inhabit shallow water and are commonly trodden on causing penetration of the dorsal spines into the foot. These wounds are extremely painful and treatment is the same as for stingray barbs as described above.

INFECTIOUS DISEASES

Malaria is common in New Guinea and there have been occasional outbreaks in Australia. Transmission is via mosquito vector, and prevention is preferable to cure. Malaria prophylaxis, prevention and treatment are covered elsewhere in this book.

Australia and New Zealand are rabies free countries. However Australia is home to the Lyssavirus, which is related to the rabies virus. The infection has been passed to humans from Australian bats and is treated in a similar manner to rabies. Good wound cleaning and rapid evacuation to a centre where vaccination is available is the wilderness management of bat related injury in Australia.

COLD WATER IMMERSION

Both hypothermia and submersion injury are described in other sections of this manual, however the problems specific to cold-water immersion (CWI) also warrant discussion. The physics of heat transfer are described in the sections on heat and cold induced injuries. In the context of cold water immersion the predominant issue is that of accelerated heat loss via conduction and convection.

Cold water immersion is particularly relevant to the New Zealand wilderness as it is a significant cause of wilderness related death. Most CWI deaths will be reported as drownings, and indeed New Zealand has one of the highest per capita drowning rates of any developed nation. The NZ death toll from drowning is on average over 100 per year of which 60% are recreational. It is consistently the third highest cause of unintentional death, after road vehicle crashes and accidental falls. When the first European settlers came to New Zealand drowning was so prevalent it became known as the "New Zealand Disease". Although submersion is often the final result of CWI, there are other pathophysiological processes to be understood. These include:

- Cold Water Shock
- Swim Failure
- Immersion Hypothermia
- Circum-Rescue Collapse

Water has a thermal conductivity of 25 times that of air, and it takes 3500 times as much heat to raise the temperature of a volume of water compared to the same volume of air. Convection can greatly facilitate conductive heat loss by movement of molecules in either a gas or a liquid. We are probably most familiar with convective heat loss in the context of wind chill, but it is equally important in running water. The velocity of a cold river can multiply the deleterious effects of cooling significantly. The temperature of thermally neutral water, when heat production balances heat loss in a nude subject, is about 33^0 to 35^0C (91^0-95^0 F). Although the definition of cold water varies, for practical purposes 25^0C (77^0F) is usually considered the temperature at which immersion hypothermia is a risk. At this temperature a body will cool one hundred times faster than in air of the same temperature. All NZ rivers and most NZ lakes are below this temperature all year round.

Cold Water Shock

The initial risk on sudden immersion into cold water is not from hypothermia. The cold-shock response occurs in the first few seconds to minutes of immersion, and its severity is dictated by the extent and rate of skin cooling. Core temperature is preserved during this phase (clothing can mitigate the severity of the response). Rapid skin cooling leads to a gasp response accompanied by an inability to breath-hold and hyperventilation. If the victim's head is submerged during entry into the cold water the gasp response may induce a submersion injury (if sufficient water is aspirated 'wet drowning' will occur, but even small volumes of water encroaching on the cords may result in laryngospasm and 'dry drowning'). Initial hyperventilation usually subsides over a few minutes; prolonged hyperventilation associated with panic can however lead to hypocapnia with associated metabolic alkalosis. This in turn can lead to numbness/paraesthesia, muscle weakness and even fainting.

The skin cooling also results in peripheral vasoconstriction with the accompanying physiological responses of tachycardia increased cardiac output and resulting increase in blood pressure. This can cause a sudden increase in myocardial workload and myocardial oxygen demand. Arrhythmias including VF or vagally mediated bradycardia (dive reflex) can occur, especially in individuals with associated cardiac comorbidities.

It has been demonstrated that previous immersions can mitigate the cold-shock response of subjects. Most importantly, entry into cold water (below 20^0C, 68^0F) should be done slowly, while keeping the head above water if at all possible. Temperature receptors are not evenly distributed across all anatomical areas, being maximally represented in the head and chest region.

Swim Failure

Having survived the initial cold-shock there continues to be a differential cooling of the peripheries in order to conserve core temperature. This phase usually lasts from the first few minutes until true hypothermia occurs (the type of clothing worn, including wetsuits etc. will dictate the precise time to onset of hypothermia, but a rough figure is 15 to 30 minutes when wearing mid-weight clothing). Peripheral vasoconstriction leads to sluggish perfusion of tissues with a build-up of metabolites. This in conjunction with the colder tissues leads to a reduction in neuromuscular function. Fingers become stiff and fine motor control is lost. This is followed by a loss in muscle power and eventually a loss in gross motor control. The ability to breath-hold can be reduced by 60% to 75%, and in combination with discoordinated swimming actions leading to frequent head submersion drowning may ensue. This is more problematic in rough water. On average, a person wearing a lifejacket and light clothing can swim about 1.85 kilometres, or just over a mile in water of 10°C. It may be better to conserve energy and adopt other survival techniques in preference to attempting a long swim to shore. Much of the original work done on swim failure came from sailors being immersed in cold seas during World War II (WWII). Survival strategies include wearing a personal flotation device (PFD) or attempting to hold on to floating debris (pulling as much of the body out of the water as possible) and adopting the heat-escape lessening position (HELP) and/or huddling together with other survivors. Pulling drawstrings tight or tucking clothing in may reduce fluid circulation close to the skin, thus reducing convective cooling. When CWI results from falls through the ice, self-rescue may be difficult as attempts to pull oneself out may simply result in more ice breaking. Under these circumstances the victim should consider placing gloved hands or even hair (including a beard if they have one) onto the ice and allowing them to freeze there. This will keep the head out of the water when hypothermia results in loss of consciousness!

Immersion Hypothermia

Most cold-water drowning result from the two mechanisms described above. Hypothermia usually only becomes significant 30 minutes to one hour after immersion. If a floatation device is worn which keeps the head above water, then even in the event of hypothermic induced loss of consciousness the victim may survive for another hour or more.

Circum-Rescue Collapse

This phenomenon was first described in sailors in WWII, and has been see as recently as survivors of Flight 1549 that landed in the Hudson River in 2009. Hypothermic victims may appear quite stable at the time of rescue, but then may faint or even suffer cardiac arrest. This may occur minutes before the rescue, at the time of rescue or within a few minutes of rewarming starting. A number of mechanisms have been suggested. Immediately before imminent rescue the victim may mentally relax, and a subsequent reduction in stress hormones may result in a drop in blood pressure with loss of consciousness and drowning. During the rescue attempt repositioning the patient from the horizontal to the vertical may result in orthostatic hypotension (vasoconstriction often fails in the cooled peripheries). There may also be some 'hydrostatic squeeze' from the surrounding water, and on pulling the victim out this benefit is lost. Perhaps more importantly, hypothermia renders the myocardium more prone to dysrhythmias including VF arrest. Rough handling of a survivor on extraction can lead to sudden cardiac arrest. The core temperature continues to decline after removal from cold water ("after-drop"), and on re-warming sudden redistribution of blood to the extremities may result in a 'reperfusion injury' with distribution of cardiotoxic metabolites to the central circulation. Sadly up to 20% of those recovered alive subsequently die from circum-rescue complications that may occur hours after a successful rescue. At the time of rescue, if possible the victim should be kept horizontal and rough handling should be avoided. Further heat loss should be minimized until active rewarming can be started

QUESTIONS

1. **If bitten by a snake in Australasia, which is the most important first aid treatment?**
    a. Apply a pressure dressing to the limb and immobilize the victim
    b. Attempt to remove any venom from the wound by suction and making the wound bleed
    c. Clean the wound and apply an antibiotic dressing
    d. Start a course of antibiotics as soon as possible

2. **You are in the Australian outback where you are bitten by a spider with a red stripe on its back. Which of the following is correct?**
    a. A pressure dressing should be applied to the wound and the victim immobilized
    b. It is probably not a venomous spider
    c. The wound should be cleaned and the victim evacuated if any symptoms develop
    d. Treatment should be started with antibiotics and simple analgesics

3. **Immersion into cold water (below 20⁰C 68⁰F) may immediately result in which of the following?**
    a. An inability to stay afloat within minutes
    b. An uncontrolled gasp
    c. Ventricular fibrillation
    d. All of the above

4. **With respect to Cold Water Immersion (CWI), which one of the following statements is incorrect?**
    a. In near freezing water the eventual cause of death is likely to be hypothermia
    b. The best way to enter cold water is to remove excess clothing and jump in quickly.
    c. Survivors of CWI may suffer cardiac arrest immediately before rescue
    d. Victims can still survive CWI related hypothermia even after loss of consciousness.

Answers:
1. **a**
2. **c**
3. **d**
4. **b**

CHAPTER 20

Wilderness Medicine in Western Europe

This chapter will train you on specific issues related to wilderness medicine in Western Europe:

Venomous snakes
Wild animals
Spider bites
Ticks
Mosquitos
Marine animals
Infectious diseases
Plants
Cold water immersion

Objectives:

- Recognize specific problems related to Wilderness Medicine practice in Western Europe
- To be aware of venomous animal and insect bites and stings and the wilderness management of these
- Be aware of the phases of cold water immersion and the management of this

CASE 1

You are hiking in the Ardennes, Belgium, when one of your group of ten trekkers steps on a brown coloured snake with a zigzag dorsal pattern down the back which turns around and bites him on his lower leg. The snake then rapidly moves off into the nearby undergrowth. It is afternoon and you are on a dirt road track, two-hour hike from the nearest small town. You have a cellphone with you.

1. What are the first priorities for treating this wound?
2. How would you prevent spread of the venom?
3. What would be the best way to evacuate the victim?

CASE 2

10 days after a camping trip to the Spanish coast one of your friends calls you to tell you he is not feeling very well.

1. What additional information would you like to know?
2. Which prevention methods could have been used?
3. Does he need to go to hospital?

CASE 3

You are kayaking in Norway, Scandinavia where the water temperature is 5°C. You are half way across the lake when you capsize and you are unable to get back into your kayak.

1. How long are you likely to survive in the water?
2. How long before hypothermia sets in?
3. Are you safe once rescued?

BACKGROUND

Western Europe is the region comprising the most western countries of Europe, one of the world's seven continents. It is bordered by the Arctic Ocean to the north, the Atlantic Ocean to the west, the Mediterranean Sea to the south, and the border. This large geographic region contains unique fauna and flora. The climate varies from sub-arctic to Mediterranean and Alpine region. Some of the typical animals in the Arctic tundra (the northernmost and coldest of European habitats) include reindeer, arctic fox, brown bear, ermine, lemmings, partridges, snowy owl and the alpine areas provide a habitat to the wolf and lynx.

ANIMAL BITES

Venomous snakes

Background
Venomous species are not common in Europe and are far from being the most dangerous in the world. The only truly venomous snakes in Europe all belong to the Viper family. One of them is the common adder (Vipera berus) and is extremely widespread it can be found throughout most of western Europe from France and Italy up to north of the Arctic Circle. The venomous viper species are not regarded as especially dangerous. The snake is not aggressive and usually bites only when alarmed or disturbed. A few fatal cases have been reported, mostly children.

Clinical manifestations of Adder envenomation
- Local symptoms include immediate and intense pain. The pain may spread within a few hours, along with tenderness and inflammation.
- Soft tissue swelling outward form the bite
- Gastrointestinal symptoms; incontinence of urine and faeces
- Other symptoms can include: sweating, fever, lightheadedness, loss of consciousness, urticaria, angioedema, bronchospasm vasoconstriction, tachycardia
- Shock and cardiovascular failure if left untreated

Treatment and evacuation
The treatment and evacuation recommendation for all victims of bites can be found in chapter 14; snakes, pit vipers.

Wild animals

General

- The incidence of wild animal bites is difficult to ascertain, as many minor wilderness bites and attacks are not reported
- The Lynx, though very rare, can be found in the forests of northern Scandinavia and the coastal wetlands of southern Spain and many places in between.
- Bears can still be found across most of Europe
- Also wild boar, deer, moose, otters, beavers, mountain goats, pine martens, polecats, wolverines and even bison can all still be found.

Bears, wolves and lynx

The number of brown bears, wolves, wolverines and lynxes are rising in Europe and are found in nearly one-third of mainland Europe. Only Belgium, Denmark, The Netherlands and Luxembourg have no breeding populations of at least one large carnivore species. Attacks from bears and wolves are relatively rare, but frequent enough to be of concern for those who are in their habitats. Attacks from a lynx are even more rare and to date there were no reports of lynx spontaneously attacking humans in Europe. The polar bear is not covered in this chapter as it lives in the arctic beyond the borders of Europe.

Wild boar

Wild boar, also known as wild pig, is native across much of Northern and Central Europe and the Mediterranean Region. Attacks on humans are not common but when they occur the boar will charge at them. Most of the damage is inflicted by the boar's tusk creating lacerations of the upper legs.

Moose

Moose live in northern Europe and are unlikely to hurt people directly, fatalities indirectly are more common (car and train crashes). If a moose does charge at you, you should run from it, as they are more prone to stop chasing you.

Prevention

- For prevention see chapter 14: wild animals
- Most animals do not attack unless provoked!!

Treatment

- The treatment of wild animals is similar to the treatment of a domestic animal attack (see chapter 14: domesticated animals).
- In general, large animals should raise more suspicion of blunt and penetrating trauma, including deep arterial damage, nerve damage and internal organ damage.
- Antibiotic choice follows that of domestic attacks, with exception of attacks that occur in natural bodies of fresh water.

INSECT BITES

Spider Bites

Background

Though many people fear spiders and many spiders are venomous, only a few are dangerous to humans. As spider venom is evolved for small invertebrates and not human beings. Many spiders do not have fangs large enough to penetrate human skin. Due to the change in climate and international commerce, importations of other spiders and also more venomous spiders are likely to occur.

The following venomous spiders are native in Europe:

- Comb-footed Spiders (family Theridiidae)-for example: the widow Spiders
- Recluse Spiders, Violin Spiders, Fiddleback Spiders (Loxosceles)
- Yellow Sac Spider, Long-legged Sac Spider (Cheiracanthium punctorium)

Most venomous spiders in Europe belong to the Theridiidae family. The species belonging to the widow spiders occurring in the warmer parts of Southern Europe are thought to be far less dangerous to man than the infamous 'black widow', and their bites are comparable to a bee sting. The approximately 100 described species of Loxosceles spiders do not generally occur in Europe. At least two species of the recluse spiders can be found in the Mediterranean region of southern Europe.

Clinical signs

- For clinical signs of a black widow bite see chapter 14: spiders
- The initial bite is usually painless and symptoms develop hours later
- The majority of bites remain local and heal within three weeks without serious complication or medical intervention.
- The European species are thought to be less venomous than the feared American Brown Recluse spider. However In more serious cases, the bite may become necrotic. •Cheiracanthium punctorium is found from central Europe to Central Asia. The bite is similar to a wasp sting, perhaps a bit more severe, although susceptible persons can have stronger reactions, like nausea and, very rare, necrosis of the skin.

Treatment

- *Catch the spider, if possible, as even a smashed spider can sometimes be identified under the microscope by an experienced entomologist*
- Cleanse the bite with soap and water.
- Elevate the extremity and loosely immobilize it.

Place a cold compress and give oral analgesics for pain control.

Hospital management is only necessary if systemic symptoms occur.

Evacuation

There is no need to evacuate the victim in the absence of systemic symptoms.

Tick Borne Disease

Ticks can be abundant in woodlands all across Europe from early spring to late autumn. They live on sucking blood from animals and occasionally bite humans. Ticks are not the cause of disease but is infected with a virus or bacterium. The pathogen can be transmitted through the tick's bite and cause disease in humans.

There are two common tick-borne diseases in Europe:

Tick-borne encephalitis (TBE): The TBE virus can infect the brain and cause tick-borne encephalitis.

Lyme borreliosis is caused by a bacterium, the spirochete Borrelia burgdorferi, which lives in the stomach of ticks and can be transmitted when humans are bitten by infected ticks.

Crimean Congo haemorrhagic fever (CCHF) and Tick-borne relapsing fever (TBRF) have also been reported but are extremely rare in Europe.

Clinical signs

About 25% of the people infected with the TBE virus fall ill and develop symptoms of encephalitis which include high fever, severe headache, and sometimes paralysis and convulsions. Most patients will recover but up to one third will suffer long-term complications.

The clinical presentation of borrelia infection ranges from no symptoms at all to a characteristic skin rash called erythema migrans and meningitis with neurological symptoms.

Prevention

See chapter 14: ticks

Treatment

For general treatment and tick removal see chapter 14: ticks and chapter 15: tick-borne diseases

There is no specific treatment for TBE but there is an effective vaccine that prevents infection.

Lyme borreliosis is effectively treated and cured with doxycycline

Evacuation

See chapter 14: ticks

Mosquitos

While the number of mosquito-borne diseases in Europe is currently low, there is an increasing trend in their global incidence and geographical distribution due to climate change and other variables. It is estimated that over the last two decades nearly one third of all recorded events related to emerging infectious diseases were vector-borne. Increased number of imported infections of malaria and chikungunya has also been blamed on international travellers, aid workers or immigrants returning from the endemic areas. Native mosquitos can spread: Malaria, Sindbis fever and the West Nile fever. Invasive mosquitos in Europe can spread: Chikungunya, Dengue fever, Japanese encephalitis, Viral haemorrhagic fevers, Yellow fever and the Zika virus infection.

Prevention, treatment
See chapter 14: mosquitos

Sand flies

Sand flies can occur in Europe and particularly the Mediterranean region, and in recent years, their range has increased and will still increase in the coming years due to prediction in climatic changes. They have piercing mouthparts capable of taking blood. Most species feed at dusk and during the night. Sand flies are tiny insects 1.5–3.5 mm in length, with a hairy appearance, large black eyes and long, stilt-like legs. They can be distinguished from other small flies by their wings, which are hairy and extended at a 40° angle over the body when the fly is at rest or blood-feeding. They are vectors of human and canine leishmaniasis, and sand fly fevers caused by phleboviruses.

Prevention
- sand flies are susceptible to insecticides, such as pyrethroids, and residual spraying of houses and animal shelters is an effective control strategy
- The use of protective clothing, insect repellents and insecticide-impregnated bed nets
- Measures such as resurfacing walls to cover cracks and holes, demolition and removal of uninhabited buildings and removal of organic waste and unwanted vegetation can help to discourage sand fly breeding.

Treatment
- Incubation period of leishmaniasis can vary between 10 days and a few years, with an average of 2-6 months. Treatment recommendations for systemic symptoms after suspected sand fly bites vary depending on the area of travel and suspicion for infection. Severity of symptoms after an leishmaniasis infection may vary from very mild to deadly (especially visceral leishmaniasis).
- Incubation period of phleboviruses is 2-9 days. Phleboviruses such as the Toscana virus, Naples virus and Sicilian virus, infection may result in Pappataci fever, an illness with mild fever, headache and

myalgia. In serious cases that go undiagnosed, acute meningitis, meningoencephalitis and encephalitis may occur. There is no specific treatment for infection, so treatment is supportive.

Evacuation
■ There is no need to evacuate the victim in the absence of systemic symptoms.

The oak processionary

The oak processionary *(Thaumetopoea processionea)* is a moth whose caterpillars can be found in oak forests. They are widely distributed in central and southern Europe, and are occasionally found as far north as Sweden. In the southern countries of Europe the populations are controlled by natural predators. Their range is expanding northward, possibly or partly as a result of global warming.

The moths may pose a human irritant because of their poisonous setae (hairs), which may cause skin irritation and asthma. The larvae construct communal nests of white silk from which they crawl at night in single file, head to tail in large processions to feed on foliage in the crowns of trees, returning in the same manner. The backs of older caterpillars are covered with up to 63,000 pointed defensive bristles containing an urticating toxin (thaumetopoein or closely related compounds). Transmission of the hairs can be airborne, by ground contact via plants or grass or even by water contact in stillwater e.g. garden ponds. The toxicity of the hairs remains active beyond the normal life cycle of the moth and in some cases can remain a problem for several seasons.

Clinical signs
The setae break off readily, become airborne and can cause epidemic caterpillar dermatitis (lepidopterism), manifested as a papular rash, pruritus, conjunctivitis and, if inhaled, pharyngitis and respiratory distress, including asthma or even anaphylaxis. However, there have been no known deaths related to or caused by such exposures to this toxin.

Treatment
It has been found that the skin irritation itching effects of contact with these hairs can be largely eliminated by the use of cetirizine-based antihistamines in tablet form.

INFECTIOUS DISEASES

Leptospirosis

Background

Leptospirosis is an infection with the spirochete bacteria leptospira spp., which is spread through the urine of infected animals. Rats, mice, and moles are important primary hosts, a wide range of other mammals are able to carry and transmit the disease as secondary hosts. Humans who get in contact with contaminated water, food or soil can become ill in 2 days to 4 weeks.

Clinical signs

The illness usually begins with flu-like symptoms (fever, chills, myalgias, intense headache, vomiting, diarrhoea, abdominal pain, red eyes, rash). Sometimes there is a second phase of the disease, also known as Weil's disease, is characterized by meningitis, liver damage (causing jaundice), and renal failure. Cardiovascular problems are also possible.

Treatment

Human therapeutic dosage of drugs is as follows: doxycycline 100 mg orally every 12 hours for 1 week or penicillin 1–1.5 MU every 4 hours for 1 week.

PLANTS

Hogweed (Acanthus)

Heracleum is a genus of about 60 species (depending on taxonomic interpretation) of herbs in the carrot family Apiaceae. They are found throughout the temperate northern hemisphere and in high mountains as far south as Ethiopia Common names for the genus or its species include hogweed.

For clinical presentation, treatment and prevention see chapter 12: dermatology, toxicodendrons

Cyanobacteria or Blue-green algae

Cyanobacteria are among the world's most ancient inhabitants. They are single-celled organisms that live in fresh, brackish, and marine water, and use sunlight to make their own food. In warm, nutrient-rich environments, microscopic cyanobacteria can grow quickly, in Northern Europe this is usually only the case during the summer months. The cyanobacteria create blooms that spread across the water's surface and may become visible. Because of the color, texture, and location of these blooms, the common name for cyanobacteria is blue-green algae.

Humans can be exposed to cyanobacterial toxins by drinking untreated water that contains the toxins, swimming in water that contains high concentrations of cyanobacterial cells, or breathing air that contains cyanobacterial cells or toxins (while watering a lawn with contaminated water, for example).

Adverse health effects associated with exposure to high concentrations of cyanobacterial toxins include stomach and intestinal illness; trouble breathing; allergic responses; skin irritation; liver damage; and neurotoxic reactions, such as tingling fingers and toes.

The only documented and scientifically substantiated human deaths due to cyanobacterial toxins have been due to exposure during dialysis. People exposed through drinking-water and recreational-water have required intensive hospital care.

COLD WATER IMMERSION

Background
In Northern Europe water can be quite cold even in spring and summer. Hypothermia can occur during warmer months, although its onset will take longer.

Clinical signs
There are four phases of cold water immersion:

1. Cold Shock Response
2. Cold Incapacitation
3. Hypothermia
4. Circum-rescue Collapse

Cold Shock Response lasts for only about a minute after entering the water and refers to the affect that cold water has on the respiratory rate. Initially, there is **an automatic gasp reflex** in response to rapid skin cooling. If the head goes underwater, water may be breathed into the lungs during the gasp. A second component of the Cold Shock Response involves **hyperventilation**. Although this physiological response will subside, panic can cause a psychological continuance of hyperventilation. Prolonged hyperventilation, results in low levels of arterial pCO2, this causes vasoconstriction in the brain, which may lead to loss of consciousness. Then there is **vasoconstriction**, which will cause increased workload for the heart, which may result cardiac arrest, especially in people with known history of heart disease.

Cold Incapacitation occurs within 5 – 15 minutes in cold water. Vasoconstriction decreases blood flow to the skin and extremities in an effort to preserve heat in the core. Muscle and nerve fibres do not function properly anymore.

Hypothermia -While it varies with water temperature and body mass, <u>it can take 30 minutes or more</u> for most adults to become even mildly hypothermic in ice water. Knowing this is vitally important in a survival situation, since people would be far less likely to panic if they knew that hypothermia would not occur quickly.

Circum-rescue Collapse can happen just before, during or after rescue. Once rescue is imminent, is in progress, or has just taken place, a mental relaxation occurs, creating a decreased output of stress hormones. Blood pressure can drop and muscles can fail, causing collapse and in some extreme cases, even cardiac arrest and death. The key thing to remember is that heart function is dramatically impacted by the way that a victim is handled and removed from the water. Knowing what NOT to do can make a life-saving difference.

Treatment

The first key consideration in the performance of any rescue is to ensure your own safety to avoid worsening an already tense, dangerous situation. Make sure that you're wearing the proper flotation and, where cold water is involved, appropriate thermal protection.

The two most critical components of the extraction are:

Be **gentle** and keep the victim **horizontal.** Because of the stress on the heart, any rough handling can trigger **ventricular fibrillation**. Horizontal extraction keeps blood flowing more uniformly throughout the body. Extracting a victim vertically can cause blood to pool in the legs resulting in a massive drop in blood pressure.

If in a protected environment, remove wet clothing, dry them and rewarm and insulate the victim. If available, wrap a vapour barrier (plastic sheeting) around the insulated victim to prevent further evaporative and convective heat loss and to keep the insulating materials dry, protecting them from the environment. If no dry clothing is available or you are in an unprotected environment, leave the victim's clothing on. In this case, wrap the vapour barrier against the wet clothing to prevent evaporative heat loss, and to prevent the insulating material from getting wet and losing its effectiveness.

For further treatment of hypothermia see chapter 7.

QUESTIONS

1. **If bitten by a snake in Europe, which is the most important first aid treatment?**
   a. Clean the wound and apply an antibiotic dressing
   b. Attempt to remove any venom from the wound by suction and making the wound bleed
   c. Apply a pressure dressing to the limb and immobilize the victim
   d. Start a course of antibiotics as soon as possible

2. **Which of the following is true regarding the oak processionary?**
   a. They are uncommon in southern Europe
   b. They do not have any natural predators
   c. Transmission of the hairs is airborne
   d. The treatment consists of cetirizine-based antihistamines in tablet form

3. **With respect to Cold Water Immersion (CWI) which of the following statements is incorrect?**
   a. In near freezing water the eventual cause of death is likely to be hypothermia
   b. The best way to enter cold water is to remove excess clothing and jump in quickly.
   c. Survivors of CWI may suffer cardiac arrest immediately before rescue
   d. Victims can still survive CWI related hypothermia even after loss of consciousness.

Answers:
1. c
2. d
3. b

APPENDIX

Legal Concerns in the Wilderness

The welfare of the people is the ultimate law
– Marcus Tullius Cicero

When encountering an accident victim or a person experiencing some other medical emergency in the back country, one's instinct is to provide medical care. In fact, medical professionals are directed by their national and international associations to provide emergency medical care. According to the World Medical Association's International Code of Medical Ethics, "... a physician shall give emergency care as a humanitarian duty ..." In addition, physicians should "respond to the best of their ability in cases of emergency where first aid treatment is essential" (Op. 8.11, Council of Ethical and Judicial Affairs, AMA). The most important aspect of treating a patient in the wilderness is providing optimal care in any given situation. Sadly, because of an increasingly litigious world, concerns about legal liability are always a concern of a well-meaning caregiver. Those liability concerns, however, can be eliminated or reduced by both understanding and following a few legal principles. This chapter presents those legal principles by examining Good Samaritan laws, contract laws, tort laws and defenses to a tort law claim. The goal of law is to provide certainty and predictability in order for citizens to conduct themselves properly. This legal review demonstrates that the law is rational, helps to define what actions are necessary in an emergency situation, and protects those providers who do their jobs well and provide care in accordance with accepted standards.

GOOD SAMARITAN LAWS

Most laws, such as Good Samaritan laws, have an intended purpose. In this case, when citizens have an emergent injury, society wants to encourage those with the ability to help and render to aid, to do so. The law provides liability protection to remove the deterrent of litigation as long as someone is not grossly negligent.

A. Affirmative Obligation to Help

In the United States, the most extreme reactions to this common law rule are found in Minnesota, Rhode Island and Vermont, where each has enacted a statute requiring a person to render aid, under certain conditions, to a stranger found in an emergency situation. Actual fines may be imposed if there is a failure to render aid. The Minnesota statute, quoted in part below, is a good example of this type of legislation.

> A person at ... an emergency who knows that another person is exposed to or has suffered grave physical harm shall, to the extent that the person can do so without danger ... to self or others, give reasonable assistance to the exposed person ...

The Province of Quebec in Canada and virtually every country on the European Continent have similar statutory requirements. Therefore, when traveling the back country in Europe, Quebec, Minnesota, Rhode Island and Vermont, remember that one is obligated to give reasonable aid and assistance to a stranger suffering or exposed to grave physical harm or otherwise found in an emergency situation. Depending on the circumstances and the particular jurisdiction's law, that obligation might be satisfied by immediately reporting the situation to the proper authorities who can provide help and aid to the victim. Most jurisdictions that impose an affirmative obligation to render emergency care generally also have a limitation of liability statute as described below.

B. Limitation of Liability

In all of the U.S. and many other common law jurisdictions (Canada, Alberta, British Colombia, Nova Scotia and Ontario) have enacted Good Samaritan laws, which provide that, under certain circumstances, a person who voluntarily renders emergency care will not be liable for ordinary negligence or simple carelessness. Although these statutes differ in language among jurisdictions, all are very similar in purpose, rest upon the same fundamental principles and have the same requirements. The Utah statute quoted below is a good example of these laws.

A person who renders emergency care at or near the scene of, or during an emergency, gratuitously and on good faith, is not liable for any civil damages or penalties as a result of any act or omission by the person rendering the emergency care, unless the person is grossly negligent or caused the emergency.

Examples of potential gross negligence by a physician would be removing an object out of an impaled person, giving a medication that the patient had stated an allergy to, or pulling a person with a likely neck injury out of a car by their head. In short, literally no one would perform in this way.

For a provider to be protected under the Good Samaritan Doctrine, in any jurisdiction, the following five general guidelines must be met:

1. **The person rendering emergency care must not have caused the emergency, either in whole or in part.** For example, if you run over someone or cause them to fall over a cliff, then you are not protected from being litigated against later for the injury and outcome.
2. **The person rendering emergency care must act in "good faith."** (The care provider must sincerely intend to help and must have a reasonable opinion that the care should not be postponed until the patient is hospitalized.)
3. **The emergency care must be provided gratuitously, without any compensation.** (The care provider should not accept anything in return for rendering the emergency care. One should never send a bill for services if they intend to utilize Good Samaritan law.)
4. **The provider must not commit gross negligence when rendering emergency care.** (To list all possible acts or omissions that might constitute gross negligence is impossible. Be advised, however, that once initiating emergency aid in the back country and then either terminating treatment or transferring care of the patient to an inadequately trained person before the patient is adequately stabilized or evacuated to a medical facility can be considered abandonment constituting gross negligence.)
5. **The person rendering emergency care must not have a preexisting duty to care for the patient.** (For example, a guide would have a preexisting duty to render emergency care to a customer where that customer had contracted with the guide to be taken on a hike and the guide had agreed to provide care to the customer in case of injury while hiking. In this situation, the Good Samaritan law would not apply to the guide in the event of injury to the customer during the hike.)

The nuances of Good Samaritan laws vary among jurisdictions. For example, Pennsylvania's Good Samaritan law covers only those who have received some training in first aid and then only to the extent trained. Courts in certain other states have suggested that Good Samaritan law protections apply only if the care given is limited to that necessary at the emergency scene. Consequently, in a back country emergency a person might decide to render only such aid as one is competent to provide and then only to the extent required at the scene. Multiple states do not allow Good Samaritan laws to apply in a hospital setting as the environment provides the resources to provide accepted medical care. A higher standard of care may be present if the care is provided with the resources of an EMS vehicle and its equipment or in a field/ship clinic setting.

If any one of the five conditions above is not satisfied, then the Good Samaritan law, with all its protections, will not apply. While there are many ways in which these principles can be violated (inadvertently accepting payment or rendering aid in a clumsy manner amounting to gross negligence), the most frequent violation arises from the presence of a preexisting duty on the part of the care giver to provide aid to the patient. A preexisting duty usually exists because of contract law.

CONTRACT LAW

A contract is an agreement, or in effect a promise, between two or more parties for performing, or not performing, certain specified acts in exchange for adequate consideration. To be a legally binding contract, there has to be 3 elements: (1) an offer, (2) acceptance of the offer, and (3) some form of consideration must be exchanged. Consideration is defined as any benefit or item of value received by parties that reasonably and fairly induces them to enter the contract. Contracts can be either "express" or "implied-in-fact." The terms of an express contract are explicitly stated in words, either written or oral, leaving little or no doubt as to its existence and terms. An implied contract is not expressly set forth, either orally or in writing. Rather, the existence and terms of an implied contract are created by conduct or circumstances that "imply-in-fact" a contract exists. For example, if someone delivers milk to a doorstep and the other party leaves an envelope with payment, even though there may not be a formal contract, both parties are behaving like there is one in place.

Contracts, letter agreements, and even brochures from summer camps, expedition companies or adventure guides sometimes expressly state they have a trained person available to provide medical care to customers in emergencies arising during the adventure activity. Alternatively, the oral sales presentation or even the brochure may well "imply" that the summer camp, expedition company or adventure guide will provide such medical aid to customers under its care. Whether express or implied, a court may find that the complaining customer stayed at the camp or took the adventurous expedition in part because the company or guide contractually agreed to provide medical aid during back country emergencies, thereby creating a preexisting duty on the part of the company or guide. Thus the Good Samaritan law will not be of protection from liability.

If the Good Samaritan law does not apply, because one or more of the principles are broken, then litigation would possibly able to be pursued under contract law or tort law. In a famous legal case, *Guilmet v. Campbell* (385 Michigan. 57, 188 N.W.2d 6-1 1971), a patient sued his surgeon who operated on him for an ulcer and guaranteed that he would be able to "eat as you please and throw away your pillbox." The patient remained symptomatic after surgery. The jury did not allow an award for malpractice but did allow an award for breach of contract. Thus it would behoove a medical provider on an expedition, to avoid being involved in a contract which in any way gives the belief or guarantees that safety and health are ensured during the trip.

Litigation could also proceed under the area of tort law.

TORT LAW

Tort law sets civil standards for people's behavior, imposing on everyone the duty to exercise reasonable care to avoid causing harm or injury to others and providing legal recourse and the possible recovery of money damages for those who suffer harm or injury as a result of a breach of this duty. Torts are legally defined civil (non-criminal) wrongs that might result in harm or injury and, thereby, constitute the basis for a claim (or law suit) by the harmed or injured party against the person who allegedly committed the tort. An injured party can claim under any of three general categories of torts: (1) an intentional tort (where one person intentionally harms or injures another); (2) a strict liability tort (making and selling an obviously defective product); and (3) a negligent tort (a careless and unintentional act, such as an automobile accident, which harms or injures another person or another person's property). Among harms or injuries suffered by a party for which it could recover a monetary award in tort litigation are compensation for (1) lost income and lost or damaged property, (2) pain and suffering and (3) reasonable medical expenses. Although a person allegedly harmed or injured when receiving emergency aid in the back country might conceivably claim an intentional tort, most often law suits arising from such circumstances claim that the tort of "negligence" occurred.

In order to prove that a person who provided emergency medical care in back country (the "defendant") committed a tort of negligence, the person who claims to have been harmed or injured by that emergency medical care (the "plaintiff") must prove the following four elements of a negligence claim.

Four Elements of a Negligence Claim

1. Duty to Provide Care at the Standard of Care
The plaintiff must demonstrate that the defendant had a duty to provide aid to the plaintiff which met a specified standard of care. Normally, a health care provider will not be held to have been negligent if good care is given in accordance with the prevailing standards of the medical profession. The issue then becomes, "what are the prevailing standards?" Although training courses such as this are making

great progress in defining and refining the standard of care in wilderness medicine, that standard is not yet well established in the law. When in doubt, courts will rely upon the traditional legal definition of the standard of care, which is the "behavior of a reasonably prudent person in the same or similar circumstances." In applying the traditional legal definition, courts commonly look to the following factors to determine the applicable standard of care:

1. The defendant's education
2. The defendant's training
3. Government or organization medical protocols that apply to the particular situation
4. Industry practice
5. Private business protocols that might apply

A duty to provide aid meeting a specified standard of care also generally requires that the informed consent of the patient be obtained before treatment is given. A parent or guardian must provide that consent when the patient is a child. Informed consent can be given only if the patient is first advised of the medical problem, the proposed course of treatment, any potential risks associated with that course of treatment and what to expect if no treatment is given. Then the patient, or parent or guardian, must give actual consent. A care provider might rely upon "implied consent" in an emergency situation where most would reasonably assume that the patient would have agreed to the care offered under the emergency circumstances if they were able to. For example, an injured traveler may be unconscious and unable to give consent but most would assume that anyone would want help in this situation so "implied consent" is utilized.

2. Failure to Perform the Duty

The plaintiff must next prove the defendant failed to perform the duty of providing aid consistent with the specified standard of care. This proof can take several forms. In most wilderness medicine litigations, the plaintiff asserts that the defendant failed to act at all (an omission) when the defendant had a preexisting duty to provide care to the plaintiff. The plaintiff might, however, claim the defendant provided care (a commission) that did not meet the prevailing medical standard or did not perform as would a reasonable person with defendant's background, education and training. The premature termination of care or the transfer of care to a less qualified provider before the patient has been stabilized or evacuated can, as mentioned above, be considered abandonment and constitute negligence or even gross negligence. Consequently, one must remain well informed of prevailing medical standards and protocols and be well trained in wilderness medicine to ensure that any care provided meets applicable standards.

3. Loss or Injury

The plaintiff must next demonstrate that he or she sustained a loss or injury, which can include loss or damage to property, medical expenses, fright, emotional trauma, personal injury, pain and suffering, and loss of life.

4. Causation

Finally, the plaintiff must demonstrate that the loss or injury sustained was caused or contributed to (the "proximate cause") by the defendant's failure to perform the duty of providing aid meeting the specified standard of care.

DEFENSES TO A TORT LAW CLAIM

Defendant can defeat plaintiff's claim by demonstrating that plaintiff failed to carry the burden of proof on one or more of the four elements of a negligence claim. For example, defendant might demonstrate that he or she satisfied the duty of performing in accordance with the applicable standard of care or that plaintiff's loss or injury was caused by another person or event. The best strategy always is to keep a contemporaneous, complete and accurate written record of the events surrounding and the medical care given in response to a back country or wilderness emergency. Such records should include dates and times, a patient history, a description of the scene, your physical assessment, treatment given and any changes in the patient while in your care. Experience teaches that such a record is an essential element in any successful defense.

JURISDICTION

Another consideration with regards to law and wilderness expeditions would involve jurisdiction. It is important for a provider to understand, if there is any legal action, under what laws, the issue will be argued. Laws can widely vary from country to country and even state to state. Knowing ahead of time, what the jurisdiction is will allow for maximum protection from litigation and optimal conduct. The jurisdiction may be spelled out when the contract/agreement is signed by the customer before the journey. For example a statement such as "both parties agree that any litigation will utilize the laws of California in resolving a dispute" could be included. Otherwise a trek in Utah, with a customer from Nevada, using a company from Arizona, can open the door to argument over whose laws apply. Or a dive expedition on a boat in international waters with a citizen from the U.S. and a physician from France, on a boat registered in Norway, can open the same host of considerations.

MALPRACTICE INSURANCE

Finally, providers would be wise to investigate, before undertaking a trip, whether they will be covered by their usual insurance provider when rendering support during expeditions in various jurisdictions. This is especially important when they are accompanying a group as contractually provided medical support as the Good Samaritan laws will be of no protection, as mentioned above.

CHAPTER 22

Wilderness Nutrition

As a wilderness healthcare provider it is important to gain an understanding of how to meet nutritional and hydration needs. Proper nutrition will aid in maintaining both the physical strength and mental stamina required for the environmental extremes you may face in wilderness rescue situations.

In this chapter you will learn how to plan and meet your nutritional needs, and that of your patients by achieving these objectives:

- Recognize the importance of adequate nutrition for the rescuer(s) and patient(s).
- Understand how to plan food and fluid intake to achieve your total daily energy and fluid requirements.
- Identify appropriate nutrition protocols for refeeding the starved rescue victim, as well as other medical situations where nutrition is an important concern.

ENERGY REQUIREMENTS

Caloric requirements for wilderness rescuers and users vary depending on gender, body type and size. Additionally, type, intensity, and duration of physical activity are important considerations in determining daily nutrition requirements.

■ **Total daily energy expenditure** is made up of four primary components: resting metabolic rate, thermic effect of food, thermic effect of exercise, and non-exercise activity thermogenesis.

  ☐ Resting metabolic rate (RMR): baseline energy requirement to maintain normal bodily functions at rest. Basal metabolic rate (BMR) is often used interchangeably with RMR. RMR is an estimate of BMR. It is commonly used for practical purposes, and is typically 10% greater than BMR.

  ☐ Thermic effect of food (TEF): energy necessary to absorb, transport, store, and metabolize food.

  ☐ Thermic effect of exercise (TEE): energy used to support exercise. TEE can increase if a person engages in physical activity or exercise.

  ☐ Non-exercise activity thermogenesis (NEAT): energy used to produce heat in response to overfeeding, shivering in cold temperatures, and spontaneous non-exercise activity such as fidgeting.

■ **The Harris Benedict** equation is commonly used to estimate RMR in healthy individuals (use kilograms and centimeters in the equation):

  ☐ Males: 66.5 + (13.75 x wt) + (5.003 x ht) - (6.775 x age)

  ☐ Females: 655.1 + (9.563 x wt) + (1.850 x ht) - (4.676 x age)

■ To estimate total daily energy needs, RMR is multiplied by an activity factor:

  ☐ **Very Light Activity** (mostly sedentary):

    RMR x 1.3 for males and females = total calories needed per day

  ☐ **Light Activity** (easy, short (1-3 hours) and slow day hike, easy climbing or skiing):

    RMR x 1.5 for females or 1.6 for males = total calories needed per day

  ☐ **Moderate Activity** (moderate intensity exercise of longer duration; brisk day hiking, skiing or climbing with little or no extra pack weight; equivalent to jogging 5-6 miles):

    RMR x 1.6 for females or 1.7 for males = total calories needed per day

  ☐ **Heavy Activity** (hard exercise; moderate to high intensity exercise of longer duration such as hiking, climbing, skiing that involves hills and carrying a heavy pack; equivalent to jogging 9-13 miles):

    RMR x 1.9 for females or 2.1 for males = total calories needed per day

  ☐ **Exceptional Activity** (very hard exercise; training for an ultra-endurance event, long, strenuous day of variable terrain hiking, scrambling, backcountry skiing or climbing with a heavy pack; equivalent to jogging 14-17 miles):

    RMR x 2.2 for females or 2.4 for males = total calories needed per day

■ **Sample RMR calculation:**
   ☐ Male: 35 years old, 170 pounds 6'0": 66.5 + (13.75 x 77.11kg) + (5.003 x 182.88cm) - (6.775 x 35) = 1,805 kcal/day x appropriate activity factor = total calories needed per day
   ☐ Female: 35 years old, 135 pounds, 5'6":   655.1 + (9.563 x 61.23kg) + (1.850 x 167.64cm) - (4.676 x 35) = 1,387 kcal/day x appropriate activity factor = total calories needed per day

MACRONUTRIENTS

Water is essential to sustain life, and adequate hydration is critical in the wilderness setting. Water serves as a transport medium, maintains body temperature and muscular functioning. It also acts as a solvent for chemical reactions, a lubricant and shock absorber, and cleanses and removes waste product.

■ **Daily requirements:** the amount of fluid you need per day varies greatly by the amount of activity performed, environmental conditions, and the amount of water in your foods.

■ **Fluid Dietary Recommended Intake (DRI):** sedentary males and females 19-50 years old 3.7 Liters (L)/day for males, 2.7 L/day for females. Wilderness users may have higher fluid needs, especially in hot weather, high altitude, and during high intensity and/or long duration physical activity.

■ **General guidelines**
   ☐ Pre-hydrate: drink 14-20 oz (plus an additional 8-16 oz in a hot environment).
   ☐ During physical activity in the wilderness: drink 200-300 mL every 15-20 minutes.
   ☐ Recovery/Rehydrate: replace 150-200% of body weight (BW) lost. Drink 24 - 32 oz (3 - 4 cups) of fluid per pound lost. For example, if you lose two pounds of water during activity, rehydrate with 48 oz (2 x 24 oz = 48 oz) of fluid containing electrolytes (eg. sports drink).
   ☐ At altitude fluid needs are increased: insensible water losses may not be noticed by the individual, but are greater because of increased ventilation.

■ **Ideas to achieve optimal intake**
   ☐ Consider a sports drink for moderate to intense activity lasting greater than 60-90 minutes. Sports drinks:
      ● Add flavor to encourage drinking
      ● Provide carbohydrates and electrolytes
      ● Aid in rehydration
   ☐ Electrolytes help retain fluid by drawing water into cells. An electrolyte supplement or sports drink with electrolytes is beneficial if you are drinking a large volume of fluid, and/or sweating heavily. This is especially important for rehydration following exercise.
   ☐ Recommended sports drink composition: Carbohydrate concentration is typically between 5–8%, sodium concentration between 500–700 mg/L, and potassium concentration varies between 120-600 mg/L.

□ To rehydrate, if you don't have a sports drink with you, it's easy to make your own. For example, first bring 16 oz of water to a boil then steep with one caffeine free lemon bag. Dissolve two tablespoons of sugar and 1/8th teaspoon of salt in the tea and let it cool. Mix the tea with four tablespoons of orange juice. Eight ounces of this drink has 60 calories, 15 g carbohydrates, 130 mg sodium and 62 mg potassium.

■ **Maintain a fluid balance**

□ Be familiar with your sweat rate. Calculate your sweat rate by weighing yourself before and after physical activity. Add the amount of fluid consumed during exercise and also add any urine amount to the losses.

● Example: Pre-exercise weight (72.7kg) – Post-exercise weight (70.4kg) = 2.3kg = 2.3L= 2300ml. Total fluid consumed during exercise = 32 oz = 960ml. 2300ml + 960ml = 3250 ml = total fluid loss. Divide by total hours to determine hourly sweat rate.

□ Are you a heavy or light sweater, what is your body type, and what is your exercise intensity? Keep in mind heat acclimatization increases water loss, but lessens sodium loss.

□ Before you plan to be physically active, or are preparing for a wilderness rescue, drink before you are thirsty to prevent dehydration.

□ Although it's important to drink enough water, you can also drink too much. This can result in hyponatremia, when blood sodium levels are less than 135 mmol/L. In order to prevent hyponatremia, include sufficient dietary sodium in your diet, ingest sodium during activity in the wilderness by eating salty foods and drinking a sports drink, and drink according to your sweat rate.

■ **Dehydration**

□ A good test to see if you are getting enough fluid is to ensure that your urine output is clear to pale yellow and that you are voiding frequently.

□ Remember that vitamins such as riboflavin and certain foods such as asparagus, carrots, and beets can also affect urine color and reliability of this test.

Carbohydrates are the body's preferred source of fuel. They are the main source of energy for moderate and high intensity physical activity in extreme environmental conditions such as heat, cold, and high altitude. Adequate glycogen stores, and intake of carbohydrate during exercise delays fatigue, decreases perceived effort, and improves concentration and reaction time. Carbohydrates are a required energy source for the brain, as well as red and white blood cells.

■ **Daily requirements:** the minimum level of glycogen required to maintain adequate glycogen stores for an active individual is 5 g/kg of BW per day.

■ **General guidelines**

□ For physical activity, including wilderness rescue recommended carbohydrate intake is between 6-10 g/kg of BW per day.

□ For moderate intensity and duration (30-60 minutes) daily carbohydrate recommendation is 6-8 g/kg of BW. This would apply to a rescue mission lasting between 30-60 minutes that requires hiking, running and/or traveling and working in technical terrain.

☐ For moderate intensity activity lasting longer than 60 minutes, daily carbohydrate recommendations are between 7-10 g/kg of BW. This would apply to a rescue mission lasting longer than 60 minutes that requires hiking, running, and or/traveling and working in technical terrain.

☐ During exercise longer than 60 minutes or if inadequate pre-exercise nutrition (eg. no breakfast or lunch) recommended carbohydrate intake is 30 to 60 g/hr based on the maximal oxidation rate of glucose. Carbohydrates during exercise helps maintain blood glucose concentration and delays central fatigue. They may also help spare glycogen stores.

☐ After exercise the recommended intake is 1-1.5 g/kg/of BW within 30-60 minutes (approximately 50-100 g, equivalent to 1-2 sports bars or 32 oz of sports drink). If you will be hiking/exercising the next day, repeat intake above two hours later to maximize glycogen stores.

☐ Carbohydrate recommendations vary with exercise intensity and duration and must be replenished daily for optimal performance.

TIP: it may be difficult to consume as many carbohydrates as recommended, and it's important that your diet is composed of a variety of nutrients, not just carbohydrates. Adjust your diet appropriately, and focus on timing of meals. Make sure to eat before, during, and immediately after physical activity and always keep some easily digested carbohydrates in your 24-hour kit/backpack such energy gels, honey, jelly and hard candies.

■ **Ideas to achieve optimal intake**

☐ Two to four hours before physical activity, consume a meal or snack that is easily digested. It should contain 2-4 g/kg of BW of carbohydrate, be moderate in protein (15-20 g), and low in fat. For example, a 70kg male could eat a turkey and cheese sandwich on a whole wheat bagel, with a banana or orange, a low fat yogurt and 25-30 whole wheat crackers.

☐ While in the wilderness consume a banana, sports chews, a slice of bread with peanut butter and jelly, or fig newton cookies. You can consume a sports drink in addition to any of these foods.

☐ Following wilderness activity, choose carbohydrate and protein foods to minimize recovery time. For example, trail mix and chocolate milk or cheese, a bagel with peanut butter or tuna, or cereal with milk.

■ **Hypoglycemia**

☐ The following foods contain at least 15g and are appropriate for the treatment of hypoglycemia (refer to Chapter 10 for more on hypoglycemia)

- 4 glucose tabs/paste
- 2 Tablespoons raisins
- 5-6 LifeSavers
- 1 Tablespoons honey

- 1 Tablespoons jelly
- 1/3-3/4 cup fruit juice
- 2 Cliff Shot Blocks
- ½ medium banana

Protein builds and repairs muscle tissue, maintains fluid balance, increases immune function, promotes satiety, and serves as a minor energy source. When total calorie and/or carbohydrate intake is low and/ or glycogen is depleted protein becomes a more significant source of energy.

■ **Daily requirements**: The Recommended Dietary Allowance (RDA) for sedentary males and females is 0.8 g/kg of BW per day.

■ **General Guidelines**
   □ Athlete specific recommendations apply well to wilderness rescuers:
      - Recreational athlete: 1.0 g/kg/ of BW
      - Endurance athlete: 1.2-1.4 g/kg of BW
      - Ultra-endurance: 1.2-2.0 g/kg of BW
   □ After physical activity: recommended intake is ~ 20 g of intact protein, and 50 – 100 g carbohydrates (~ 1.0 -1.5 g/kg) in the form of sports drink with electrolytes within 30 minutes of exercise.
   □ During caloric restriction protein needs are increased to maintain lean body mass and preserve nitrogen retention. Twice the usually recommended RDA of 0.8 g/kg of BW (1.6 g/kg/d) is recommended.
   □ In the wilderness timing of meals is most important for muscle repair. Focus on small frequent meals.

■ **Ideas to achieve optimal intake**
   □ Carry chicken or tuna pouches and make your own trail mix with a combination of nuts, dried fruit, pretzels and chocolate. Bring jerky and use powdered milk and eggs to add protein to your meals.

Lipids and Fats serve as the main source of energy during prolonged low intensity exercise and are important for immune health, hormone production and fat-soluble vitamin transport. Fat provides twice as many calories per gram as carbohydrate and protein, and can help you to stay warmer at night and in cold environments. Additionally, if you have to carry a heavy pack with medical supplies, weight and space become a concern. Foods high in fat are an excellent choice as they are calorically dense.

■ **Daily requirements:** fats should make up 20-35% of your daily diet.
■ **Ideas to achieve optimal intake**
   □ Choose healthy omega-3 Fatty Acids that may help with reducing inflammation: walnuts, soy nuts, green pumpkin seeds, and fish.

☐ Choose healthy monounsaturated fatty acids (MUFA's) and polyunsaturated fatty acids (PUFA's): nuts, seeds, oils, grains, legumes, and nut butters.

☐ For general health, foods containing unsaturated and trans fats such as cookies, chips, pastries, many packaged snack foods, marbled meats, and high fat cheese should be limited. These foods have their place in the wilderness setting. Desserts can be a great way to enjoy a satisfying meal and add calories. Similarly cheese and salami can be a satisfying snack, and are also an excellent way to add calories to your daily intake.

Nutrient Density & Energy Density: nutrient density is a measure of nutrients provided per kcal of food. Foods with a high nutrient density are rich in nutrients relative to their energy (kcal) content. Nutrient density is used to assess nutritional quality of food. Examples of nutrient dense foods include whole grain bread, nonfat milk, and fruits and vegetables. Energy density compares the energy content of food with its weight. Foods that are energy dense are high in kcals, but weigh little. They are a good choice if you are trying to gain weight or are traveling in the wilderness and have limited space, but need to pack a lot of calories. Examples of energy dense foods include: cookies, nuts, chips, chocolate, oils, nut butters, and fat free snacks and pretzels.

CONSIDERATIONS FOR REFEEDING

Patients who have been chronically starved or severely malnourished, and are refed on scene may be at risk for refeeding syndrome.

■ **Refeeding Syndrome:** in a starved or severely malnourished patient the body aims to prevent muscle and protein breakdown. As glycogen stores are depleted, fatty acids become the primary source of energy. Insulin is suppressed, while glucagon and cortisol secretion is increased. When provided nutrition the body attempts to reverse its adaption to the catabolic, starved state. Insulin levels increase inhibiting gluconeogenesis and promote glycogen, fat, and protein synthesis. This shift to the anabolic state from a reliance on fat oxidation depletes critical electrolytes and micronutrients needed for carbohydrate metabolism. The uptake of glucose, phosphorus, potassium, magnesium, and thiamin into cells, leaves little in the blood. This causes hypophosphatemia, hypokalemia, hypomagnesemia, thiamine deficiency, and sodium and water retention, resulting in refeeding syndrome.

■ **Complications** are serious and may include: arrhythmia, heart failure and sudden death, kidney failure, metabolic acidosis, delirium, paralysis, muscle cramps, Wernicke-Korsakoff syndrome, and sepsis.

■ **Risk Factors:** The guidelines at the National Institute for Clinical Excellence (NICE) for patients at risk for refeeding syndrome are as follows. Guidelines may be difficult to assess in a wilderness setting, but you can evaluate physical appearance and how long the patient has been without food.

ONE or more of the following: -OR-	**TWO** or more of the following:
BMI < 16 kg/m²	BMI <18.5 kg/m²
Unintentional weight loss of > 15% in the previous 3-6 months	Unintentional weight loss of >10% in the previous 3-6 months
Little or no nutritional intake for >10 days	Little or no nutritional intake for >5 days
Low levels of potassium, phosphorus, or magnesium before refeeding.	History of alcohol abuse or drugs including insulin, chemotherapy, antacids, or diuretics.

- ■ **Wilderness nutrition refeeding protocol:** while there is no standardized care for refeeding in the wilderness setting, suggestions are listed below. Most importantly resolve any life threatening medical issues prior to addressing nutrition concerns. Begin by assessing risk for refeeding syndrome by following NICE guidelines. As a general rule, don't allow the patient to gorge. In all circumstances, make sure the patient's kidneys can process fluid by monitoring how frequently the patient is voiding. In order to appropriately feed a patient, the rescuer should:
  - ☐ Assess how long the patient has been without food and/or water
  - ☐ Assess length of transport to a medical facility
  - ☐ For both short and extended length of transport, if the patient has been without food and/or water for a shorter period of time (3-5 days) without significant weight loss and is at low risk for refeeding syndrome, the rescuer should offer small frequent feedings of normal food. Providing food will assist the patient to become ambulatory. An ambulatory patient is easier to transport than a non-ambulatory patient. Assess for dehydration and hypoglycemia and provide fluid and snacks as needed to assist the patient. Good choices include: sports drinks, juices, soups, instant oatmeal, granola bars, banana chips, and small pieces of jerky.
  - ☐ If length of time to a medical facility is short (less than a few hours) and the patient has been without food for ≥5 days and medical history suggests significant weight loss indicating risk for refeeding syndrome, administer 200-300 mg oral or IV thiamine prior to any administration of food or dextrose solution. A multivitamin can be used if thiamine is not available. If the patient is dehydrated and/or hypoglycemic restore fluid and blood glucose levels carefully with dilute Gatorade or similar drink or low concentration (10%) IV dextrose. No other food need be administered until reaching the medical facility. Alert the medical facility of possible risk for refeeding syndrome. If you don't have thiamine, or a way to monitor electrolytes, do not refeed the patient in the field. Wait until the hospital, where electrolytes can be monitored and hospital staff can properly begin refeeding the patient.
  - ☐ If length of time to a medical facility is extended beyond a few hours and the patient is at risk for refeeding syndrome, administer 200-300 mg oral or IV thiamine. Following thiamine, follow the above protocol for dehydration and hypoglycemia. Minimal food should be introduced, as refeeding should primarily be conducted at the medical facility where electrolytes can be monitored. NICE recommendations specify no more than 10 kcal/kg/d and for the critically

malnourished victim no more than 5 kcal/kg/d. High fat, high protein foods are generally well tolerated.

☐ If the length of time to a medical facility is extended beyond a few hours and the rescuer does not have thiamine or a multivitamin to administer to the patient, avoid giving any food and if necessary, provide only the lowest dextrose concentration possible to treat hypoglycemia. Refeeding syndrome has been known to occur within a few hours in some patients.

CONCLUSION

As a wilderness healthcare provider you may travel and work in stressful physical environments such as mountainous or technical terrain, high altitude and extreme temperatures. These environments increase the need for adequate nutrition. Unfortunately, stressful physical environments and crisis situations often coincide with decreased availability of food. Planning nutrition needs along with fueling and hydrating properly for wilderness rescue operations will allow you to maintain the concentration and physical stamina required for a wilderness rescue. In addition, you will be able to evaluate nutritional concerns of patients, and follow appropriate protocols of nutrition intake, refeeding and other medical situations where nutrition is an important concern.

An easy way to prepare ahead of time for a wilderness rescue is having a 24-Hour Pack ready to use. Examples of nutrition related items include:

- Adequate fluid and a means of water purification (iodine tablets, a water filter, or UV water purification pen)
- If traveling in remote areas with the likelihood of an extended rescue mission consider carrying a military ration such as the Meals Ready to Eat (MRE). They are lightweight, calorie dense, and can provide adequate nutrition for a longer duration rescue operation
- Trail mix (nuts, seeds, chocolate and granola)
- Jerky
- Hard candies
- Honey packets
- Granola or sports bars
- Sports gels
- Thiamine (oral)
- Multivitamin
- Single portion of drink mix
- Glucose tabs

Works Cited:

Askew EW. Environmental and physical stress and nutrient requirements. *American Journal of Clinical Nutrition.* 1995;61:631S–637S.

Askew EW. Nutrition and performance in hot, cold and high altitude environments, In: Wolinsky I, ed. *Nutrition in Exercise and Sport,* 3rd ed. Boca Raton, Fla: CRC Press;1997:597–619.

Askew EW. Nutrition for a cold environment *The Physician and Sportsmedicine.* 1989;18(12):77-89.

Askew EW. Nutrition, Malnutrition and Starvation. In: Auerbach PS. *Textbook of Wilderness Medicine,* 6th ed. Philadelphia, PA: Elsevier Mosby; 2012:1374-1393.

Askew EW. Nutritional Support for Expeditions In: Bledsoe GH, Manyak MJ, Towne, DA. *Expedition and Wilderness Medicine.* New York, New York: Cambridge University Press; 2008:83-97.

Askew EW. Work at high altitude and oxidative stress: antioxidant nutrients. *Toxicology.*2002;(180):107-19.

Blondin DP, Tingelstad HC, Mantha OL, Gosselin C, Haman F. Maintaining thermogenesis in cold exposed humans: relying on multiple metabolic pathways. *Comprehensive Physiology.* 2014;4(4):1383-1402.

Boateng AA, Sriram K, Meguid MM, Crook M. Refeeding syndrome: treatment considerations based on collective analysis of literature case reports. *Nutrition.* 2010;26(2):156-167.

Charney P, Malone AM. *Pocket Guide to Nutrition Assessment,* 2nd ed. American Dietetic Association: 2009.

Dunford M, Doyle JA. *Nutrition for Sport and Exercise.* 2nd ed. Belmont, CA: Wadsworth, Cengage Learning; 2012: 37-251.

Hultgren HN. *High Altitude Medicine.* Stanford, CA: Hultgren Publications; 1997.

Khan LU, Ahmed J, Khan S, Macfie J. Refeeding syndrome: a literature review. *Gastroenterology research and practice.* 2011.

Mehanna HM, Moledina J, Travis J. Refeeding Syndrome: what is it, and how to prevent and treat it *BMJ.* 2008; 226(7659):1495-1498.

Nelms MN, Sucher KP, Lacey K, Roth SL. *Nutrition Therapy & Pathophysiology* Vol 2. Belmont, CA: Wadsworth Cengage Learning; 2011:119-127.

Refeeding Syndrome: Prevention and Management. Sydney Children's Hospital Website. http://www.schn.health.nsw.gov.au/_policies/pdf/2013-7036.pdf Published June 13, 2013. Accessed May 1, 2015.

Rodriguez NR, Di Marco NM, Langley S. Position of the American Dietetic Association, Dietitians of Canada, and the American College of Sports Medicine: Nutrition and Athletic Performance. *Journal of the American Dietetic Association.* 2009;109(3):509-527.

Ryan MH. *NOLS Backcountry Nutrition : Eating Beyond the Basics.* 1st ed. Mechanicsburg, PA: Stackpole Books; 2008:5-93.

Sherman WM, Costill DL. The marathon: dietary manipulation to optimize performance. *The American Journal of Sports Medicine.* 1984;12(1):44-51.

Thompson JJ, Manore M, Vaughan L. *The Science of Nutrition.* 2nd ed. San Francisco, CA: Pearson Benjamin Cummings; 2011:323-332.

INDEX

Made in the USA
Las Vegas, NV
24 April 2022

47933782R00208